A TEXTBOOK OF

MODERN TOXICOLOGY

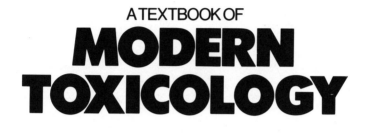

A TEXTBOOK OF
MODERN TOXICOLOGY

ERNEST HODGSON • PATRICIA E. LEVI

Toxicology Program
North Carolina State University
Raleigh, North Carolina

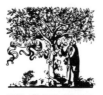

ELSEVIER
New York • Amsterdam • London

Elsevier Science Publishing Co., Inc.
52 Vanderbilt Avenue, New York, New York 10017

Sole distributors outside the United States and Canada:

Elsevier Science Publishers B.V.
P.O. Box 211, 1000 AE Amsterdam, The Netherlands

Library of Congress Cataloging in Publication Data

Hodgson, Ernest, 1932–
  A textbook of modern toxicology.

  Includes bibliographies and index.
  1. Toxicology. I. Levi, Patricia. II. Title.
RA1211.H62   1987   615.9   86–24392
ISBN 0–444–01131–5

Current printing (last digit):
10 9 8 7 6 5 4 3 2 1

Manufactured in the United States of America

CONTENTS

Preface xix

1. INTRODUCTION TO TOXICOLOGY 1
Ernest Hodgson

1.1 Definition and Scope, Relationship to Other Sciences,
    and History 1
    1.1.1 Definition and Scope 1
    1.1.2 Relationship to Other Sciences 5
    1.1.3 History of Toxicology 6
1.2 Sources of Toxic Compounds 7
    1.2.1 Synthetic Organic Compounds 7
        1.2.1.1 Air, Water, and Food Pollutants 7
        1.2.1.2 Chemical Additives in Food 8
        1.2.1.3 Chemicals in the Workplace 8
        1.2.1.4 Drugs of Abuse 9
        1.2.1.5 Therapeutic Drugs 10
        1.2.1.6 Pesticides 12
        1.2.1.7 Solvents 14
        1.2.1.8 Polycyclic Aromatic Hydrocarbons 15
        1.2.1.9 Cosmetics 15
    1.2.2 Naturally Occurring Toxins 16
        1.2.2.1 Mycotoxins 16
        1.2.2.2 Microbial Toxins 17
        1.2.2.3 Plant Toxins 18
        1.2.2.4 Animal Toxins 18
    1.2.3 Inorganic Chemicals 19
1.3 Environmental Movement of Toxicants 21
1.4 Suggested Further Reading 22

2. **ABSORPTION AND DISTRIBUTION OF TOXICANTS** 23
   Frank E. Guthrie and Ernest Hodgson

   2.1 Introduction 23
   2.2 Membranes 24
   2.3 Ionization 26
   2.4 Partition Coefficient 27
   2.5 Mechanisms of Entry 28
        2.5.1 Passive Transport 28
        2.5.2 Filtration 29
        2.5.3 Special Transport 29
        2.5.4 Endocytosis 29
   2.6 Rate of Penetration 30
   2.7 Routes of Penetration in Mammals 32
        2.7.1 Skin Penetration 32
        2.7.2 Gastrointestinal (GI) Penetration 36
        2.7.3 Respiratory Penetration 38
   2.8 Distribution 40
   2.9 Toxicodynamics 46
   2.10 Suggested Further Reading 50

3. **METABOLISM OF TOXICANTS** 51
   Ernest Hodgson

   3.1 Introduction 51
   3.2 Phase-One Reactions 51
        3.2.1 The Endoplasmic Reticulum, Microsomes,
               and Monooxygenations 52
        3.2.2 The Cytochrome P-450–Dependent Monooxygenase
               System 52
               3.2.2.1 Distribution of Cytochrome P-450 54
               3.2.2.2 Multiplicity of Cytochrome P-450 and Purification
                        and Reconstitution of Cytochrome P-450–
                        Dependent Monooxygenase Systems 56
               3.2.2.3 Microsomal Cytochrome P-450–Dependent
                        Monooxygenase Reactions 57
                        3.2.2.3a Epoxidation and aromatic
                                  hydroxylation 59
                        3.2.2.3b Aliphatic hydroxylation 60
                        3.2.2.3c Aliphatic epoxidation 60
                        3.2.2.3d Dealkylation: 0-, N- and
                                  S-dealkylation 60
                        3.2.2.3e N-Oxidation 61
                        3.2.2.3f Oxidative deamination 61
                        3.2.2.3g S-Oxidation 62
                        3.2.2.3h P-Oxidation 63
                        3.2.2.3i Desulfuration and ester cleavage 63
                        3.2.2.3j Methylenedioxy (benzodioxole) ring
                                  cleavage 64
        3.2.3 The Microsomal FAD-Containing Monooxygenase 64

3.2.4 Nonmicrosomal Oxidations 65
    3.2.4.1 Alcohol Dehydrogenases 65
    3.2.4.2 Aldehyde Dehydrogenase 67
    3.2.4.3 Amine Oxidases 67
        3.2.4.3a Monoamine oxidases 67
        3.2.4.3b Diamine oxidases 67
3.2.5 Cooxidation During Prostaglandin Biosynthesis 68
3.2.6 Reduction Reactions 69
    3.2.6.1 Nitro Reduction 69
    3.2.6.2 Azo Reduction 70
    3.2.6.3 Disulfide Reduction 70
    3.2.6.4 Ketone and Aldehyde Reduction 70
    3.2.6.5 Sulfoxide Reduction 70
3.2.7 Hydrolysis 70
3.2.8 Epoxide Hydration 72
3.2.9 DDT-Dehydrochlorinase 72
3.3 Phase-Two Reactions 73
3.3.1 Glycoside Conjugation 73
    3.3.1.1 Glucuronides 73
    3.3.1.2 Glucosides 75
3.3.2 Sulfate Conjugation 75
3.3.3 Methyltransferases 76
    3.3.3.1 *N*-Methylation 76
    3.3.3.2 *O*-Methylation 77
    3.3.3.3 *S*-Methylation 77
    3.3.3.4 Biomethylation of Elements 78
3.3.4 Glutathione Transferases and Mercapturic Acid Formation 78
3.3.5 Cysteine Conjugate β-Lyase 81
3.3.6 Acylation 81
    3.3.6.1 Acetylation 82
    3.3.6.2 *N,O*-Acyltransferase 82
    3.3.6.3 Amino Acid Conjugation 82
    3.3.6.4 Deacetylation 83
3.3.7 Phosphate Conjugation 83
3.4 Suggested Further Reading 83

4. MODIFICATION OF METABOLISM 85
Ernest Hodgson

4.1 Introduction 85
4.2 Nutritional Effects 85
4.2.1 Protein 86
4.2.2 Carbohydrates 86
4.2.3 Lipids 86
4.2.4 Micronutrients 86
4.2.5 Starvation and Dehydration 87
4.3 Physiological Effects 87
4.3.1 Development 87

4.3.2 Sex Differences 89
4.3.3 Hormones 90
    4.3.3.1 Thyroid Hormone 90
    4.3.3.2 Adrenal Hormones 90
    4.3.3.3 Insulin 90
    4.3.3.4 Other Hormones 90
4.3.4 Pregnancy 91
4.3.5 Disease 91
4.3.6 Diurnal Rhythms 91
4.4 Comparative and Genetic Effects 91
    4.4.1 Variations Among Taxonomic Groups 92
        4.4.1.1 In Vivo Toxicity 93
        4.4.1.2 In Vivo Metabolism 93
        4.4.1.3 In Vitro Metabolism 98
    4.4.2 Selectivity 102
    4.4.3 Genetic Differences 102
        4.4.3.1 In Vivo Toxicity 103
        4.4.3.2 Metabolite Production 103
        4.4.3.3 Enzyme Differences 104
4.5 Chemical Effects 105
    4.5.1 Inhibition 106
        4.5.1.1 Types of Inhibition: Experimental Demonstration 106
        4.5.1.2 Synergism and Potentiation 111
        4.5.1.3 Antagonism 112
    4.5.2 Induction 113
        4.5.2.1 Specificity of Monooxygenase Induction 113
        4.5.2.2 Mechanism and Genetics of Induction in Mammals 115
        4.5.2.3 Effect of Induction 116
        4.5.2.4 Induction of Xenobiotic-Metabolizing Enzymes Other Than Monooxygenases 117
    4.5.3 Biphasic Effects: Inhibition and Induction 117
4.6 Environmental Effects 118
    4.6.1 Temperature 118
    4.6.2 Ionizing Radiation 118
    4.6.3 Light 119
    4.6.4 Moisture 119
    4.6.5 Altitude 119
    4.6.6 Other Stress Factors 119
4.7 General Summary and Conclusions 119
4.8 Suggested Further Reading 120

5. ELIMINATION OF TOXICANTS 123
Frank E. Guthrie and Ernest Hodgson

5.1 Introduction 123
5.2 Renal Excretion 124
    5.2.1 Glomerular Filtration 124
    5.2.2 Tubular Reabsorption 124

5.2.3   Tubular Secretion   125
5.2.4   Factors Affecting Renal Excretion   125
5.3   Hepatic Excretion   126
   5.3.1   Bile Formation and Secretion   126
   5.3.2   Enterohepatic Circulation   128
5.4   Pulmonary Excretion   128
5.5   Minor Routes of Elimination   129
   5.5.1   Sex-linked Routes   129
      5.5.1.1   Milk   129
      5.5.1.2   Eggs   130
      5.5.1.3   Fetus   130
   5.5.2   Alimentary Elimination   130
   5.5.3   Obscure Routes   131
5.6   Suggested Further Reading   131

6. TOXIC ACTION 133
Patricia E. Levi

6.1   Role and Formation of Reactive Metabolites   133
   6.1.1   Metabolic Activation: Definition   133
   6.1.2   Activation Enzymes   133
   6.1.3   Chemical Classes of Reactive Metabolites   134
   6.1.4   Fate of Reactive Metabolites   134
      6.1.4.1   Binding to Cellular Macromolecules   134
      6.1.4.2   Lipid Peroxidation   134
      6.1.4.3   Trapping and Removal: Role of Glutathione   134
   6.1.5   Specific Examples of Activation Reactions   136
      6.1.5.1   Aflatoxin B_1 136
      6.1.5.2   Acetylaminofluorene   136
      6.1.5.3   Acetaminophen   137
      6.1.5.4   Cycasin   137
   6.1.6   Factors Affecting Toxicity of Reactive Metabolites   138
6.2   Acute Toxicity   139
   6.2.1   Introduction   139
   6.2.2   Nervous System Toxicants   139
      6.2.2.1   Cholinesterase Inhibitors: Insecticides, Nerve Gases   139
      6.2.2.2   Other Nervous System Toxicants   141
          6.2.2.2a   Tubocurarine   141
          6.2.2.2b   Botulinum toxins   142
          6.2.2.2c   Tetradotoxin   142
          6.2.2.2d   Batrachotoxin   142
   6.2.3   Inhibitors of Oxidative Phosphorylation   142
      6.2.3.1   Electron Transport Inhibitors   142
          6.2.3.1a   Cyanide   142
          6.2.3.1b   Other inhibitors   143
      6.2.3.2   Uncouplers of Oxidative Phosphorylation   144
   6.2.4   Lethal Synthesis: Fluoroacetate   144
6.3   Chronic Toxicity   145
   6.3.1   Carcinogenesis   145

6.3.1.1   Historical Perspective 145
6.3.1.2   Carcinogenic Process 147
    6.3.1.2a   Initiation 147
    6.3.1.2b   Promotion 147
    6.3.1.2c   Essential features of initiation and promotion 148
    6.3.1.2d   Examples of promoters 149
    6.3.1.2e   Cocarcinogenesis 149
6.3.1.3   Genotoxic and Epigenetic Carcinogens 150
6.3.1.4   Activation of Carcinogens and Binding to Macromolecules 150
6.3.1.5   DNA Repair 152
6.3.1.6   Radiation Carcinogenesis 152
6.3.1.7   Oncogenes and a Common Pathway 153
6.3.2   Mutagenesis 154
    6.3.2.1   Introduction 154
    6.3.2.2   Point Mutations: Base-Pair Transformation 154
        6.3.2.2a   Chemical transformation 155
        6.3.2.2b   Incorporation of abnormal base analogs 155
        6.3.2.2c   Alkylating agents 155
    6.3.2.3   Frameshift Mutations 156
    6.3.2.4   DNA Repair 156
    6.3.2.5   Chromosome Aberrations 158
    6.3.2.6   Relationship of Mutagenesis to Carcinogenesis 158
6.3.3   Teratogenesis 159
    6.3.3.1   Introduction 159
    6.3.3.2   General Principles of Teratology 159
        6.3.3.2a   Genetic factors/influences 159
        6.3.3.2b   Critical periods 160
        6.3.3.2c   Initiating mechanisms 160
        6.3.3.2d   Consequences of abnormal development 162
        6.3.3.2e   Access to embryo and fetus 162
        6.3.3.2f   Dose–response relationship 163
    6.3.3.3   Teratogenic Mechanisms 163
        6.3.3.3a   Mutation 163
        6.3.3.3b   Chromosomal abnormalities 163
        6.3.3.3c   Mitotic interference 164
        6.3.3.3d   Interference with nucleic acid function 164
        6.3.3.3e   Nutritional deficiencies 164
        6.3.3.3f   Deficient or altered energy supply 164
        6.3.3.3g   Changes in osmolarity 165
        6.3.3.3h   Ultrastructural changes in cell membrane 165
        6.3.3.3i   Enzyme inhibition 165
    6.3.3.4   Human Teratogenesis: Some Specific Examples 165
        6.3.3.4a   Folic acid antagonists 165

6.3.3.4b   Androgenic hormones 165
6.3.3.4c   Thalidomide 166
6.3.3.4d   Alcohol 166
6.3.3.4e   Methyl mercury 167
6.3.3.4f   Infectious diseases 167
6.3.3.4g   Transplacental carcinogenesis 168
6.3.4 Organ Toxicity 168
6.3.4.1 Hepatotoxicity 168
6.3.4.la   Susceptibility of liver 168
6.3.4.lb   Types of liver injury 168
6.3.4.lc   Mechanisms 170
6.3.4.ld   Carbon tetrachloride 171
6.3.4.le   Bromobenzene 172
6.3.4.lf   Acetaminophen 172
6.3.4.2 Nephrotoxicity 174
6.3.4.2a   Susceptibility of the kidney 174
6.3.4.2b   Metals 175
6.3.4.2c   Antibiotics 175
6.3.4.2d   Reactive metabolites 176
6.3.4.3 Pulmonary Toxicity 177
6.3.4.3a   Susceptibility of the lungs 177
6.3.4.3b   Toxic responses of the lungs 177
6.3.4.3c   Metabolic activation of toxicants 178
6.3.5 Behavioral Effects 179
6.3.5.1 Introduction and Definition 179
6.3.5.2 Behavioral Teratology 180
6.3.5.3 Behavioral Testing 181
6.3.5.4 Summary 181
6.4 Suggested Further Reading 182

7. TOXICITY OF CHEMICALS 185
Patricia E. Levi

7.1 Introduction 185
7.2 Chemical Pollutants in the Air 185
7.2.1 History 185
7.2.2 Types of Air Pollutants 186
7.2.2.1 Unpolluted Air 186
7.2.2.2 Gaseous Pollutants 187
7.2.2.3 Particulate Pollutants 187
7.2.3 Sources of Air Pollutants 188
7.2.3.1 Natural 188
7.2.3.2 Man-Made 189
7.2.4 Human Health Effects 189
7.2.5 Environmental Effects 190
7.2.5.1 Vegetation, Crops, and Forests 190
7.2.5.2 Domestic Animals 191
7.2.5.3 Materials and Structures 191
7.2.5.4 Atmospheric Effects 191

    7.2.5.5 Acidic Deposition 192

7.3 Chemical Pollutants in the Soil and Water 192
    7.3.1 Introduction 192
    7.3.2 Sources of Chemical Pollutants 193
    7.3.3 Pollutants and Their Effects 193
        7.3.3.1 Metals 193
        7.3.3.2 Pesticides 194
        7.3.3.3 Inorganic Nutrients 194
        7.3.3.4 Petroleum 194
        7.3.3.5 Acids 195
        7.3.3.6 Other Organic Chemicals 195

7.4 Chemical Additives and Pollutants in Food 195
    7.4.1 Introduction and Legal Aspects 195
    7.4.2 Reasons for Using Food Additives 196
    7.4.3 Color Additives 196
    7.4.4 Antioxidants 198
    7.4.5 Preservatives 199
    7.4.6 Flavorings 201
    7.4.7 Artificial Sweeteners 201
    7.4.8 Nonintentional Additives 202

7.5 Chemicals in the Workplace 202
    7.5.1 Introduction 202
    7.5.2 Routes of Exposure 204
    7.5.3 Occupational Carcinogenesis 204
    7.5.4 Examples of Toxic Industrial Substances 205
        7.5.4.1 Metals 205
        7.5.4.2 Benzene 207
        7.5.4.3 Asbestos and Other Fibers 207

7.6 Pesticides 208
    7.6.1 Introduction 208
    7.6.2 Classes of Pesticides 208
        7.6.2.1 Organochlorine Insecticides 208
        7.6.2.2 Organophosphorus Insecticides 208
        7.6.2.3 Carbamate Insecticides 210
        7.6.2.4 Botanical (Natural) Insecticides 211
        7.6.2.5 Herbicides 212
        7.6.2.6 Fungicides 213
        7.6.2.7 Rodenticides 213
        7.6.2.8 Fumigants 213

7.7 Therapeutic Drugs 213
    7.7.1 Barbiturates (Barbitals) 214
    7.7.2 Benzodiazepines 215
    7.7.3 Tricyclic Antidepressants 216
    7.7.4 Amphetamines 216
    7.7.5 Narcotic Analgesics (Opiates) 217
    7.7.6 Anticonvulsants (Phenytoin and Diphenylhydantoin) 218
    7.7.7 Isoniazid 219
    7.7.8 Lithium 220

7.8   Other Drugs (Including Drugs of Abuse)   220
    7.8.1   Cocaine   220
    7.8.2   Phencyclidine (PCP)   221
    7.8.3   Lysergic Acid Diethylamide (LSD)   222
    7.8.4   Mescaline/Peyote   223
    7.8.5   Psilocybin   223
    7.8.6   Dimethyltryptamine (DMT)   224
    7.8.7   Marijuana   224
7.9   Solvents   224
    7.9.1   Aliphatic Hydrocarbons   225
    7.9.2   Aliphatic Halogenated Hydrocarbons   225
        7.9.2.1   Chloroform   225
        7.9.2.2   Carbon Tetrachloride   226
        7.9.2.3   Methylene Chloride   226
        7.9.2.4   Methyl Chloride   226
        7.9.2.5   Trichloroethylene   227
        7.9.2.6   Vinyl Chloride   227
    7.9.3   Alcohols   227
        7.9.3.1   Methanol   228
        7.9.3.2   Isopropyl Alcohol   228
        7.9.3.3   Higher Saturated Alcohols   229
    7.9.4   Glycols and Derivatives   229
        7.9.4.1   Ethylene Glycol   229
        7.9.4.2   Propylene Glycol   230
        7.9.4.3   Glycol Ethers   230
    7.9.5   Aromatic Hydrocarbons   230
        7.9.5.1   Benzene   230
        7.9.5.2   Toluene   230
        7.9.5.3   Xylene   230
7.10   Suggested Further Reading   231

8.   MEASUREMENT OF TOXICITY   233
Ernest Hodgson
8.1   Introduction   233
8.2   Experimental Administration of Toxicants   235
8.3   Chemical and Physical Properties   238
8.4   Exposure and Environmental Fate   239
8.5   In Vivo Tests   239
    8.5.1   Acute Toxicity   239
        8.5.1.1   LD50 and LC50   239
        8.5.1.2   Eye Irritation   243
        8.5.1.3   Dermal Irritation and Sensitization   244
    8.5.2   Subchronic Tests   245
        8.5.2.1   Ninety-Day Feeding Tests   246
            8.5.2.1a   Experimental (nonbiological) variables   246
            8.5.2.1b   Biological variables   247
            8.5.2.1c   Results   247

8.5.2.2 Thirty-Day Dermal Tests 251
8.5.2.3 Thirty-Day to Ninety-Day Inhalation Tests 251
8.5.3 Chronic Tests 251
8.5.3.1 Chronic Toxicity and Carcinogenicity 252
8.5.3.2 Reproductive Toxicity and Teratogenicity 253
8.5.3.2a Fertility and general reproductive
performance: Single-generation tests 253
8.5.3.2b Fertility and general reproductive
performance: Multigeneration tests 255
8.5.3.2c Teratology 256
8.5.3.2d Effect of chemicals in late pregnancy and
lactation (perinatal/postnatal effects) 260
8.5.4 Special Tests 260
8.5.4.1 Neurotoxicity (Including Delayed
Neuropathy) 261
8.5.4.2 Potentiation 262
8.5.4.3 Toxicokinetics and Metabolism 262
8.5.4.4 Behavior 263
8.5.4.5 Covalent Binding 265
8.5.4.6 Immunotoxicity 266
8.6 In Vitro and Other Short-Term Tests 268
8.6.1 Introduction 268
8.6.2 Prokaryote Mutagenicity 269
8.6.2.1 Ames Test 269
8.6.2.2 Related Tests 270
8.6.3 Eukaryote Mutagenicity 271
8.6.3.1 Mammalian Cell Mutation 271
8.6.3.2 Drosophila Sex-Linked Recessive Lethal Test 271
8.6.3.3 Related Tests 272
8.6.4 DNA Damage and Repair 273
8.6.4.1 Unscheduled DNA Synthesis in Mammalian
Cells 273
8.6.4.2 Related Tests 274
8.6.5 Chromosome Aberrations 274
8.6.5.1 Sister Chromatid Exchange (SCE) 274
8.6.5.2 Micronucleus Test 275
8.6.5.3 Dominant Lethal Test in Rodents 276
8.6.5.4 Related Tests 276
8.6.6 Mammalian Cell Transformation 277
8.6.7 General Considerations and Testing Sequences 277
8.7 Ecological Effects 278
8.7.1 Laboratory Tests 279
8.7.2 Simulated Field Tests 280
8.7.3 Field Tests 280
8.8 Risk Analysis 281
8.9 The Future of Toxicity Testing 283
8.10 Suggested Further Reading 283

9. THE MEASUREMENT OF TOXICANTS 287
Ross B. Leidy and Ernest Hodgson

9.1 Introduction 287
9.2 Chemical and Physical Methods 288
    9.2.1 Sampling 288
        9.2.1.1 Air 288
        9.2.1.2 Soil 291
        9.2.1.3 Water 291
        9.2.1.4 Tissues 292
            9.2.1.4a Environmental studies 292
            9.2.1.4b Experimental studies 292
            9.2.1.4c Forensic studies 293
    9.2.2 Extraction 294
        9.2.2.1 Blending 294
        9.2.2.2 Shaking 294
        9.2.2.3 Washing 294
        9.2.2.4 Continuous Extraction 294
    9.2.3 Separation and Identification 295
        9.2.3.1 Solvent Partitioning 295
        9.2.3.2 Chromatography 296
            9.2.3.2a Paper 296
            9.2.3.2b Thin-layer chromatography 296
            9.2.3.2c Column: adsorption, hydrophobic, ion
                     exchange 296
            9.2.3.2d Gas-liquid chromatography (GLC) 297
            9.2.3.2e High-performance liquid chromatography
                     (HPLC) 301
        9.2.3.3 Spectroscopy 301
            9.2.3.3a AA spectroscopy 302
            9.2.3.3b Mass spectroscopy (MS) 303
            9.2.3.3c IR spectrophotometry 303
            9.2.3.3d Ultraviolet/visible spectrophotometry 304
            9.2.3.3e Nuclear magnetic resonance (NMR) 304
            9.2.3.3f Other analytical methods 304
    9.2.4 Data Handling 305
9.3 Bioassay 305
9.4 Suggested Further Reading 307

10. PREVENTION OF TOXICITY 309
Ernest Hodgson

10.1 Introduction 309
10.2 Legislation and Regulation 309
    10.2.1 Federal Government: United States 309
    10.2.2 State Governments 312
    10.2.3 Legislation and Regulation in Other Countries 312
10.3 Prevention in Different Environments 313
    10.3.1 Home 313

10.3.2 Workplace 314
10.3.3 Pollution of Air, Water, and Land 315
10.4 Education 316
10.5 Suggested Further Reading 317

11. DIAGNOSIS AND TREATMENT OF TOXICITY 319
Ernest Hodgson

11.1 Introduction 319
11.2 Diagnosis 319
    11.2.1 Introduction 319
    11.2.2 Case History 319
    11.2.3 Systemic Examination 322
11.3 Nonspecific Therapy 323
    11.3.1 First Aid and Emergency Management 323
    11.3.2 Life Support 325
    11.3.3 Nonspecific Maintenance Therapy 325
11.4 Specific Therapy 328
    11.4.1 Categories of Specific Therapy 328
    11.4.2 Specific Examples 328
        11.4.2.1 Methanol 329
        11.4.2.2 Cyanide 329
        11.4.2.3 Heavy Metals (Lead and Mercury) 331
        11.4.2.4 Carbon Monoxide 331
        11.4.2.5 Organophosphorus Cholinesterase Inhibitors 332
        11.4.2.6 Carbamate Cholinesterase Inhibitors 332
        11.4.2.7 Bromide 332
11.5 Chronic Toxicity 332
11.6 Suggested Further Reading 333

12. LITERATURE OF TOXICOLOGY 335
Ernest Hodgson

12.1 Introduction 335
12.2 Textbooks 335
12.3 Monographs, Conference Proceedings, Review and Primary Research Journals 336
    12.3.1 General Toxicology 336
        12.3.1.1 Monographs 336
        12.3.1.2 Conference Proceedings 337
        12.3.1.3 Review Journals 337
        12.3.1.4 Primary Research Journals 337
    12.3.2 Agricultural Chemicals 338
        12.3.2.1 Monographs 338
        12.3.2.2 Conference Proceedings 338
        12.3.2.3 Review Journals 338
        12.3.2.4 Primary Research Journals 338
    12.3.3 Analytical Toxicology 338
        12.3.3.1 Monographs 338
        12.3.3.2 Conference Proceedings 339
        12.3.3.3 Primary Research Journals 339

12.3.4   Behavioral Toxicology   339
    12.3.4.1   Conference Proceedings   339
    12.3.4.2   Primary Research Journals   339
12.3.5   Biochemical Toxicology   339
    12.3.5.1   Monographs   339
    12.3.5.2   Conference Proceedings   339
    12.3.5.3   Review Journals   340
    12.3.5.4   Primary Research Journals   340
12.3.6   Carcinogenesis, Mutagenesis, and Teratogenesis   340
    12.3.6.1   Monographs   340
    12.3.6.2   Conference Proceedings   340
    12.3.6.3   Primary Research Journals   341
12.3.7   Clinical and Human Toxicology   341
    12.3.7.1   Monographs   341
    12.3.7.2   Primary Research Journals   341
12.3.8   Drugs and Cosmetics   341
    12.3.8.1   Monographs   341
    12.3.8.2   Conference Proceedings   342
    12.3.8.3   Review Journals   342
    12.3.8.4   Primary Research Journals   342
12.3.9   Environmental Toxicology   342
    12.3.9.1   Monographs   342
    12.3.9.2   Conference Proceedings   342
    12.3.9.3   Review Journals   342
    12.3.9.4   Primary Research Journals   343
12.3.10   Food Additive Toxicology   343
    12.3.10.1   Monographs   343
    12.3.10.2   Conference Proceedings   343
12.3.11   Forensic Toxicology   343
    12.3.11.1   Monographs   343
    12.3.11.2   Conference Proceedings   344
12.3.12   Legislative and Societal Aspects of Toxicology   344
    12.3.12.1   Monographs   344
    12.3.12.2   Conference Proceedings   344
    12.3.12.3   Review Journals   344
    12.3.12.4   Primary Research Journals   344
12.3.13   Metal Toxicology   344
    12.3.13.1   Monographs   344
12.3.14   Nutritional Toxicology   345
    12.3.14.1   Monographs   345
    12.3.14.2   Primary Research Journals   345
12.3.15   Occupational Health and Industrial Hygiene   345
    12.3.15.1   Monographs   345
    12.3.15.2   Review Journals   345
    12.3.15.3   Primary Research Journals   345
12.3.16   Organ Toxicity   346
    12.3.16.1   Monographs   346
    12.3.16.2   Conference Proceedings   346
    12.3.16.3   Primary Research Journals   346

12.3.17   Physical Agents 346
    12.3.17.1   Monographs 346
    12.3.17.2   Conference Proceedings 346
    12.3.17.3   Primary Research Journals 346
12.3.18   Toxins 347
    12.3.18.1   Monographs 347
    12.3.18.2   Conference Proceedings 347
    12.3.18.3   Primary Research Journals 347
12.3.19   Veterinary Toxicology 347
    12.3.19.1   Monographs 347
    12.3.19.2   Conference Proceedings 347
    12.3.19.3   Primary Research Journals 347
12.4   Journals in Related Areas 348
12.5   International Documents, Government Documents, and Miscellaneous Sources of Information 348
    12.5.1   International Documents 348
    12.5.2   National Documents 349
12.6   Abstracts, Indexes, and Computer Services 350
    12.6.1   Abstracting Services 350
    12.6.2   Indexes 350
    12.6.3   Computer Data Bases 351
12.7   Personal Information Storage and Retrieval Systems 352
12.8   Conclusions 355
12.9   Suggested Further Reading 355

GLOSSARY 357
INDEX 375

PREFACE

Although there are some excellent reference works in general toxicology, such as Casarett and Doull's *Toxicology* (edited by Doull, Klaassen, and Amdur) and *Principles and Methods in Toxicology* (edited by Hayes), there is still a scarcity of textbooks designed for student and teacher to use in the classroom setting. In preparing the current volume we have attempted to fill that particular niche. At North Carolina State University we have taught a course in general toxicology that is open to graduate students as well as undergraduates at the senior level. In our opinion, toxicology is, in most instances, not a suitable course for an undergraduate, as some knowledge of chemistry, biochemistry, and physiology is an essential prerequisite. However, with proper guidance, all of the material in the present text is appropriate for biology, chemistry, or biochemistry majors in their senior year. For graduate students it is intended to lay the foundation for subsequent, specialized courses in toxicology, such as those in biochemical toxicology, chemical carcinogenesis, regulatory toxicology, etc.

We share the view that an introductory text must present all of the necessary fundamental information, but in as uncomplicated a manner as possible. To enhance readability, references have been deleted from the text. While this may result in a text which appears simple to the advanced student, or one which is unsuitable as a reference work, a list of suggested further reading at the end of each chapter will permit students to extend their knowledge in any area of interest.

Clearly the amount of material, and the detail with which some of it is presented, is more than needed for the average general toxicology course. This is done, however, to permit each instructor the opportunity to select and emphasize those areas of toxicology that they feel need additional emphasis. The obvious biochemical bias of some sections is deliberate and based on the philosophy that progress in toxicology depends most on further understanding of the fundamental basis of toxic action at the cellular and molecular levels.

The efforts of Karen Clark, who prepared the manuscript through all its many revisions, are greatly appreciated, as are those of Drs. Frank E. Guthrie and Ross Leidy for their contributions to Chapters 2, 5, and 9. Thanks are due also to many reviewers, but particularly to the students of the 1984 and 1985 classes in general toxicology at NCSU. Finally we thank Yale Altman and others at Elsevier whose fine work and unfailing good humor made the final stages of the project possible.

Ernest Hodgson
Patricia E. Levi

Raleigh, North Carolina

chapter one

INTRODUCTION TO TOXICOLOGY

Ernest Hodgson

1.1 DEFINITION AND SCOPE, RELATIONSHIP TO OTHER SCIENCES, AND HISTORY

1.1.1 Definition and Scope

Having defined toxicology as that branch of science that deals with poisons and a poison as any substance that causes a harmful effect when administered, either by accident or design, to a living organism, we leave simplicity behind. Many complications exist, both in bringing more precise definition to the meaning of poison, and in the measurement of toxic effect. Broader definitions of toxicology such as "the study of the detection, occurrence, properties, effects, and regulation of toxic substances," although more descriptive, do not resolve the difficulties. It is to the complications, and to the basic science behind them and their resolution, that this textbook is devoted. Taken together, they circumscribe the perimeter of the science of toxicology.

Toxicology exists in the service of society, not only in the sense of protecting human and other organisms from the deleterious effects of toxicants, but also to serve directly by developing better selective toxicants. Thus, the study of comparative toxicology and selective toxicity contributes to the development of better and more selective anticancer drugs, pesticides, and so forth.

It must be emphasized at the outset that poison is a quantitative concept. Almost any substance is harmful at some dose and, at the same time, is harmless at a very low dose. Between these two limits there is a range of possible effects, from subtle long-term chronic toxicity to immediate lethality. Vinyl chloride may be taken as an example; it is a potent hepatotoxicant at high doses, a carcinogen with a long latent period at lower doses, and is apparently without effect at very low doses. Clinical drugs are even more poignant examples because, although therapeutic and highly beneficial at some doses, they are not

1

without deleterious side effects and are frequently lethal at higher doses. Aspirin (acetylsalicylic acid), for example, is a relatively safe drug at recommended doses and is taken by millions of people. At the same time, chronic use can cause deleterious effects on the gastric mucosa, and it is fatal at a dose of about 0.2–0.5 g/kg. Some 15% of reported accidental deaths from poisoning in children are due to salicylates, particularly aspirin.

The importance of dose is clearly seen with metals that are dietary essentials but are toxic at higher doses. Thus, iron, copper, magnesium, cobalt, manganese, and zinc can be present at too low a level in the diet (deficiency), at an appropriate level (maintenance), or at too high a level (toxic).

The definition of a poison, or toxicant, also involves a quantitative biological aspect because a compound, highly toxic to one species or genetic strain, may be relatively harmless to another. For example, carbon tetrachloride, a potent hepatotoxicant in many species, is relatively harmless to the chicken, whereas certain strains of rabbit can eat *Belladonna* with impunity. Compounds may also be toxic under some circumstances but not others or, perhaps, toxic in combination with another compound but nontoxic alone. The methylenedioxyphenyl insecticide synergists, such as piperonyl butoxide, are of low toxicity to either mammals or insects when administered alone but are, by virtue of their ability to block xenobiotic-metabolizing enzymes, capable of causing dramatic increases in the toxicity of other compounds.

The measurement of toxicity is also complex. Toxicity may be acute or chronic, and may vary from one organ to another as well as with the age, sex, diet, physiological condition, or health status of the organism. Even the simplest measure of toxicity, the LD50 (the dose required to kill 50% of a population of an organism under stated conditions), is highly dependent on the extent to which many of the above variables are controlled, and LD50 values, as a result, vary markedly from one laboratory to another.

The toxicity of a particular compound may vary with the portal of entry into the body, whether through the alimentary canal, the lungs, or the skin. Even experimental methods such as injection may give rise to highly variable results; thus, the toxicity from intravenous (IV), intraperitoneal (IP), intramuscular (IM), or subcutaneous (SC) injection of a given compound may be quite different. Toxicity may vary as much as tenfold with the route of administration.

The scope of toxicology can be described in a number of ways. Loomis (1974) divides the subject into environmental, economic, and forensic toxicology. The first is concerned with residues, pollution, and industrial hygiene; the second is concerned with the development of chemicals such as drugs, pesticides, and food additives; and the third deals with diagnosis, treatment, and medicolegal aspects. Although this classification is useful, it does not give adequate weight to the modern mechanistic approach concerned with events at the fundamental level that occur during metabolism, mode of toxic action, etc., nor does it do justice to the current wide scope of the subject.

Any attempt to define the scope of toxicology, including that which follows, must take into account the fact that the various subdisciplines are not mutually exclusive and frequently are heavily interdependent. Due to overlapping of mechanisms, chemical classes, use classes and effects, clear division into subjects of equal importance is not possible.

A. Mechanisms of Toxic Action. This includes the consideration—at the fundamental level of organ, cell, and molecular function—of all events leading to toxicity in vivo: uptake, distribution, metabolism, mode of action, and excretion. Important aspects include the following:

1. *Biochemical toxicology* considers events at the biochemical and molecular level, including enzymes that metabolize xenobiotics, generation of reactive intermediates, interaction of xenobiotics or their metabolites with macromolecules, etc.

2. *Behavioral toxicology* deals with the effect of toxicants on animal and human behavior, which is the final integrated expression of nervous function at the intact animal level. This involves both peripheral and central nervous systems as well as effects mediated by other organ systems such as the endocrine glands.

3. *Nutritional toxicology* deals with the effects of diet on the expression of toxicity and the mechanisms for these effects.

4. *Carcinogenesis* is of tremendous current interest and includes the chemical and biochemical events that lead to the large number of effects on cell growth collectively known as cancer.

5. *Teratogenesis* is also of much current interest and includes the chemical and biochemical events that lead to deleterious effects on the developmental process.

6. *Mutagenesis* is concerned with toxic effects on the genetic material and the inheritance of these defects.

7. *Organ toxicity* considers effects at the level of organ function, eg, neurotoxicity, hepatotoxicity, and nephrotoxicity.

B. Measurement of Toxicants and Toxicity. These important aspects deal primarily with analytical chemistry, bioassay, and applied mathematics, and are designed to provide the methodology to answer certain critically important questions. Is the substance likely to be toxic? What is its chemical identity? How much of it is present? How can we assay its toxic effect and what is the minimum level at which this toxic effect can be detected? This aspect of toxicology includes a number of important fields:

1. *Analytical toxicology* is a branch of analytical chemistry that is concerned with methods for the identification and assay of toxic chemicals and their metabolites in biological and environmental materials.

2. *Toxicity testing* involves the use of living systems to estimate toxic effects. It covers the entire gamut from short-term tests for genotoxicity such as the Ames test and cell culture techniques to the use of intact animals for acute toxicity tests and for lifetime or multigeneration chronic toxicity tests. The term bioassay is properly used only to describe the use of living organisms to quantitate the amount of a particular toxicant present.

3. *Toxicological pathology* is that branch of pathology which deals with the effects of toxic agents as manifested by changes in subcellular, cellular, tissue, or organ morphology.

4. *Structure-activity study* is a subdiscipline of toxicology that deals with the relationship between chemical and physical properties of xenobiotics and toxicity and, particularly, the use of such relationships for the prediction of toxicity.

5. *Biomathematics and statistics* are important subjects, related to a number of areas of toxicology. They deal with data analysis, the determination of significance, and the formulation of risk estimates and predictive models. The latter is particularly important in epidemiology and environmental toxicology.

6. *Epidemiology,* as it applies to toxicology, is closely related to the previous subject and is of great importance since it deals with the study of toxicity as it actually occurs, rather than in an experimental setting.

C. Applied Toxicology. This includes various aspects of toxicology as they occur in the field, including:

1. *Clinical toxicology* is the diagnosis and treatment of human poisoning.

2. *Veterinary toxicology* is the diagnosis and treatment of the poisoning of animals other than humans, particularly livestock and companion animals but not excluding feral species. An important concern of veterinary toxicology is the possible transmission of toxins to the human population in meat, fish, milk, and other foodstuffs.

3. *Forensic toxicology* concerns medicolegal aspects, including the detection of poisons in clinical and other samples.

4. *Environmental toxicology* is concerned with the movement of toxicants and their metabolites in the environment and in food chains and the effect of such toxicants on individuals and populations.

5. *Industrial toxicology* is a specific area of environmental toxicology that deals with the work environment. Because of the large number of industrial chemicals and possibilities for exposure as well as a number of specific laws that govern such situations, this subject is well developed.

D. Chemical Use Classes. This includes the toxicological aspects of the development of new chemicals for commercial use. In some of these use classes, toxicity, at least to some organisms, is a desirable trait; in others, it is an undesirable side effect. Use classes are not composed entirely of synthetic chemicals; many natural products are isolated and used for commercial and other uses and must be subjected to the same toxicity testing as synthetic compounds. Examples include the insecticide pyrethrin, the clinical drug digitalis, and psilocibin, a drug of abuse.

1. *Agricultural chemicals* include many compounds, such as insecticides, herbicides, fungicides, and rodenticides, in which toxicity to the target organism is a desired quality whereas toxicity to "nontarget" species is to be avoided. Development of such selectively toxic chemicals is one of the applied roles of comparative toxicology.

2. *Clinical drugs* are properly the province of pharmaceutical chemistry and pharmacology. Only toxic side effects and testing for them fall within the science of toxicology.

3. *Drugs of abuse* are chemicals taken for psychological or other effects that cause dependence and toxicity. Many of these are illegal, but some are of clinical significance when used correctly.

4. *Food additives* are of concern to toxicologists only when toxic or being tested for possible toxicity.

5. *Industrial chemicals* are so numerous that testing for toxicity and

controlling exposure to those known to be toxic is a large field of toxicology.

6. *Naturally occurring substances* include many phytotoxins, myco-toxins, and inorganic minerals, all occurring naturally in the environment.

7. *Combustion products* are not properly a use class but a large and important class of toxicants, generated primarily from fuels and other industrial chemicals.

E. Regulatory Toxicology. These aspects, concerned with the formulation of laws, and regulations authorized by laws, are intended to minimize the effect of toxic chemicals on human health and the environment. They involve:

1. *Legal aspects* are concerned with the formulation of laws and regulations and their enforcement. In the United States, the latter generally falls under such government agencies as the Environmental Protection Agency (EPA), the Food and Drug Administration (FDA), and the Occupational Safety and Health Administration (OSHA). Similar government departments exist in many other countries.

2. *Risk assessment,* which is the definition of risks, potential risks, and the risk–benefit equations necessary for regulation of toxic substances.

1.1.2 Relationship to Other Sciences

Toxicology should be viewed as a science and human activity in a spectrum of sciences and human activities. At one end of this spectrum are those sciences that contribute their methods and philosophical concepts to serve the needs of toxicologists, either in research or in the application of toxicology to human affairs. At the other end of the spectrum are those sciences and human activities to which toxicology contributes.

Most important in the first group are chemistry, biochemistry, pathology, physiology, and epidemiology, whereas such sciences as immunology, biomathematics, and ecology are also important, but to a more limited extent.

In the group to which toxicology contributes heavily are such aspects of medicine as forensic medicine, clinical toxicology, pharmacy and pharmacology, public health, and industrial hygiene. Toxicology also contributes in an important way to veterinary medicine and to such aspects of agriculture as the development and safe use of agricultural chemicals. The contributions of toxicology to environmental studies is one of the most rapidly expanding areas of the subject.

Clearly, toxicology is preeminently an applied science, dedicated to the enhancement of the quality of life and the protection of the environment. It is also much more. Frequently, the perturbation of normal life processes by toxic chemicals enables us to learn more about the life processes themselves. The use of uncoupling agents such as dinitrophenol to study oxidative phosphorylation or the use of α-amanitin to study RNA polymerases are but two of many examples of this principle. The field of toxicology has expanded enormously in recent years, both in the numbers of toxicologists and in the amount of accumulated knowledge. This expansion has been accompanied by a change from a purely descriptive science to one which uses the whole range of methodology of experimental science to investigate the mechanisms behind toxic events. Many investigators have finally realized that only through the latter method will further real progress be made.

1.1.3 History of Toxicology

Much of the early history of toxicology has doubtless been lost, like all early history. Much that has survived is of almost incidental importance in manuscripts dealing primarily with medicine. Some, however, was more specifically concerned with toxic action, and many records deal with the use of poisons either for judicial execution, political assassination, or suicide. It is also undoubtedly true that toxicology must rank as one of the oldest practical sciences because humans, from the very beginning, needed to avoid the numerous toxic plants and animals in their environment.

The papyrus *Ebers,* an Egyptian papyrus dating from about 1500 BC, which must rank as the earliest surviving pharmacopeia, and the surviving medical works of Hippocrates, Aristotle, and Theophrastus, published during the period 400–250 BC, all included some mention of poisons. The early Greek poet Nicander treats, in two poetic works, of animal toxins (Therica) and antidotes to plant and animal toxins (Alexipharmica). The earliest surviving attempt to classify plants according to their toxic and therapeutic effects is that of Dioscorides, a Greek employed by the Roman Emperor Nero about AD 50.

There appear to have been few advances in either medicine or toxicology between the time of Galen (AD 131–200) and Paracelsus (1493–1541). It was the latter who, despite frequent confusion between fact and mysticism, laid the groundwork for the later development of modern toxicology. He clearly was aware of the dose–response relationship. His statement: "All substances are poisons; there is none that is not a poison. The right dose differentiates a poison and a remedy," is properly regarded as a landmark in the development of the science. His belief in the value of experimentation also represents a break with much earlier tradition.

Although Orfila, writing in the early nineteenth century, is generally regarded as the father of modern toxicology there were some important developments in the eighteenth century. Probably the best known is the publication of Ramazzini's *Diseases of Workers* in 1700, which has led to his recognition as the father of occupational medicine. The correlation between the occupation of chimney sweeps and scrotal cancer by Percival Pott in 1775 is also noteworthy.

Orfila, a Spaniard working at the University of Paris, clearly identified toxicology as a separate science and wrote the first book, in 1815, devoted exclusively to it. (An English translation, published in 1817, was entitled *A General System of Toxicology or, a Treatise on Poisons, Found in the Mineral, Vegetable and Animal Kingdoms, Considered in Their Relations with Physiology, Pathology and Medical Jurisprudence.*) Workers of the later nineteenth century who produced treatises on toxicology include Christison, Kobert, and Lewin. Since then, advances have been numerous—too numerous to list. They have increased our knowledge of the chemistry of poisons, the treatment of poisoning, the analysis both of toxicants and toxicity, as well as mode of action and detoxication. Many of them will be outlined in the pages to follow.

It is clear, however, that during the last two or three decades, toxicology has entered a phase of rapid development and has changed from a science that was almost entirely descriptive to one in which the study of mechanisms enjoys a considerable vogue. There are many reasons for this, including the development of new analytical methods since 1945, the emphasis on drug testing following the thalidomide tragedy, the emphasis on pesticide testing following the publication of Rachel Carson's *Silent Spring,* and public concerns with hazardous waste disposal.

1.2 SOURCES OF TOXIC COMPOUNDS

1.2.1 Synthetic Organic Compounds

Some of the compounds mentioned are natural products and are included in this section in cases in which they are closely related, by use or chemistry, to a large class of synthetic chemicals. Otherwise, they may appear in Section 1.2.7.

1.2.1.1 Air, Water, and Food Pollutants

Both the nature and source of air pollutants vary with the location; open country remote from industry or heavy traffic will clearly differ from the center of a large city or an area downwind from a coal-fired power plant or other industry. In general, however, the principal air pollutants are CO, oxides of nitrogen, oxides of sulfur, hydrocarbons, and particulates. The principal sources are transportation, industrial processes, electric power generation, and the heating of homes and buildings.

Of the organic constituents, hydrocarbons such as benzo(a)pyrene are produced by incomplete combustion and are probably associated primarily with the automobile. The hydrocarbons are usually not present at levels high enough to cause a directly measurable toxic effect but are important in the formation of photochemical air pollution. This pollution is formed as a result of interactions between oxides of nitrogen and hydrocarbons in the presence of ultraviolet (UV) light, the resultant reactions giving rise to such lung irritants such as peroxyacetyl nitrate, acrolein, and formaldehyde.

Particulates are a heterogeneous mixture, often in the form of smoke; they are important as carriers of adsorbed hydrocarbons as well as being irritants to the respiratory system. The distribution of such particles in the atmosphere, as well as in the respiratory tract, is largely a function of their size.

Water pollution by toxic chemicals comes from run-off from urban streets or of agricultural chemicals from cultivated fields, from sewage, or from specific industrial sources such as refineries, smelters, or chemical plants. Although some sources are diffuse and difficult to control, others are from specific point sources and can be controlled at the point of origin.

Agricultural chemicals found in water may include insecticides such as chlorinated hydrocarbons, organophosphates, and carbamates (see Section 1.2.1.6). The chlorinated hydrocarbons such as DDT, chlordane, and dieldrin, previously of most concern because of their persistence, are now less important because of curtailed use in the United States and some other countries. Other pesticides include herbicides, fungicides, nematocides, and rodenticides. Fertilizers, although less of a toxic hazard, contribute to such environmental problems as eutrophication. In some cases, the point source for agricultural chemicals is the manufacturing operation. The contamination of the James river in Virginia with kepone (chlordecone) is a case in point.

Low molecular weight halogenated hydrocarbons such as chloroform, dichloroethane, and carbon tetrachloride may enter water directly or may be formed as a result of the chlorination of precursors during water purification. Chlorinated aromatics such as the polychlorinated biphenyls (PCBs), chlorophenols, and even the highly toxic 2,3,7,8-tetrachlorodibenzo-*p*-dioxin (TCDD) are commonly found in water, as are the phthalate ester plasticizers, such as di-2-ethylhexylphthalate and di-*n*-butylphthalate. Detergents, such as the alkyl benzene sulfonates, are common contaminants of water that arise from domestic effluent. Since the discovery of insecticides such as aldicarb or soil fumigants such as ethylene dibromide in ground water drawn from wells, this form of water pollution has become a new concern. A number of toxic inorganics, mentioned in Section 1.2.3, have also been found in water.

Food contaminants, as opposed to food additives, are those compounds included inadvertently in foods, either raw, cooked, or processed. They include a wide variety of products ranging from bacterial toxins such as the exotoxin of *Clostridium botulinum,* mycotoxins such as aflatoxins from *Aspergillus flavus,* plant alkaloids, animal toxins, pesticide residues, and residues of animal food additives such as diethylstilbestrol and antibiotics, to a variety of industrial chemicals such as PCBs and polybrominated biphenyls.

1.2.1.2 Chemical Additives in Food

Chemicals are added to food for a number of reasons: as preservatives, either antibacterial, antifungal, or antioxidants; to change physical characteristics, particularly for processing; to change taste; to change color; and to change odor. In general, food additives have proven to be safe and without chronic toxicity. Many were introduced when toxicity testing was relatively unsophisticated, however, and some of these have been subsequently shown to be toxic. Table 1.1 gives examples of different types of organic food additives. Inorganics, the most important of which are nitrate and nitrite, are discussed later. Certainly hundreds, and possibly thousands, of food additives are in use worldwide, many with inadequate testing. The question of synergistic interactions between these compounds has not been adequately explored. Not all toxicants in food are synthetic; many examples of naturally occurring toxicants in the human diet are known, including carcinogens and mutagens (see Section 1.2.2.3).

1.2.1.3 Chemicals in the Workplace

In an industrial society, the number of possible chemicals in the workplace is extremely high, and many of these chemicals are known to have deleterious biological effects. Regulation and control of industrial chemicals are discussed in Chapter 10.

Among the inorganics are metals such as lead, copper, mercury, zinc, cadmium, and beryllium, as well as fluorides, carbon monoxide, etc.

The organic compounds include aliphatic hydrocarbons (eg, hexane), aromatic hydrocarbons (eg, benzene, toluene, xylene), halogenated hydrocarbons

TABLE 1.1
Examples of Organic Chemicals Used as Food Additives

Function	Class	Example
Preservatives	Antioxidants	Butylatedhydroxyanisole Ascorbic acid
	Fungistatic agents	Methyl *p*-benzoic acid Propionates
	Bactericides	Sodium nitrite
Processing aids	Anticaking agents	Calcium silicate Sodium aluminosilicate
	Emulsifiers	Propylene glycol Monoglycerides
	Chelating agents	EDTA Sodium tartrate
	Stabilizers	Gum ghatti Sodium alginate
	Humectants	Propylene glycol Glycerol
Flavor and taste modification	Synthetic sweeteners	Saccharin Mannitol Aspartame
	Synthetic flavor	Piperonal Vanillin
Color modification	Synthetic dyes	Tartrazine (FD&C Yellow 5) (a pyrazolone dye) Sunset Yellow (a monoazophenyl naphthalene dye)
Nutritional supplements	Vitamins	Thiamin Vitamin D_3
	Amino acids	Alanine Aspartic acid
	Inorganics	Manganese sulfate Zinc sulfate

(eg, dichloromethane, trichloroethane, trichloroethylene, vinyl chloride), alcohols (eg, methanol, ethylene glycol), esters [eg, methylmethacrylate, di-(2-ethylhexyl)phthalate], organometallics (eg, tributyltin acetate), amino compounds (eg, aniline), nitro derivatives (eg, nitrobenzene), and many others. In addition, there are many manufactured products, such as the pesticides summarized in Section 1.2.1.6 and the intermediates that occur in their synthesis.

1.2.1.4 Drugs of Abuse

All drugs are toxic at some dose and at such doses have deleterious effects on humans. Drugs of abuse either have no medicinal function or are taken at dose levels higher than would be required for therapy. Many, when properly prescribed and taken, are of clinical importance. In the latter case, the benefits, in the opinion of the physician, outweigh the risks.

Although some drugs of abuse may affect only higher nervous functions — mood, reaction time, and coordination — many produce physical dependence and have serious physical effects, with fatal overdoses being a common occurrence.

The drugs of abuse include central nervous system (CNS) depressants such as ethanol, methaqualone (quaalude), and secobarbital; central nervous system stimulants such as cocaine, methamphetamine (speed), caffeine, and nicotine; opioids such as heroin, morphine, and meperidine (demerol); and hallucinogens such as lysergic acid diethylamide (LSD), phencyclidine (PCP), and tetrahydrocannabinol, the most important active principle of marijuana. A further complication of toxicological significance is that many drugs of abuse are synthesized in illegal, inadequately equipped laboratories with little or no quality control. The resultant products are therefore often contaminated with compounds of unknown, but conceivably dangerous, toxicity.

The structures of some of these compounds are shown in Figure 1.1.

1.2.1.5 Therapeutic Drugs

Essentially all therapeutic drugs can be toxic, producing deleterious effects at some dose. The danger to the individual depends on several factors, including the nature of the toxic response, the dose necessary to produce the toxic response, and the relationship between the therapeutic dose and the toxic dose. Drug toxicity is affected by all factors that affect the toxicity of other xenobiotics, including individual (genetic) variation, diet, age, and the presence of other exogenous chemicals.

Even when the risk of toxic side effects from a particular drug has been evaluated, it must be weighed against the expected benefits. The use of a very dangerous drug with only a narrow tolerance between the therapeutic and toxic doses may still be justified if it is the sole treatment for an otherwise fatal disease. On the other hand, a relatively safe drug may be inappropriate if safer compounds are available or if the condition being treated is trivial. One must also keep in mind that the dramatic expansion of the pharmaceutical industry between 1935 and 1965 placed a large number of drugs in use, many of which have not been tested for toxicity by methods now considered adequate.

The three principal classes of cytotoxic agents used in the treatment of cancer all contain known carcinogens, eg, Melphalen, a nitrogen mustard, adriamycin, an antitumor antibiotic, and methotrexate, an antimetabolite. Diethylstilbestrol (DES), a drug formerly widely used, has been associated with cancer of the cervix and vagina in the offspring of treated women.

Other toxic effects of drugs can be associated with almost every organ system. The stiffness of the joints accompanied by optic nerve damage (SMON subacute myelo-optic neuropathy) that was common in Japan in the 1960s was apparently a toxic side effect of chloroquinol (Enterovioform), an antidiarrhea drug. Teratogenesis can also be caused by drugs, with thalidomide the most alarming example. Skin effects (dermatitis) are common side effects of drugs, for example, in the case of topically applied corticosteroids.

1. Central Nervous System Depressants

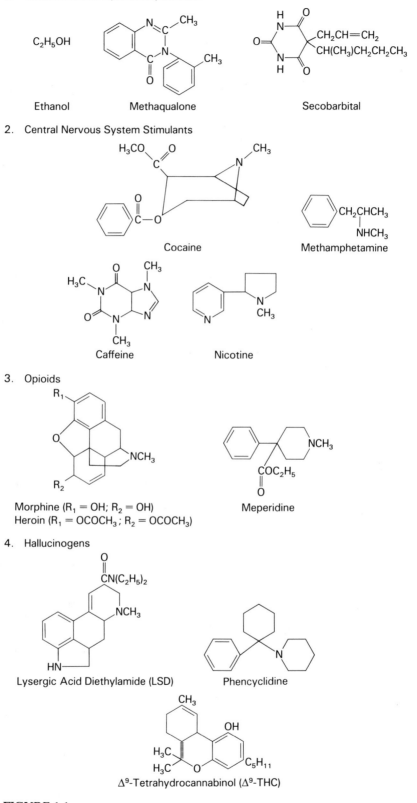

Ethanol   Methaqualone   Secobarbital

2. Central Nervous System Stimulants

Cocaine   Methamphetamine

Caffeine   Nicotine

3. Opioids

Morphine (R$_1$ = OH; R$_2$ = OH)
Heroin (R$_1$ = OCOCH$_3$; R$_2$ = OCOCH$_3$)

Meperidine

4. Hallucinogens

Lysergic Acid Diethylamide (LSD)   Phencyclidine

Δ^9-Tetrahydrocannabinol (Δ^9-THC)

FIGURE 1.1.
Some common drugs of abuse.

A number of toxic effects on the blood have been documented, including agranulocytosis caused by chlorpromazine, hemolytic anemia caused by methyldopa, and megaloblastic anemia caused by methotrexate. Toxic effects on the eye have also been noted, and range from the retinotoxicity caused by thioridazine to glaucoma caused by systemic corticosteroids.

It should be emphasized that, in general, toxic side effects are not common and may occur only in susceptible individuals or populations. At the same time, the wide variety of such effects and their frequent severity argue against indiscriminate or unnecessary use of therapeutic drugs.

1.2.1.6 Pesticides

Pesticides are developed to control a wide variety of pests, to increase the production of food and fiber, and to facilitate modern agricultural production methods. By the very nature of their use in pest control, they are common contaminants of the environment, food and water, and domestic structures. Although selective toxicity toward target organisms is a desirable quality, it is not absolute, and most pesticides are toxic to a greater or lesser extent toward nontarget organisms, including humans. Thus, in an attempt to control unwanted toxic side effects and, at the same time, obtain the benefits to be derived from their use, a considerable body of law and regulation concerned with their registration and use has developed.

The various classes of pesticide are shown in Table 1.2; some of the important structures are shown in Figure 1.2.

TABLE 1.2
Classification of Pesticides, with Examples

Class	Principal Chemical Type	Example Common Name (Chemical Name)
Algicide	Organotin	Brestar (triphenyltin acetate)
Fungicide	Dicarboximide	Captan (N-trichloromethylthio)-4-cyclohexene-1,2-dicarboximide)
	Chlorinated aromatic	Pentachlorophenol
	Dithiocarbamate	Maneb ((ethylene*bis* (dithiocarbamato))manganese)
	Mercurial	Phenylmercuric acetate
Herbicide	Amides, Acetamides	Propanil (N-(3,4-dichlorophenyl)-propanamide)
	Bipyridyl	Paraquat (N,N'-dimethyl-γ,γ'-dipyridylium)
	Carbamates, Thiocarbamates	Barban ((3-chlorphenyl)carbamic acid 4-chloro-2-butynyl ester)
	Phenoxy	2,4-D (2,4-dichlorophenoxyacetic acid)
	Dinitrophenol	DNOC (4,6-dinitro-o-cresol)
	Dinitroaniline	Trifluralin (2,6-dinitro-N,N-dipropyl-4-trifluoromethyl aniline)
	Substituted urea	Monuron (N'-(4-chlorophenyl)-N,N-dimethylurea)

TABLE 1.2 *(Continued)*

Class	Principal Chemical Type	Example Common Name (Chemical Name)
	Triazine	Atrazine (6-chloro-*N*-ethyl-*N'*-(1-methylethyl)-1,3,5-triazine-2,4-diamine)
Nematocide	Halogenated alkane	Ethylene dibromide (EDB) (This is a misnomer; compound is 1,2-dibromoethane)
Molluscide	Chlorinated hydrocarbon	Bayluscide (2,5-dichloro-4'-nitrosalicylanilide ethanolamine)
Insecticide	Chlorinated hydrocarbons DDT analogs	DDT (1,1,1-trichloro-2,2-*bis* (*p*-chlorophenyl)ethane)
	Chlorinated alicyclic Cyclodiene	BHC (hexachlorocyclohexane) Aldrin (1,2,3,4,10,10-hexachloro-1,4,4a,5,8,8a-hexahydro-1,4,5,8-dimethanonaphthalene)
	Chlorinated terpenes	Toxaphene (complex mixture of chlorinated terpenes)
	Organophosphate	Parathion (*O*,*O*-diethyl *O-p*-nitrophenyl phosphorothioate
	Carbamate	Carbaryl (1-naphthyl-*N*-methylcarbamate)
	Thiocyanate	Lethane 60 (2-thiocyanatoethyl laurate)
	Dinitrophenols	DNOC (4,6-dinitro-*o*-cresol)
	Fluoroacetates	Nissol (2-fluoro-*N*-methyl-*N*-(1-naphthyl) acetamide)
	Botanicals Nicotinoids	Nicotine (1-methyl-2-(3-pyridyl)-pyrrolidine)
	Rotenoids	Rotenone (1,2,12,12a-tetrahydro-8,9-dimethoxy-2-(1-methylethenyl-(1)benzopyrano (3,4b)furo(2,3h)(1) benzopyran-6(6H)-one)
	Pyrethroids	Fenvalerate (cyano(3-phenoxyphenyl)-methyl-4-chloro-α-(1-methylethyl)benzene-acetate)
	Juvenile hormone analogs	Methoprene (isopropyl(2E,4E) 11-methoxy-3,7,11-trimethyl-2,4-dodecadienoate)
	Growth regulators	Dimilin (*N*(((4-chlorophenyl)-amino)carbonyl)-2,6-difluorobenzamide)
	Inorganics Arsenicals	Lead arsenate
	Fluorides	Sodium fluoride
	Microbials	Thuricide (68,000-dalton protein from *Bacillus thuringensis*) Avermectin

(Continued)

TABLE 1.2 *(Continued)*

Class	Principal Chemical Type	Example Common Name (Chemical Name)
Insecticide synergists	Methylenedioxyphenyl	Piperonyl butoxide (α-(2-(2-butoxyethoxy)ethoxy)-4,5-methylenedioxy-2-propyl-toluene)
	Dicarboximides	MGK-264 (*N*-(2-ethylhexyl)-5-norbornene-2,3-dicarboximide
Acaricides	Organosulfur compounds	Ovex (*p*-chlorphenyl *p*-chlorobenzenesulfonate)
	Formamidine	Chlordimeform (*N'*-(4-chloro-2-methylphenyl)-*N,N*-dimethyl-methanimidamide)
	Dinitrophenols	Dinex (2-cyclohexy-4,6-dinitro-phenol)
	DDT analogs	Chlorobenzilate (ethyl-4,4'-di-chlorobenzilate)
Rodenticides	Anticoagulants	Warfarin (3-(α-acetonylbenzyl)-4-hydroxycoumarin)
	Botanicals	
	Alkaloids	Strychnine sulfate
	Glycosides	Scillaren A and B
	Fluorides	Sodium fluoroacetate
	Inorganics	Thallium sulfate
	Thioureas	ANTU (α-naphthylthiourea)

1.2.1.7 Solvents

Although solvents are more a feature of the industrial environment, they are also found in the home. In addition to cutaneous effects of solvents, such as defatting and local irritation, many have systemic toxic effects, including effects on the nervous system or, as with benzene, on the blood-forming elements. Commercial solvents are frequently complex mixtures and may include nitrogen or sulfur-containing organics—gasoline and other oil-based products are excellent examples of this.

The common solvents fall into the following classes:

1. Aliphatic hydrocarbons, such as hexane. These may be straight or branched chain compounds and are often present in mixtures.
2. Halogenated aliphatic hydrocarbons. The best known examples are methylene dichloride, chloroform, and carbon tetrachloride, although chlorinated ethylenes are also widely used.
3. Aliphatic alcohols, such as methanol and ethanol.
4. Glycols and glycol ethers such as ethylene and propylene glycols. Use in antifreeze gives rise to considerable exposure of the general public. The glycol ethers, such as methyl cellosolve, are also widely used.
5. Aromatic hydrocarbons. Benzene is probably the one of greatest concern, but others, such as toluene, are also used.

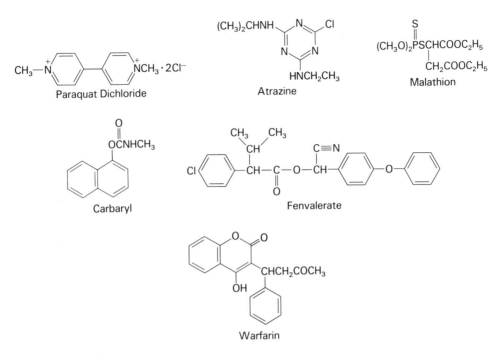

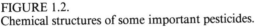

FIGURE 1.2.
Chemical structures of some important pesticides.

1.2.1.8 Polycyclic Aromatic Hydrocarbons

Although some natural products such as coal and crude oil contain polycyclic aromatic hydrocarbons, they are generally associated with incomplete combustion of organic materials and are found in smoke from wood, coal, oil, tobacco, etc., as well as in tar and broiled foods. Because some of them are carcinogens, they have been studied intensively from the point of view of metabolic activation, interaction with DNA, and chemical carcinogenesis. Some of these compounds are heterocyclic, containing nitrogen atoms in at least one of the rings.

The chemical structures of a selection of the most studied polycyclic aromatic hydrocarbons are shown in Figure 1.3.

1.2.1.9 Cosmetics

The most common deleterious effects of cosmetics are occasional allergic reactions and contact dermatitis. The highly toxic and/or carcinogenic azo or aromatic amine dyes are no longer in use; neither are the organometallics, which were used in even earlier times. Bromates, used in some cold-wave neutralizers may be acutely toxic if ingested, as may the ethanol used as a solvent in hair dyes and perfumes.

Thioglycolates and thioglycerol used in cold-wave lotion and depilatories and sodium hydroxide used in hair straighteners are also toxic on ingestion. Used as directed, cosmetics appear to present little risk of systemic poisoning,

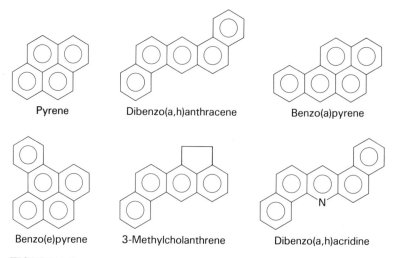

Pyrene   Dibenzo(a,h)anthracene   Benzo(a)pyrene

Benzo(e)pyrene   3-Methylcholanthrene   Dibenzo(a,h)acridine

FIGURE 1.3.
Examples of carcinogenic polycyclic aromatic hydrocarbons.

due in part to the deletion of ingredients now known to be toxic and in part to the small quantities absorbed.

1.2.2 Naturally Occurring Toxins

1.2.2.1 Mycotoxins

The range of chemical structures and biological activity among the broad class of fungal metabolites is large and cannot be summarized briefly.

> However narrowly they are defined, the mycotoxins do not constitute a chemical category and they have no molecular features in common. All that can be found among their variety is a series of structurally related groups, which emerge most clearly and rationally when they are considered alongside other fungal products and classified in terms of biosynthetic pathways rather than structural features as such. (Bu'Lock 1980)

The reader is referred to P.S. Steyn (ed), 1980, for such a treatment.

Mycotoxins of most interest are those found in human food or in the feed of domestic animals. They include the ergot alkaloids produced by *Claviceps* sp., aflatoxins and related compounds produced by *Aspergillus* sp., and the tricothecenes produced by several genera of fungi imperfecti, primarily *Fusarium* sp.

The ergot alkaloids (Figure 1.4) are known to affect the nervous system and to be vasoconstrictors. Historically, they have been implicated in epidemics of both gangrenous and convulsive ergotism (St Anthony's fire), although such epidemics no longer occur in humans due to increased knowledge of the cause and to more varied modern diets. Outbreaks of ergotism in livestock do still occur frequently, however. These compounds have also been used as abortifacients. The ergot alkaloids are derivatives of ergotine, the most active being, more specifically, amides of lysergic acid.

Aflatoxins are products of species of the genus *Aspergillus,* particularly *A*

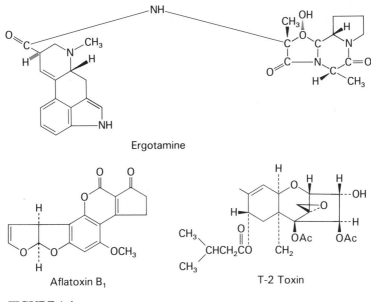

FIGURE 1.4.
Selected mycotoxins.

flavus, a common fungus found as a contaminant of grain, maize, peanuts, etc. First implicated in poultry diseases such as Turkey-X disease, they were subsequently shown to cause cancer in experimental animals and, from epidemiological studies, in humans. Aflatoxin B_1, the most toxic of the aflatoxins, must be enzymatically activated to exert its carcinogenic effect (see Section 6.1.5.1).

Tricothecenes are a large class of sesquiterpenoid fungal metabolites produced particularly by members of the genera *Fusarium* and *Tricoderma.* They are frequently acutely toxic, displaying bactericidal, fungicidal, and insecticidal activity, as well as causing various clinical symptoms in mammals, including diarrhea, anorexia, and ataxia. They have been implicated in natural intoxications in both humans and animals, such as Abakabi disease in Japan and Stachybotryotoxicosis in the USSR, and are the center of a continuing controversy concerning their possible use as chemical warfare agents.

Mycotoxins may also be used for beneficial purposes. The mycotoxin avermectin is currently generating considerable interest both as an insecticide and for the control of nematode parasites of domestic animals.

1.2.2.2 Microbial Toxins

The term microbial toxin is usually reserved by microbiologists for toxic substances produced by microorganisms that are of high molecular weight and have antigenic properties; toxic compounds produced by bacteria that do not fit these criteria are referred to simply as poisons. Many of the former are proteins or mucoproteins and may have a variety of enzymatic properties. They include some of the most toxic substances known, such as tetanus toxin, botulinus toxin, and diphtheria toxin. Bacterial toxins may be extremely toxic to mammals and may affect a variety of organ systems, including the nervous system and the cardiovascular system. A detailed account of their chemical nature and mode of action is beyond the scope of this volume.

The range of poisonous chemicals produced by bacteria is also large. Some examples are shown in Figure 1.5.

Again, such compounds may also be used for beneficial purposes, for example, the insecticidal properties of *Bacillus thuringiensis,* due to a toxin, have been utilized in agriculture for some time.

1.2.2.3   Plant Toxins

The large array of toxic chemicals produced by plants (phytotoxins), usually referred to as secondary plant compounds, are often held to have evolved as defense mechanisms against herbivorous animals, particularly insects and mammals. These compounds may be repellent, but not particularly toxic, or they may be acutely toxic to a wide range of organisms. They include sulfur compounds, lipids, phenols, alkaloids, glycosides, and many other types of chemicals. Many of the common drugs of abuse (Figure 1.1) such as cocaine, caffeine, nicotine, morphine, and the cannabinoids are plant toxins. Some further examples are shown in Figure 1.6. Many chemicals that have been shown to be toxic are constituents of plants that form part of the human diet. For example, the carcinogen safrole and related compounds are found in black pepper. Solanine and chaconine, which are cholinesterase inhibitors and possible teratogens, are found in potatoes, and quinones and phenols are widespread in food. Livestock poisoning by plants is still an important veterinary problem in some areas.

1.2.2.4   Animal Toxins

Some species from practically all phyla of animals produce toxins. Some are passively venomous, often following inadvertent ingestion, whereas others are actively venomous, injecting poisons through specially adapted stings or mouthparts. It may be more appropriate to refer to the latter group only as venomous, referring to the former simply as poisonous. The chemistry of animal toxins extends from enzymes and neurotoxic and cardiotoxic peptides and proteins to many small molecules such as biogenic amines, alkaloids,

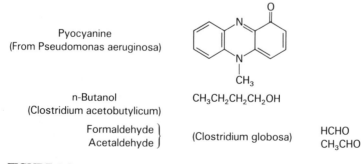

Pyocyanine
(From Pseudomonas aeruginosa)

n-Butanol
(Clostridium acetobutylicum) $CH_3CH_2CH_2CH_2OH$

Formaldehyde ⎫
Acetaldehyde ⎭   (Clostridium globosa)   HCHO
                                                       CH_3CHO

FIGURE 1.5.
Some selected poisons from bacteria.

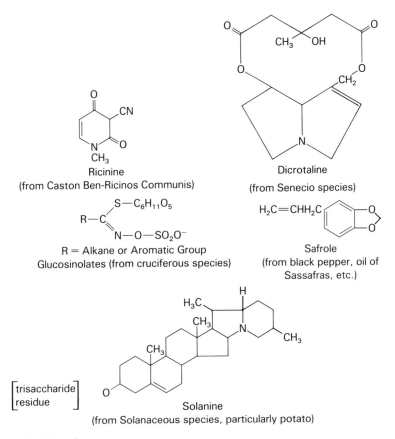

Ricinine
(from Caston Ben-Ricinos Communis)

Dicrotaline
(from Senecio species)

R = Alkane or Aromatic Group
Glucosinolates (from cruciferous species)

Safrole
(from black pepper, oil of
Sassafras, etc.)

trisaccharide residue

Solanine
(from Solanaceous species, particularly potato)

FIGURE 1.6.
Selected examples of plant toxins.

glycosides, terpenes, and others. In many cases, the venoms are complex mixtures that include both proteins and small molecules and depend on the interaction of the components for the full expression of their toxic effect. For example, bee venom contains a biogenic amine, histamine, three peptides, and two enzymes (Table 1.3). The venoms and defensive secretions of insects may also contain many relatively simple toxicants or irritants such as formic acid, benzoquinone, and other quinones, or terpenes such as citronellal.

Snake venoms have also been extensively studied; their effects are due, in general, to toxins that are peptides with 60–70 amino acids. These toxins are cardiotoxic or neurotoxic and their effects are usually accentuated by the phospholipases, peptidases, proteases, and other enzymes present in venoms. These enzymes may affect the blood clotting mechanisms and damage blood vessels.

Some other well-known animal toxins are shown in Figure 1.7.

1.2.3 Inorganic Chemicals

In addition to the inorganic air pollutants such as nitrogen oxides and oxides of sulfur, probably the most important inorganic toxicants are metals.

Some of the most important toxic metals are beryllium, used in the steel

TABLE 1.3
Some Components of Bee Venom

Compound	Effect
Biogenic Amine	
Histamine	Pain
	Vasodilation
	Increased capillary permeability
Peptides	
Apamine	CNS effects
Melittin	Hemolytic
	Serotonin release
	Cardiotoxic
Mast cell degranulating peptide	Histamine release from mast cells
Enzymes	
Phospholipase A	Increased spreading and penetration of tissues
Hyaluronidase	

Saxitoxin
(Produced by dinoflagelates — taken up by molluscs)

Tetrodotoxin
(Produced by puffer fish and other fishes)

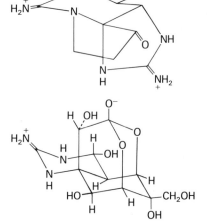

Batrachotoxin A
(Produced by poison-dart frogs)

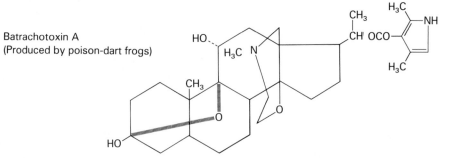

FIGURE 1.7.
Selected animal toxicants.

industry; cadmium, exposure to which occurs in welding and soldering and through tobacco smoking; and mercury, which is used in the electronics industry and in fungicides. Epidemics of mercury poisoning have resulted from the use of mercury compounds in the pulp and paper industries and in plastic manufacturing. Another metal of particular importance is lead, used in leaded gasoline and batteries and formerly in paint. Lead poisoning has been common in children, particularly in slum housing, and has been diagnosed frequently in livestock. Lead is still a widespread contaminant of water, air, and a common component of gasoline.

Certain metals, such as mercury, can be converted into more toxic alkyl derivatives by bacteria in the environment. Organic lead compounds, such as tetraethyl lead, can be absorbed readily through the lungs and skin.

In food and animal feeds, nitrite and nitrate are the toxic inorganic chemicals of most concern.

1.3 ENVIRONMENTAL MOVEMENT OF TOXICANTS

Chemicals released into the environment rarely remain in the form, or at the location, of release. Agricultural chemicals used as sprays may drift from the point of application as air contaminants or enter run-off water as water contaminants. Many of these chemicals are susceptible to bacterial and fungal degradation and are rapidly detoxified, frequently being broken down to compounds that can enter the carbon, nitrogen, and oxygen cycles. Others, particularly halogenated organics, are recalcitrant to a greater or lesser degree to metabolism by microorganisms and persist in the soil as contaminants; they may enter biological food chains and move to higher trophic levels or persist in the processed crop as postharvest food contaminants. For example, DDT and its principal metabolite DDE were involved in all of these routes and can still be detected in many locations years after the use of DDT was discontinued. Soil fumigants, such as ethylene dibromide (EDB), have now been found in ground water. Similarly, industrial chemicals released in waste water may also become widely disseminated.

Although most transport between inanimate phases of the environment results in wider dissemination but, at the same time, dilution of the toxicant in question, transfer between living creatures may result in an increased concentration or bioaccumulation. Lipid soluble toxicants are readily taken up by organisms following exposure in air, water, or soil. Unless rapidly metabolized, they persist in the tissues long enough to be transferred to the next trophic level. At each level, the lipophilic toxicant tends to be retained while the bulk of the food is digested, utilized, and excreted, thus increasing the toxicant concentration. At some point in the chain, the toxicant can become deleterious, particularly if the organism at that trophic level is more susceptible than those at the level proceeding it. Examples of such food chains are:

$$
\left(\begin{array}{c} \text{Soil} \\ \text{Residues} \end{array}\right)
\begin{array}{l}
\nearrow \quad \text{Soil invertebrates} \rightarrow \text{predatory invertebrates} \rightarrow \\
\qquad \text{terrestrial vertebrates} \rightarrow \text{predatory birds or mammals} \\
\\
\searrow \quad \text{Terrestrial plants} \rightarrow \text{herbivorous animals} \rightarrow \text{predatory} \\
\qquad \text{birds or mammals}
\end{array}
$$

It seems fairly certain that the reproductive failure in certain raptorial birds such as the sparrow hawk, brought about by egg shell thinning, was due to the uptake of DDT through the food chain and their particular susceptibility to this type of toxicity.

It is clear that such transport can occur through both aquatic and terrestrial food chains, although in the former, higher members of the chains, such as fish, can accumulate large amounts of toxicants directly from the medium. This accumulation occurs because of the large area of the gill filaments, their intimate contact with the water, and the high flow rate of water over them. Given these characteristics and a toxicant with a high partition coefficient between water and lipid membranes, considerable uptake is inevitable.

1.4 SUGGESTED FURTHER READING

Ames, B.W. Dietary carcinogens and anticarcinogens. Science 1983; 221:1256–1264.

Ariens, E.J., Simonis, A.M., Offermeier, J. Introduction to General Toxicology. New York: Academic Press, 1976, 230 pp.

Bennett, G., Vourakis, C., Woolf, D.S. (eds.). Substance Abuse. Pharmacological, Developmental and Clinical Perspectives. New York: Wiley, 1983, 453 pp.

Doull, J., Klaassen, C.D., Amdur, M.O. (eds.). Casarett and Doull's Toxicology. 2nd ed. New York: Macmillan, 1980, 778 pp.

Esser, H.O., Moser, P. An appraisal of problems related to the measurement and evolution of bioaccumulation. Ecotoxicol. Environ. Safety 1982; 6:131–148.

Gilman, A.G., Goodman, L.S., Gilman, A. (eds.). Goodman and Gilman's The Pharmacological Basis of Therapeutics. 7th ed. New York: Macmillan, 1985, 1843 pp.

Guthrie, F.E., Perry, J.J. (eds.). Introduction to Environmental Toxicology. New York: Elsevier, 1980, 484 pp.

Habermehl, G.G. Venomous Animals and Their Toxins. Berlin: Springer-Verlag, 1981, 195 pp.

Hayes, A.W. (ed.). Principles and Methods of Toxicology. New York: Raven Press, 1982, 750 pp.

Hayes, W.J. Pesticides Studied in Man. Baltimore: Williams & Wilkins, 1982.

Hodgson, E., Guthrie, F.E. (eds.). Introduction to Biochemical Toxicology. New York: Elsevier, 1980, 437 pp.

Loomis, T.A. Essentials of Toxicology. 2nd ed. Philadelphia: Lea & Febiger, 1974, 223 pp.

Matsumura, F. Toxicology of Insecticides. New York: Plenum Press, 1975, 503 pp.

Steyn, P.S. (ed.). The Biosynthesis of Mycotoxins: A Study in Secondary Metabolism. New York: Academic Press, 1980.

Thomson, W.T. Agricultural Chemicals Book I. Insecticides. 1979–1980 rev. San Francisco: Thomson Publications, 1979, 234 pp.

Timbrell, J.A. Principles of Biochemical Toxicology. London: Taylor and Francis, 1982, 249 pp.

Wexler, P. Information Resources in Toxicology. New York: Elsevier, 1982, 333 pp.

chapter two

ABSORPTION AND DISTRIBUTION OF TOXICANTS

Frank E. Guthrie and Ernest Hodgson

2.1 INTRODUCTION

Until the middle part of this century, the skin and other body barriers were believed to be relatively effective in preventing potential poisons from entering the body. We now know that almost every toxicant can pass through one or more portals of entry, although there may be considerable differences in rate; thus, given time, few, if any, chemicals will be excluded from entry. Toxicants, however, are usually metabolized between the time of entry and transport to the site of action, so that they may become either less harmful or activated to more toxic compounds. It should be emphasized that toxicants do not pass through the body on a single linear pathway. Different routes of metabolism and modes of action are possible, and these routes are dependent on the organ to which that portion of the dose was distributed, the simultaneous presence of other toxicants, the dose level, and many other factors. Not only are these various pathways dynamically related to each other, but their relative contribution to the overall fate of the toxicant can vary as a result of both extrinsic and intrinsic factors.

Each portal of entry permits a different rate of penetration and may also cause different metabolic patterns. In general, the respiratory system offers the most rapid route of entry and the dermal the least rapid, although overall entry depends both on the amount present and the saturability of the epithelium involved.

Many of the opportunities for entry into the body are related to the form of the toxicant and its location in the environment. Although a chemical in the vapor phase may have very high probability for respiratory entry, if it is associated exclusively with water insofar as its contact with the target organism is concerned, the problem becomes primarily one of gastrointestinal (GI) toxicity for terrestrial animals and dermal and gill uptake for aquatic animals. If a chemical is strongly bound to an organic or inorganic component of the environment, there is little likelihood that it will be absorbed while it is in that strongly bound form. Opportunities for transfer from one form (or substrate) to another make poisoning difficult to predict, however. For example, some very volatile compounds that could cause serious problems through lung entry have been found to be transported in water for considerable distances. They become GI problems during the transport phase and may again become respiratory poisons at termination of transport. For this reason, volatile toxic compounds do not always disappear as might be expected and may become chronic hazards at points far removed from their original entry into the environment. For example, a volatile compound placed "safely" in a metal drum in a waste dump may enter ground water following leakage from a rusting drum. Eventually, it could become a chronic problem in a house that, although built several miles from the disposal dump, still receives small amounts of effluent on a continuing basis.

As will be discussed later, the events occurring during toxic action are very dynamic. A chemical may enter the body only to be metabolized and eliminated prior to toxic action. On the contrary, the toxicant may be absorbed, transported to the site of action, and quickly effect an adverse action. Toxicokinetics refers to the rates of all metabolic processes related to the expression of toxic endpoints and includes the relationship between such rates and their integration into formal models that provide a mathematical description of all or any part of the overall process. Often overlooked is the fact that the acute and chronic actions of a toxicant are often exerted on different systems. Many chlorinated hydrocarbons affect the nervous system following relatively high, acute doses. The same chemicals given in small, chronic amounts for long periods have no important actions on the nervous system but, in time, may have carcinogenic actions on such organs as the liver.

The major routes of entry are respiratory, gastrointestinal, and dermal. Depending on the chemical form and access of the organism to the chemical, the importance of a particular route may be either inconsequential or of key importance. If the chemical enters the body, it is then transported. The circulatory system offers an ideal transport system because it can easily move water-soluble as well as lipid-soluble compounds by virtue either of the aqueous medium or the proteins it contains. These proteins may serve to bind the toxicants for release at some tissue distant from the site of entry. Such transport may carry a toxicant to a site of toxic action, to a site of metabolism, to a site of storage, or to organs of elimination. All these events occur simultaneously, and the resulting dynamic flux makes the study of movement quite complex.

2.2 MEMBRANES

Toxicants pass a number of barriers during entry into the body as well as entering tissues and cells. Such barriers include structures that vary from the relatively thick areas of the skin to the relatively thin lung membranes. In all cases, the membranes of tissue, cell, and cell organelle are basically similar and are described by the unifying cell membrane concept.

The basic model, first postulated by Davson and Danielli in 1935, still remains the generalized concept, with relatively few modifications. The major difference in presently accepted models and the earlier one is the now well-documented fluidity of membranes. The lipid constituents in the membrane permit considerable movement of macromolecules, and membrane constituents may move appreciably within membranes (Figure 2.1). Although membrane biochemistry has been largely conducted with RBC stroma, sufficient experiments have been carried out with other cell types to suggest a basic similarity. Specialized animal and plant cells show the greatest divergence from the general concept.

All membranes appear to be bimolecular lipid leaflets, which are usually oriented to proteins in a variety of ways. Leaflets are oriented on opposing sides of the membrane so that they are approximately mirror images of each other. The average width of a membrane is 75 Å; Figure 2.1 illustrates one such membrane.

Several types of lipids are found in membranes, but phospholipids and cholesterol predominate. Sphingolipids comprise the primary minor component. Phosphatidylcholine, phosphatidylserine, and phosphatidylethanolamine are the primary phosphatides, and their two fatty acid hydrocarbon chains (typically 16–18 carbon atoms, but varying from 12 to 22) comprise the nonpolar region. Some of the fatty acids are unsaturated and contribute appreciably to fluidity of the membrane.

Proteins, which have many physiological roles in normal cell function, are intimately associated with lipids and may be variously located throughout lipid bilayers. Hydrophobic forces are responsible for maintaining the structural integrity of proteins and lipids within membranes but, as Figure 2.1 shows, movement within the membranes may occur.

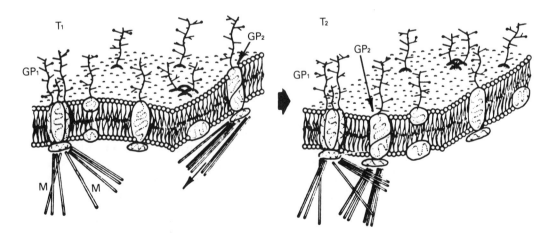

FIGURE 2.1.
Modified version of the fluid mosaic model of membrane structure. T1 and T2 represent different time points. Certain integral glycoproteins (GP1) may be "anchored" by microfilaments (M); other integral glycoproteins (GP2) may move within the membrane in an energy-dependent process; other components are uncoupled and free to diffuse laterally within the lipid bilayer. Source: Nicholson, Biochem. Biophys. Acta 1976; 457:61. Used by permission.

The ratio of lipid to protein varies from 5 : 1 for the myelin membrane to 1 : 5 for the inner structure of the mitochondria. A more important feature with regard to the extent and rate of absorption may be the proportion of the membrane surface that is comprised of lipid bilayers. One hundred percent of the myelin membrane surface is lipid bilayer, whereas the inner membrane of the mitochondria may have only 40% lipid bilayer surface.

For ready movement of small molecules such as water through membranes, the presence of pores of approximately 4 Å has been postulated. Thus, certain molecules that ordinarily would be excluded may rapidly traverse the charged, highly lipid barrier. In specialized membranes such as those associated with the kidney, pore size may be as large as 45 Å, permitting the ready transfer of molecules with molecular weights approaching 50,000 daltons.

The amphipathic nature of the membrane produces a barrier for ionized, highly polar compounds—although not an absolute barrier. The importance of nonionic, lipid-soluble characteristics of a xenobiotic will be discussed later. It is worthy of note that differences between membranes, such as the presence of different lipids, the amount of surface lipid, differences in size and shape of proteins, or physical features of bonding may cause differences in permeability between membranes. It has also been suggested that a miniscule portion (<0.05 %) of the membrane surface has characteristics different from the rest of the membrane. If correct, this may account for different permeabilities to toxicants.

2.3 IONIZATION

Membranes are much less permeable to compounds in the ionized state than to those in the nonionized form. This was shown many years ago, when it was found that alkaloids such as strychnine which were ionized as a result of introduction into the strongly acid stomach area did not show toxic effects if the digestive tract was ligated between stomach and intestine. On the other hand, when the alkaloids were allowed to pass to the more alkaline intestine and thus became nonionized, toxicity became apparent because the toxic alkaloid was easily absorbed. This is not an important criterion for most toxicants because they are incapable of being ionized and are thus unaffected by pH. A small number of toxicants, however, such as alkaloids and organic acids, are ionizable, and their penetration may be appreciably altered by pH.

The amount in the ionized or nonionized form depends upon the pK_a (negative logarithm of the acidic dissociation constant) of the potential toxicant and the pH of the bathing medium. When the pH of a solution is equal to the pK_a of the dissolved compound, one half exists in the ionized and one half exists in the nonionized form. The degree of ionization is given by the Henderson-Hasselbach equation:

$$\log \frac{\text{nonionized form}}{\text{ionized form}} = pK_a - pH \text{ (for weak acids)}$$

$$\log \frac{\text{ionized form}}{\text{nonionized form}} = pK_a - pH \text{ (for weak bases).}$$

Because the nonionized form of a weak electrolyte is the diffusable molecule, weak organic acids diffuse most readily in acid and organic bases in alkaline

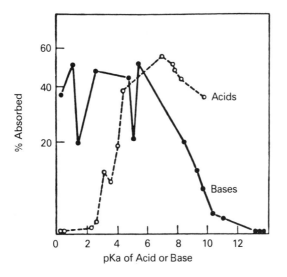

FIGURE 2.2.
Absorption of acids and bases from the rat colon. Source: Schanker, Ch. 2 in Concepts in Biochemical Pharmacology. Berlin: Springer-Verlag, 1971. Used by permission.

environments (Figure 2.2). In almost all cases, some degree of penetration occurs even when toxicants are not in the most lipid-soluble form, and even a small amount of absorption may produce serious effects with highly toxic compounds. There are the usual exceptions to the generalizations concerning ionization, because such compounds as pralidoxime (2-PAM), paraquat, and diquat are absorbed to an appreciable extent in the ionized forms. The mechanisms allowing these exceptions are not understood.

2.4 PARTITION COEFFICIENT

A second parameter influencing penetration is the relative lipid solubility of the potential toxicant. The lipid solubility of a compound is measured by the partition coefficient, which is a measure of the compounds partitioning between aqueous and lipid phases (concentration in lipid phase/concentration in water phase). Thus, a high partition coefficient indicates greater lipophilicity. The lipid solvent used for measurement is usually octanol because it best mimics the carbon chain of phospholipids, but many other systems have been reported (chloroform/water, ether/water, olive oil/water). Obviously, each may give a different value, and there is often little consistency in correlations between penetration and partition coefficients derived from different solvent systems.

The correlation between high partition coefficient and rapid penetration has probably been more generally accepted than is warranted. In particular, many early studies showed good correlations between high partition coefficients and rapid penetration, such as the classic study of Callander (Figure 2.3), this relationship became generally accepted. Chemically related groups of compounds such as an analogous series of alcohols show the best correlation. A number of studies have shown a less positive correlation, however, and many

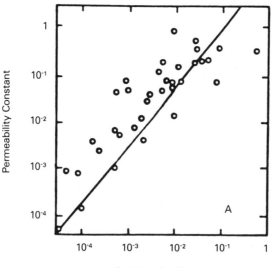

FIGURE 2.3.
Relationship between oil/water partition coefficient and cell membrane permeability for the marine plant *Chara ceratophylla*. Source: Modified from Collander. Trans. Faraday Soc. 1937; 33:989.

recent studies have indicated that this generalization is obscured by other factors. Although lipid solubility is clearly necessary for initial uptake, once the toxicant has entered the membrane other factors complicate further penetration. For example, too high a lipid solubility may reduce penetration through the highly lipid membrane by restricting exit, a polar region may need to be traversed during penetration, different regions of the external parts of the organ being penetrated may have different membrane characteristics, etc. Chemical similarity of penetrants, size of molecule, and conformational similarities are other parameters that add to penetration similarities and differences among compounds, and measuring these characteristics is somewhat complex. Thus, a moderate degree of water solubility is often a facilitating factor in increased penetration, nevertheless, some very lipid soluble compounds such as DDT, polychlorinated biphenyls (PCBs), and synthetic pyrethroids are able to penetrate, in many cases without difficulty. If a large molecule has high water solubility, the penetration rate is invariably low.

2.5 MECHANISMS OF ENTRY

The mechanism of the movement of toxicants across membranes, particularly initial entry, has been a poorly researched area in general although considerable work has been done in the specific case of drugs. There appear to be four primary mechanisms that allow toxicants to traverse membranes.

2.5.1 Passive Transport

For most toxicants, this mechanism appears to predominate. Simple diffusion of compounds with appropriate water/lipid partition coefficients largely determines the rate of movement, which may vary considerably among compounds, and this rate is not always predictable. Compounds in the ionized form do not move readily in this fashion due to ionic interactions among xenobiotics, lipids, and proteins. The ionized form also tends to be less lipid soluble, a factor necessary for membrane diffusion.

2.5.2 Filtration

There are often pores in the membrane that allow compounds with molecular weights of ≤ 100 daltons to traverse more quickly. Larger molecules are excluded except in more highly porous tissues, such as kidney and liver. Because many toxicants are relatively large molecules, this pathway is often of limited importance.

2.5.3 Special Transport

A number of special transport systems, particularly in the gastrointestinal tract, aid in transport of endogenous compounds across membranes. Such processes may require energy and permit passage against a concentration gradient (active transport) or may not require energy and be unable to move compounds against a gradient (facilitated transport). Although the results may differ, the mechanisms are somewhat similar and will be discussed together. In both cases, a carrier protein that associates with the toxicant is postulated. This protein furthers the movement from one side of the membrane to the other and, on the other side, the chemical dissociates from the protein, which is then free to take up another molecule of the compound. Such penetration is more rapid than simple diffusion and, in the case of active transport, may proceed beyond the point at which concentrations are equal on both sides of the membrane.

These mechanisms may be important in those relatively rare instances in which toxicants have chemical or structural similarities to endogenous chemicals that rely on special transport mechanisms for normal physiological uptake and can thus utilize the same system. For example, 5-fluorouracil is transported by the pyrimidine transport system. Lead may be more quickly moved by a transport system that aids the penetration of calcium. As stated, such special transport mechanisms are most manifest in GI absorption. These mechanisms become of much greater importance in the elimination of toxicants, however, in which special transport is important in the removal of xenobiotics and their metabolites. An important characteristic of the special transport systems, when operative, is that they allow movement of compounds with lesser lipid solubility, compounds that would ordinarily be expected to move very slowly through highly lipid membranes.

2.5.4 Endocytosis

Pinocytosis (for liquids) and phagocytosis (for solids) are specialized transport processes in which the membrane invaginates or flows around a toxicant, allowing more ready transfer across membranes. Only in such isolated instances as absorption of carrageenens (mol wt $\sim 40,000$) in the gut have these mechanisms been found to be important in initial entry. Once inside the body, however, endocytosis is a rather common mechanism, and engulfment of compounds in the lung is common (lung phagocytosis).

2.6 RATE OF PENETRATION

For a single vehicle and solvent system, the rate of penetration of nonpolar, nonionized toxicants is believed to follow Fick's law of diffusion. One assumption of this pattern is that the concentration at the application site is much higher than the absorbed concentration, which can be considered negligible because it is removed quickly. Thus,

$$K = \frac{A(C)}{d}$$

where C = concentration, A = surface area directly related to transfer, d = thickness of membrane, and K = diffusion constant.

This equation may be expanded to the more experimentally useful equation

$$J = \frac{K_m C v D_m}{\delta}$$

where J = absorption rate per unit area at steady state (flux), K_m = vehicle partition coefficient, Cv = concentration of penetrant, D_m = diffusion constant of penetrant in stratum corneum, and δ = the thickness of the membrane (eg, stratum corneum in skin). The rate of absorption, then, depends on two easily controlled, externally determined factors (partition coefficient and concentration of penetrant) and two innate factors (diffusion constant and stratum corneum thickness). Permeability constants for human skin range from 1×10^{-6} to 5×10^{-2} cm/h.

The above equation implies conditions of steady-state penetration, not attained until a lag phase has occurred. A plot of the logarithm of the amount unpenetrated v time should be linear, indicating first-order kinetics.

This ideal situation may be an oversimplification except in the most rigid, nonphysiological terms, and deviations from first-order kinetics may be commonplace. When the absorption of a series of pesticides was compared in mice, no single equation seemed appropriate. Statistical tests of first-, second-, and third-order models generally showed significant departures from these kinetic models. Empirical models that used transformed responses (log P and arc sine $\sqrt{P}$ where P = percentage unpenetrated) and regressed on log (time) were much more effective in linearizing the response–time relationship, and the resulting $t_{0.5}$ estimates were then comparable because a single model fit was sufficient for all toxicants. Possible explanations for these variations from simple diffusion include differential shunts within the highly lipid membrane, contribution of appendagical shunts, effects of the carrier necessary for application, injury to surface membranes, hydration of the stratum corneum, binding of the penetrant to the stratum corneum, regional variations in skin permeability, etc.

When first-order kinetics hold, a simple relationship exists between the penetration constant, K, and $t_{0.5}$ (time necessary for half of the applied dose to penetrate):

$$K = \frac{0.693}{t_{0.5}}$$ and the units of K are percentage of change/time unit.

When first-order kinetics do not apply, the only relevant number is $t_{0.5}$ itself, since the units of K change for any model other than first order.

When oral and dermal administration were compared in in vivo experiments, the half-time penetration rates were found to vary considerably (Table 2.1). It is obvious that in these experiments no useful correlation between partition coefficients, animal species, or route of administration could be found. Although such comparisons may be interesting, it is perhaps not surprising to find large differences among animals because the skin or cuticle are very different and, even among higher animals, one would have great difficulty in assuming that a skin area was similar (smooth v hairy skin, or skin of a mammal v that of a bird). Furthermore, comparisons of dermal application v GI application have quite dissimilar patterns. A GI application will always be complicated by the much greater surface area of the gut as opposed to skin, immediate diffusion of the toxicant in the liquid of the GI tract, and the possibilities of binding of the administered dose to extraneous material in the gut contents. Thus, it is prudent to consider measurements of the penetration rates of toxicants derived from different animals or from different routes of application as estimates which may contain large errors.

TABLE 2.1
Comparison Between Physical Properties and Penetration of Pesticides in Mice

Chemical Class / Toxicant	Mol Wt	H_2O Solution (ppm)	Partition Coefficient Olive oil/H_2O	T0.5 (min) Dermal	T0.5 (min) Oral	Percent Penetrated (60 min) Dermal	Percent Penetrated (60 min) Oral
Carbamate							
Carbaryl	203	40	46	12.8	17.0	71.7	68.7
Carbofuran	221	700	5	7.7	10.0	76.1	67.4
Organophosphorus							
Malathion	330	145	56	129.7	33.5	24.6	88.8
Chlorpyrifos	350	2	1,044	20.6	78.1	69.0	47.2
Parathion	292	24	1,738	66.0	33.3	31.9	56.8
Chlorinated Hydrocarbon							
DDT	355	.001	1,775	105.4	62.3	34.1	55.1
Dieldrin	384	.020	282	71.7	42.1	33.7	63.2
Miscellaneous							
Nicotine	162	Miscible	0.02	18.2	23.1	71.5	82.9
Permethrin	390	.07	360	5.9	177.6	79.7	39.1

Source: Ahdaya, S.M. et al. Pestic. Biochem. Physiol. 1981; 16:38–46; and Shah, P.V. et al. Toxicol. Appl. Pharmacol. 1981; 59:414–23.

2.7 ROUTES OF PENETRATION IN MAMMALS

Because humans are the principal target of concern, this section will be primarily devoted to animals that are usually chosen to assess toxicity to humans or to data derived from human tissue. Primary routes of entry are dermal, gastrointestinal, and respiratory. Methods for studying these different routes are numerous, but they are perhaps best developed for the study of dermal penetration because this route is subject to more direct methodology. Methods for studying respiratory absorption require highly specialized instrumentation, and the appropriate chapters of Doull et al and Lee et al listed at the end of this chapter should be consulted.

2.7.1 Skin Penetration

The skin is a complex, multilayered tissue comprising approximately 18,000 cm^2 of surface in an average human male and contributing approximately 10% of the body weight. It is a membrane that is relatively impermeable to most ions as well as aqueous solutions. It is permeable to a large number of toxicants in the solid, liquid, or gaseous phases, however. Although many cases of poisoning occur after respiratory entry, it is also apparent that many toxicants can easily gain entry through the dermal route. Many examples of poisoning by the dermal route have been reported — organophosphate pesticides in agricultural workers, chlorophenol in domestic and wild animals, and a large number of industrial solvents are a few examples.

A schematic representation of human skin is shown in Figure 2.4. Three distinct layers make up this important organ, but the epidermis is the only layer that is important in penetration of toxicants. In general, the vasculature is usually > 100 μm from the outer layer of skin. The outermost layer, the epidermis, is a multilayered tissue varying in thickness from about 0.1 to 0.8 mm. The thicker areas of the skin have a higher concentration of keratin than do the thinner areas. The basal cells of the epidermis proliferate and differentiate as they migrate outward. The columnar cells become rounded and then flattened as they move through loosely defined layers and finally to the stratum corneum, the primary barrier to penetration. This layer consists of 8–16 layers of flattened, highly keratinized cells. The layer is approximately 25- to 40-μm wide, lies parallel to the skin surface, and forms a relatively impermeable, shingle-like layer which is approximately 10-μm thick. It requires 26–28 days for cells to migrate from the basal layer to the stratum corneum, where they are eventually sloughed off. A number of appendages are associated with the skin, including hair follicles, sebaceous glands, eccrine and apocrine sweat glands, and nails. Recently, it was found that removal of the stratum corneum does not allow complete absorption; thus, it is apparent that some role, although of lesser importance, is played by other barriers.

The dermis and subcutaneous areas of the skin play a very minor role in penetration. The dermis is highly vascular, a characteristic that provides maximal opportunity for further transport once molecules have gained entry through the epidermis or through skin appendages. The blood supply of the dermis is under neural and humoral influence whose temperature-regulating

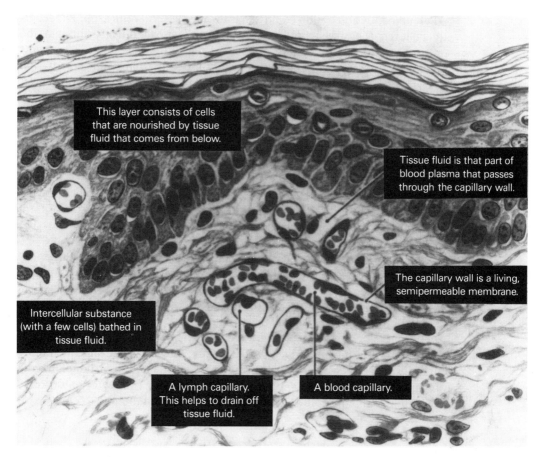

This layer consists of cells that are nourished by tissue fluid that comes from below.

Tissue fluid is that part of blood plasma that passes through the capillary wall.

The capillary wall is a living, semipermeable membrane.

Intercellular substance (with a few cells) bathed in tissue fluid.

A lymph capillary. This helps to drain off tissue fluid.

A blood capillary.

FIGURE 2.4.
Retouched photomicrograph of the skin of a pig. Source: Ham and Cormack in Histology. 8th ed. Philadelphia: Lippincott, 1979. Used by permission.

function could thus affect penetration and distribution of toxicants. The subcutaneous layer of the skin is highly lipid in nature and serves as a shock absorber, an insulator, and a reserve depot of energy. The pH of the skin varies between 4 and 7 and is markedly affected by hydration.

The skin not only serves as a passive barrier to diffusion but may also have a function in the metabolism of topically applied substances before they enter the systemic circulation. The epidermal layer accounts for the major portion of biochemical transformations in skin although the total skin activity is low (2–6% that of the liver). If activity is based on epidermis alone, however, that layer is as active as the liver or, in the case of certain toxicants, several times more active. Although skin metabolism usually deactivates, activation of some skin carcinogens is known to occur. The skin enzymes can be induced and are potentially of toxicological importance. For rapidly penetrating substances, the skin metabolic transformations are not presently considered to be of major significance, but skin may have an important first-pass metabolic function, especially for compounds that are absorbed slowly.

Percutaneous absorption could occur through several routes, but it is generally believed that most lipid-soluble toxicants move directly through the stratum corneum rather than through hair follicles or sweat ducts. Arguments in favor of transepidermal absorption are that epidermal damage or partial removal increases penetration, that epidermal penetration is markedly slower than dermal, and that the epidermal surface area is much greater than the surface area of skin appendages. Initial penetration may be aided by appendages, but absorption through the general skin surface eventually becomes more important than appendicular absorption (Figure 2.5). There is no evidence for active transport in the skin; ie, all available evidence suggests simple diffusion, whether gas, ion, or nonelectrolyte.

Variations in areas of the body cause appreciable differences in penetration of toxicants, as has been shown for both pesticides and hydrocortisone in human skin (Table 2.2). Head, neck, and axilla (where environmental exposure is greatest) are areas of increased absorption.

It is important to recognize that occlusion of the site of application by bandage, clothing, or ointment markedly increases absorption. Such action changes physical and physiological factors, affecting penetration as well as retarding mechanical abrasion of the applied compound.

Surfactants and soaps applied in conjunction with a toxicant may also affect penetration. Alterations of the stratum corneum appear to be the major factor. Organic solvents may be divided into damaging categories (acetone, methanol, ether, hexane) which alter lipids and increase permeability, or nondamaging categories (long-chain esters, olive oil, higher alcohols) which often decrease penetration. Aqueous solutions of detergents have been found to increase penetration markedly.

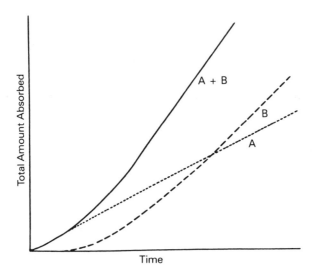

FIGURE 2.5.
Contribution of general skin surface and appendicular routes to diffusion through skin. A, diffusion via sweat ducts and hair follicles; B, general surface. Source: Dugard, Ch. 22 in Marzulli and Maibach (eds.) Dermatotoxicology and Pharmacology. 2nd ed. Washington, D.C.: Hemisphere, 1977. Used by permission.

TABLE 2.2
Penetration of Hydrocortisone in Humans at Different Anatomic Sites

Anatomic Site	Penetration Ratio
Forearm (ventral)	1.0
Foot (plantar)	0.14
Ankle (lateral)	0.42
Palm	0.83
Back	1.7
Scalp	3.5
Forehead	6.0
Scrotum	42.0

Source: Modified from Feldman, R.J., and Maibach, H.I. J. Invest. Dermatol. 1967; 48:181–183.

The choice of the most appropriate experimental animal to mimic penetration into human skin has always been controversial. Data in Figure 2.6 show in vitro and comparative in vivo results. Although a suitable animal model has not been developed for all cases, monkeys, pigs, and rats seem the better models, whereas mice and rabbits appear to absorb toxicants faster than humans do. Whereas comparison of in vivo and in vitro data with human skin does not give

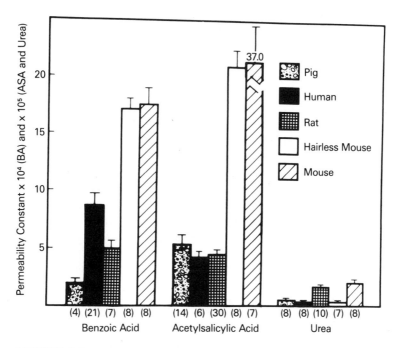

FIGURE 2.6.
Permeability constants obtained with animal and human skin. Source: Bronough et al. Toxicol. Appl. Pharmacol. 1982; 62:481. Used by permission.

consistent correlations, it has been possible to distinguish between compounds of low permeability with the much simpler in vitro system. Recent methodology has improved the in vitro technique, and it is hoped that this may become a valuable tool in absorption studies since in vivo testing in humans is becoming much more impractical for ethical and legal reasons.

Miscellaneous factors that have an effect on penetration, including concentration of toxicant, age of animal, temperature, multiple dose application, skin condition, relative humidity, surface area of applied dose, and hyperemia should be mentioned.

2.7.2 Gastrointestinal (GI) Penetration

The oral route is especially important for accidental or deliberate ingestion of toxicants. Food additives, food toxins, licking or rubbing, and airborne particles excluded from passage to the alveoli and returned to the glottis are among potential avenues for accidental ingestion. Although the buccal cavity and the rectum are sometimes used to introduce drugs, with a few exceptions ingested toxicants enter the body in the stomach or intestine. Exceptions include nicotine, which enters readily through the buccal cavity, and cocaine, which enters through the nasal mucosa.

The digestive system (Figure 2.7a) is lined by a layer of columnar cells protected by mucus, although the latter has little role in absorption. The distance from the outer membrane to the vasculature is about 40 μm, from which point further transport can easily occur. Venous blood flow from the stomach and intestine causes absorbed materials to have first pass through the liver, a route that favors metabolism. On the other hand, absorption through the skin or lungs follows more indirect routes to organs of detoxication, without a first pass directly to the liver. A major factor favoring absorption in the intestine is the presence of microvilli, which provide an extremely large surface area (Figure 2.7b).

Although it is generally conceded that absorption is more rapid via the GI than the dermal route, meager data support this assumption. As stated earlier, it is difficult to make a direct comparison experimentally, but recent tests with mice indicate that differences in penetration between the dermal and oral routes are often either relatively small or even nonexistent (Table 2.1).

The greater surface area of the intestine favors absorption at that location rather than the stomach, but is must be recognized that compounds enter the stomach first and may be readily absorbed during residence in that organ.

Appreciable differences in pH exist within the GI tract, a factor that may change permeability characteristics, as previously mentioned. The stomach tends to be much more acidic than the intestine, affecting absorption of ionized compounds. The measured pH of the GI contents may not be identical to the pH of the epithelium at the site of absorption and may explain the entrance of compounds whose pK_a would normally suggest a much slower rate.

In contrast to skin, active transport of toxicants is also known to occur in the GI tract. For toxicants with structural similarities to compounds normally taken up by active transport mechanisms, entry is enhanced. For example, cobalt is absorbed by the same active transport mechanism that normally transports iron.

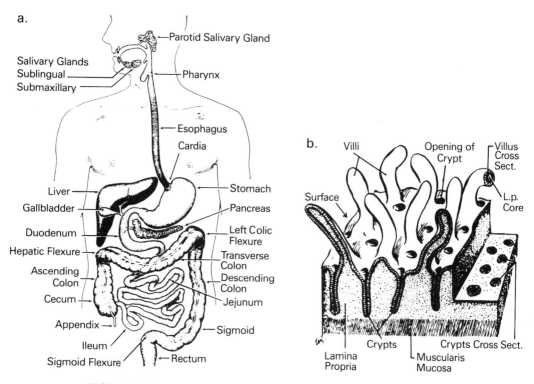

FIGURE 2.7.
(a) Alimentary canal and associated structures. Source: Scholtelius and Scholtelius in Textbook of Physiology, St. Louis: Mosby, 1973. Used by permission. (b) Schematic drawing of the lining of the small intestine. Source: Ham and Cormack in Histology, 8th ed. Philadelphia: Lippincott, 1979. Used by permission.

A feature of the GI tract that seems to contradict basic assumptions of absorption is penetration of certain very large molecules. Compounds such as bacterial endotoxins, large particles of azo dyes, and carrageenans are apparently absorbed by endocytotic mechanisms.

Some factors contributing to GI absorption require brief mention. One important factor is that dissolution of a toxicant in the gut contents greatly increases absorption because the compound must be in intimate contact with the epithelium for significant absorption to occur. Such factors as particle size, solvent effects, presence of emulsifiers, and rate of dissolution are also important. The presence of microorganisms and hydrolysis-promoting pH conditions, binding to gut contents, the rate of emptying of the stomach, the temperature of the contents, intestinal motility, dietary and health effects, and GI secretion are all related factors that may affect penetration.

An important aspect of GI absorption is enterohepatic circulation. Following secretion of conjugated metabolites from the bile duct into the intestine, a water-soluble metabolite may be altered to a less polar compound, readsorbed through the intestine, and returned to the liver. Enterohepatic circulation is discussed in greater detail in Section 5.3.2.

2.7.3 Respiratory Penetration

Although the respiratory system is an organ in unavoidable contact with contaminated air, it is also equipped with a number of mechanisms to avoid many airborne substances, especially particles. The respiratory system is especially vulnerable from two aspects, however. The rich capillary exchange at the deeper lung recesses causes a toxicant at the lung surface to be separated by only $1-2$ μm from the circulation, enabling exchange of gases in seconds or less. In addition, the surface area of the lung is large — $50-100$ m^2, some 50 times the area of the skin.

The sequences of respiration involve several interrelated air volumes that define the capacity of the lung and factors important to particle disposition and retention. Among the elements important in lung capacity is the residual volume, the amount of air retained in the lung despite maximum expiratory effort. Largely due to slow release from this volume, gaseous toxicants in the respiratory air are not cleared immediately; instead, many expirations may be necessary to rid the lung air of residual toxicant.

The rate of entry of vapor-phase toxicants is controlled by the alveolar ventilation rate, with the toxicant being presented to the alveoli in an interrupted fashion approximately 20 times/minute.

Although many definitions are used for airborne toxicants, these may be simplified to two general types. Compounds that are subject to gas laws include solvents, vapors, and gases. These are most easily carried to the alveolar areas. The second group is not subject to gas laws because they are in particulate form, and includes aerosols, clouds, particles, fumes, etc.

Entry of aerosols and particulates is governed by a number of factors that may seem to facilitate or preclude their entry. The efficiency of the system is illustrated by the fact that on average only 100 g of coal dust is found postmortem in the lungs of coal miners although they inhale at least 6,000 g during their lifetime. The parameters of air velocity and directional air change favor impaction of particles in the upper respiratory system. In addition to particle size, such factors as coagulation, sedimentation, electrical charge, and diffusion may be important. Particles of >5 μm are usually deposited in the nasopharyngeal region. Particles down to 2 μm are deposited in the tracheobronchiolar region where they are cleared upward by the mucus blanket that covers the backward-beating cilia. The removal of particles may result in half-lives of <5 hours (movement up to 1 mm/min) and 80% of lung clearance may occur in this way. Particles may be temporarily trapped in nasal passages or may move to the glottis where they are swallowed. This could permit later absorption in the GI tract.

In addition to upper pathway clearance, lung phagocytosis is very active in both upper and lower pathways of the respiratory tract and may be coupled to the mucus cilia. Phagocytes may also direct engulfed toxicants into the lymph, where they may be stored for long periods. If not phagocytized, particles ≤ 1 μm may penetrate to the alveolar portion of the lung. Some particles do not desquamate but instead proliferate to form a dust node in association with a developing network of reticulin fibers. Overall, removal of alveolar particles is markedly slower than that achieved by the directed upper pulmonary mechanisms.

For very small particles and gaseous toxicants, absorption takes place in the alveolar region (Figure 2.8). Gas in the alveoli equilibrates almost instantaneously with the blood passing through the pulmonary capillary bed. Release of gas into or out of the blood is dependent on solubility in blood. If a substance has a low solubility, only a small amount of the gas in the lung is removed by the blood. Due to low carrying capacity, the respiratory rate would not affect exchange. The rate of cardiac output would affect transfer into blood, however. The time for blood-gas to come in equilibrium with alveolar gas often exceeds ten minutes for relatively insoluble gases.

The greater portion of highly blood-soluble gases is transferred to the blood with each breath, and little is left in the alveolus. The more soluble the toxicant, the more time it will take to reach equilibrium in the blood. Thus, the time required to equilibriate with blood water will be longer than with low-solubility gases ($\simeq 1$ hour). For highly soluble gases, the principal factor limiting absorption is the rate of respiration. Increasing cardiac output does not appreciably increase rate of absorption.

A thin film of aqueous fluid wets the alveolar walls, aiding in initial absorption of toxicant from the alveolar air. In some cases, the phospholipid component of the surfactant monolayer may interact with very highly lipid toxicants to slow uptake.

There is little evidence for active transport in the respiratory system, although pinocytosis may be of importance. Although the lung is an area of

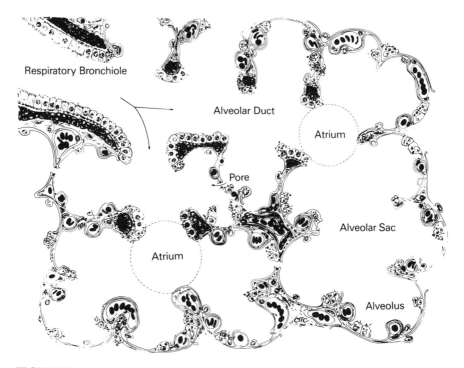

FIGURE 2.8.
Schematic representation of the respiratory unit of the lung. Source: Bloom and Fawcett in A Textbook of Histology. Philadelphia: W.B. Saunders, 1975. Used by permission.

extensive metabolic activity, detoxication mechanisms during uptake are not presently believed to be of major significance. The lung is also an important excretory organ for anesthestic gases, certain gaseous toxicants, such as dimethylsulfoxide (DMSO) and ethanol (see Chapter 5 on elimination).

2.8 DISTRIBUTION

Body fluids are distributed between three primary components: plasma water, interstitial water, and intracellular water. Vascular fluid has the important role in the distribution of absorbed toxicants. Human plasma accounts for ≈ 4% of body weight but 53% of total blood volume, whereas the interstitial tissue fluids account for 13% of body weight and intracellular fluids comprise 41%. The concentration a toxicant may achieve in the blood following exposure depends on the apparent volume of distribution. If the toxicant is distributed only in plasma, a high concentration is achieved in the vascular tissue. On the contrary, if the same quantity of toxicant is also distributed in the interstitial and intracellular water, concentrations will be much lower in the vascular system.

Following absorption, a toxicant may be distributed to the site of toxic action, transferred to a storage depot, transported to organs of detoxication or interaction, and eventually eliminated.

Although many compounds have sufficient solubility in the aqueous portion of the blood for simple solution to be the important route of distribution, toxicants are usually transported in association with plasma proteins. Cellular components, such as erythrocytes, may also be responsible for transport but usually to a minor degree. The transport of toxicants by lymph is quantitatively of little importance, since blood flow is many times faster than that of lymph. It must be recognized, however, that both erythrocytes and lymph can have important roles on occasions. Recently, it was observed that highly water soluble metabolites of toxicants are also bound to blood proteins, suggesting a role in transport to the kidney.

Studies on plasma proteins have shown the albumin fraction to be of particular importance in the binding of drugs. Because many toxicants are very lipophilic, the plasma lipoproteins also play an important role in toxicant binding.

Toxicants are often distributed and stored in specific tissues, either at sites of storage, in liver or kidney, or at the site of action (eg, binding to hemoglobin). Toxicants may be sequestered either physically, such as solubilization of lipophilic chemicals in fat or chemically by binding to tissue components, such as proteins. If a toxicant is stored in a depot removed from the site of action, such as PCBs in fat or lead in bone, no adverse effect may be manifested immediately. Although an equilibrium is established between tissue and blood, amounts escaping from the storage depot are usually very small at any given time. The large amount stored in the depot is a potential toxic hazard, however. Thus, opportunity for chronic action, or even acute action if the toxicant is suddenly mobilized, is continuous and a complication in the assessment of potential hazard.

If a compound is bound to a blood protein, it is immobilized away from the site of action. Other consequences of such binding are possible displacement of one toxicant by another perhaps more toxic chemical, facilitation of cellular absorption while bound to a lipoprotein, and dilution of the toxicant.

A ligand–protein interaction raises the apparent contradiction that although many toxicants are chemically "unreactive" in the strict sense, they can be reversibly bound to a variety of biological constituents. In the case of ligand–protein interactions important to transport, the law of mass action provides a remarkably efficient means whereby toxicants can be transported and then dissociate at various tissues.

$$T_f + \text{Free site} \underset{k_2}{\overset{k_1}{\rightleftharpoons}} T_b$$

T_f and T_b are free and bound toxicant molecules, and k_1 and k_2 are rate constants for association and dissociation. The rate constant, k_2, which governs the rate of binding to the protein, dictates the rate of toxicant release at a site of action, inaction, or storage. The ratio k_2/k_1 is identical with the dissociation constant, K_{diss}. Among a group of binding sites on proteins, those with the smallest K_{diss} values for a given toxicant bind it most tightly. In contrast to reversible binding, some potentially carcinogenic metabolites (eg, epoxides) may be covalently bound to tissue proteins, in which case there is no true distribution mechanism operative in the sense used in this section, because k_2 is nonexistent and there is no opportunity for dissociation. In addition to cytotoxicity, such covalent binding may lead to allergies or other immune responses.

Once a molecule binds to a plasma protein, it moves throughout the circulation until it dissociates, perhaps for attachment to another large molecule or at a site where the concentration of unbound ligand is low. Dissociation occurs when the affinity of another molecule or tissue component is greater than that of the plasma protein to which the toxicant was originally bound. Concentration differential, innate affinity, pH change, ionic strength, and temperature change may all be involved. Forces of association must be strong enough to establish an initial interaction but weak enough to permit dissociation at another site. As long as binding is reversible, redistribution will occur whenever the concentration of one pool (blood or tissue) is diminished. Redistribution must occur when a pool is diminished in order to maintain equilibrium.

Ligands complex with proteins in various ways. Covalent binding may have a pronounced effect on an organism due to the modification of an essential molecule, but such binding is usually a very minor portion of the total dose. Because covalent complexes dissociate very slowly (if at all), they are of no further consequence in this discussion.

Noncovalent binding is of primary importance to distribution because the ligand can dissociate more readily than it can in covalent binding. In rare cases, the noncovalent bond may be so stable that the bond is equivalent to a covalent one for all practical purposes. For example, the compound 3-hydroxy-2,4,4-triiodo-ethyl hydrocinnamic acid is bound tightly to plasma albumin for months. Types of interactions that lead to noncovalent binding under the proper physiological conditions include ionic binding, hydrogen bonding, van der Waals forces, and hydrophobic interactions.

Although drug studies have been numerous, toxicants have been neglected as chemicals of study. The major difference between drugs and toxicants is the frequent ionizability and high water solubility of drugs as compared with the nonionizability and high lipid solubility of many toxicants. Thus, experience with drugs forms an important background, but one that may not always be relevant to toxicants.

Pesticides exhibit great variation in chemical and physical features, and some recent studies seem worthy of mention. Table 2.3 shows the results of binding studies with a group of insecticides with greatly differing water and lipid solubilities. The affinity for albumin and lipoproteins is inversely related to water solubility, although the relation may be imperfect. Chlorinated hydrocarbons bind strongly to albumin but even more strongly to lipoproteins. Strongly lipophilic organophosphates bind to both protein groups, whereas the more water soluble compounds bind primarily to albumin. The most water-soluble compounds appear to be transported primarily in the aqueous phase.

Movement of highly lipid soluble compounds such as benzo(a)pyrene between different lipoproteins is known (Table 2.4), indicating the dynamic nature of binding phenomena. Such distribution may have important consequences in dictating which "pools" ultimately determine toxicity. For example, chlordecone (kepone) has partitioning characteristics that cause it to bind in the liver rather than in fatty depots as is the case with DDT. Thus, the toxicological implications may be quite different.

Many binding possibilities exist for attachment of a small molecule, such as a toxicant, to a large molecule, such as a blood protein. Although highly specific (high-affinity, low-capacity) binding is more common with drugs, examples of specific binding for toxicants seem less common. It seems probable that low-affinity, high-capacity binding describes most cases of toxicant binding. The number of binding sites can only be estimated, often with considerable error, because of the nonspecific nature of the interaction.

TABLE 2.3
Relative Distribution of Insecticides into Albumin and Lipoproteins

Chemical Class	Percent Bound Insecticide	Percent Distribution of Bound Insecticide		
Ligand		Albumin	Low-Density Lipoprotein	High-Density Lipoprotein
Chlorinated Hydrocarbon				
DDT	99.9	35	35	30
Dieldrin	99.9	12	50	38
Lindane	98.0	37	38	25
Organophosphate				
Parathion	98.7	67	21	12
Diazinon	96.6	55	31	14
Carbamate				
Carbaryl	97.4	99	<1.0	<1.0
Carbofuran	73.6	97	1.0	2.0
Aldicarb	30.0	94	2.0	4.0
Miscellaneous				
Nicotine	25.0	94	2	4

Source: From Maliwal, B.P., and Guthrie, F.E. Chem. Biol. Interactions. 1981; 35:177–188.

TABLE 2.4
Transfer of Benzo(a)pyrene among Lipoproteins

Benzo(a)pyrene			Percentage of Distribution		
Before Incubation			After Incubation		
VLDL	LDL	HDL	VLDL	LDL	HDL
100	0	0	61	35	4
0	100	0	60	36	4
0	0	100	63	34	3

VLDL, very-low-density lipoproteins; LDL, low-density lipoprotein; HDL, high-density lipoprotein. ^{14}C benzo(a)pyrene was separately incorporated into lipoprotein fractions obtained from
subject with hypertriglyceridemia. Labeled fractions were then incubated with other lipoproteins. After 21 hours, the lipoproteins were reisolated, and percentage of distribution was obtained.
Source: From Shu, H.P., and Nichols, A.V. Cancer Res. 1979; 39:1224–1230. Used by permission.

Several factors must be considered regarding the physiological and biological
significance of protein binding. The number of ligand molecules bound per
protein molecule, v, and the maximum number of binding sites, n, define the
definitive capacity of the protein. Another consideration is the binding affinity
$K_{binding}$ (or $1/K_{diss}$). If the protein has only one binding site for the toxicant, a
single value, $K_{binding}$, describes the strength of the interaction. Usually, more
than one binding site is present, each site having its intrinsic binding constant,
$k_1, k_2, \ldots, k_n$. Rarely does one find a case where $k_1 = k_2 = \cdots = k_n$,
wherein a single value would describe the affinity constant at all sites. This is
especially true when hydrophobic binding and van der Waals forces contribute
to nonspecific, low-affinity binding. Obviously, the chemical nature of the
binding site is of critical importance in determining binding characteristics.
The three-dimensional molecular structure of the binding site, the environment of the protein, the general location in the overall protein molecule, and
allosteric effects are all factors that influence binding. Studies with toxicants,
and even more extensive studies with drugs, have not yet provided an adequate
elucidation of these factors. Binding appears to be too complex a phenomenon
to be accurately described by any one set of equations.

There are many methods for analyzing binding but equilibrium dialysis is,
perhaps, the most common. The examples presented here will be greatly simplified to avoid the undue confusion engendered by a very complex subject.
Toxicant–protein complexes that utilize relatively weak bonds (energies of the
order of hydrogen bonds or less) readily associate and dissociate at physiological
temperatures, and the law of mass action applies to the thermodynamic equilibrium.

$$K_{binding} = \frac{[TP]}{[T][P]} = \frac{1}{K_{diss}},$$

where $K_{binding}$ is the equilibrium constant for association, $[TP]$ is the molar
concentration of toxicant–protein complex, $[T]$ is the molar concentration of

free toxicant, and $[P]$ is the molar concentrations of free protein. This equation does not describe the binding site(s) or the binding affinity. To incorporate these parameters and estimate the extent of binding, double-reciprocal plots $1/[TP]$ v $1/[T]$ may be used to test the specificity of binding. Regression lines passing through the origin imply infinite binding, and the validity of calculating an affinity constant under these circumstances is questionable. Figure 2.9a illustrates one such case with four pesticides, and the insert illustrates the low-affinity, "unsaturable" nature of binding in this example.

The two classes of toxicant–protein interactions encountered may be defined as (1): specific, high-affinity, low-capacity; and (2): nonspecific, low-affinity, high-capacity. The term high-affinity implies an affinity constant $(K_{binding})$ of the order of $\leq 10^8$ mol/L^{-1}, whereas low affinity implies concentra-

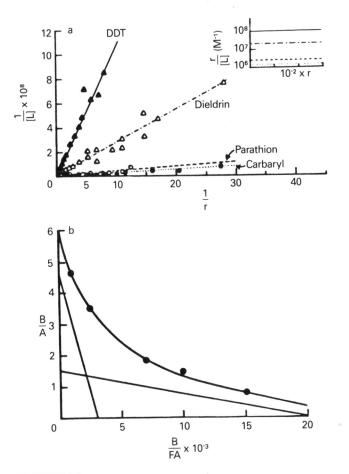

FIGURE 2.9.
Binding of toxicants to blood proteins: (a) Double-reciprocal plot of binding of rat serum lipoprotein fraction with four insecticides. Insert illustrates magnitude of differences in slope with Scatchard plot. Source: Skalsky and Guthrie. Pest. Biochem. Physiol. 1977; 7:289. (b) Scatchard plot of binding of salicylate to human serum proteins. Source: Moran and Walker, Biochem. Pharmacol. 1968; 17:153.

tions of $\geq 10^4$ mol/L^{-1}. Nonspecific, low-affinity binding is probably most characteristic of nonpolar compounds, although most cases are not as extreme as that shown in Figure 2.9a.

A well-accepted treatment for binding studies is the Scatchard equation:

$$v = \frac{n\,k[T]}{1 + k[T]},$$

which is simplified for graphical estimates to

$$\frac{v}{[T]} = k(n - v),$$

where v is the mol of ligand (toxicant) bound per mol of protein, $[T]$ is the concentration of free toxicant, k is the intrinsic affinity constant, and n is the number of sites exhibiting such affinity. When $v\,[T]$ is plotted against v, a straight line is obtained if only one class of binding sites is evident. The slope is $-k$ and the intercept on the v axis becomes n (number of binding sites). If more than one class of sites occurs (probably the most common situation for toxicants), a curve is obtained from which the constants may be obtained. This is illustrated in Figure 2.9b, for which the data show not one but two species of binding sites: one with low capacity but high affinity and another with about three times the capacity but less affinity. Commonly used computer programs usually solve such data by determining one line for the specific binding and one line for nonspecific binding, the latter being an average of many possible solutions (see suggested reading under Transport).

When hydrophobic binding of lipid toxicants occurs, as is the case for many environmental contaminants, binding is probably not limited to a single type of plasma protein. For example, the binding of the chlorinated hydrocarbon, DDT, is strongest for lipoproteins and albumin, but other proteins account for a significant part of overall transport. Similar results have been seen for several compounds with a range of physicochemical properties.

Protein-binding data are often expressed in terms of the percentage of ligand bound. A factor that must be noted, however, is that, as ligand concentration is lowered, the percentage of bound ligand increases. Thus, if a compound has a high affinity for a ligand, as often occurs with albumin, the percentage bound falls sharply when the total ligand concentration (D_T) exceeds a critical value.

Competitive binding for the same sites on a protein can have an important toxicological significance. If a toxicant competes for sites already occupied by a previously applied compound, displacement may result. The anticoagulant warfarin has an important therapeutic value in treatment of heart disease, but many fatty acids, and some drugs, also bind to the same site. Concurrently applied phenylbutazone, an antiinflammatory agent, displaces warfarin, and the resultant increase in free warfarin may appreciably increase anticoagulant effects. Many metals show competitive binding for the metal binding protein, metallothionein.

If a highly toxic compound has a very high affinity, the consequences of such interactions can be very important. For example, assume that compound A has low fractional binding (30%) and compound B displaces 10% of A from the protein. The net increase in free A is negligible (free A increases from 70–73%).

If A were 98% bound and 10% were displaced, however, free A would increase from 2 to 12%, and a severe reaction might result.

2.9 TOXICODYNAMICS

The dynamic situation involving the constantly changing events following absorption and terminating with excretion is a relatively new field of research best described by appropriate mathematical equations. For this introduction to the subject, a very simplified discussion is presented; for discussions of more complex models, the reader is directed to the suggested reading section.

Immediately on entering the body, a chemical begins changing location, concentration, or chemical identity. It may be transported independently by several components of the circulatory system, absorbed by various tissues, or stored, may effect an action, be detoxified, or be activated; the parent compound or its metabolite(s) may react with body constituents, be stored, or be eliminated—to name some of the more important actions (Figure 2.10). Each of these processes may be described by rate constants. Thus, at no time is the situation stable; but is constantly changing instead. The chemical reactions comprising biotransformation will become evident in later chapters. Such reactions include not only interactions between cellular macromolecules and parent and/or altered toxicant, but repair mechanisms also may determine the difference between an adverse and an inconsequential reaction.

The explanation of the kinetics (pharmacokinetics or toxicokinetics) involved in these processes is a highly specialized branch of toxicology. In the physiological sense, one can divide the body into "compartments" that may represent discrete parts of the whole—blood, liver, urine, etc.—or the mathematical model describing the process may be a composite representing the pooling of parts of tissues involved in distribution and bioactivation. Usually pharmacokinetic compartments have no anatomical or physiological identity; they represent all locations within the body that have similar characteristics relative to the dynamics of the particular toxicant. Simple first-order kinetics is usually accepted to describe individual rate processes for the toxicant after entry. The resolution of the model necessitates mathematical estimates (as a function of time) concerning the absorption, distribution, biotransformation, and excretion of toxicant that ultimately provide information relative to innate toxicity. Not only chemical and biological processes are involved in this complex transformation, but such physical processes as diffusion, dissolution, and physical interaction with receptor sites must also be considered.

Thus, complexity is inherent in even the simplest one-compartment case. Measurements of blood and excretory products are usually taken as the simplest and most easily determined experimental parameters. Even here, the situation quickly becomes complex. Is the radioactivity, if a labeled compound is used, the parent compound or metabolite(s)? Is the compound bound? If so, is it bound to one primary macromolecule or several? What proportion of the changes are occurring in which tissue? Many factors can perturb the dynamics of a toxicant. Some of these are rate of uptake, which can be affected by physical characteristics of the absorbing media; physiological factors, such as blood flow or peristalsis; GI functions, such as emptying and motility; differences in membranes, etc.

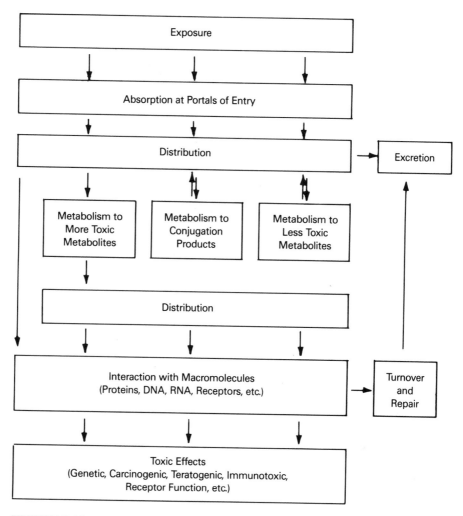

FIGURE 2.10.
Sequence of events following exposure of an animal to exogenous chemicals.

Each factor in the first phase of absorption may cause alteration of a first-order kinetic process, and as distribution and other factors come into play, the phases become the sum of a number of simultaneous and consecutive first-order reactions. A complete kinetic analysis for all routes of administration is a rarity, but the monitoring of blood and urine (and metabolites) is the most simple method of analysis and provides useful information concerning the onset and duration of toxic effects.

Several equations that measure the reaction(s) that occur have been described. One useful equation is

$$1n\ \frac{a}{a-x} = kt,$$

where a is the initial concentration, x is the amount reacted at time t, and k is a rate constant. A plot of the natural logarithm of the concentration measured at various time intervals against sampling time should yield a straight line of slope k and an intercept on the ordinate axis at $1n$ of the original concentration. Linearity of the line confirms first-order kinetics. When k has been determined in this way, $t_{0.5}$ can be determined from the relationship $t_{0.5} = \dfrac{0.693}{k}$. Proceeding from the simple to the complex situation requires appropriate modifications of the model, but by similar procedures equations for two-compartment and three-compartment models can be developed (Figure 2.11). The rapid increase in complexity is illustrated by the observation that 13 different three-compound models are possible. Examination of the selected references is recommended for the interested reader.

The use of linear pharmacokinetics to assess potential bioaccumulation and toxic hazard of 2,3,7,8-tetrachlorodibenzo-p-dioxin (TCDD) is illustrative. TCDD is an unwanted contaminant in the manufacture of several commercial compounds involving reactions of chlorinated phenols. The high toxicity and

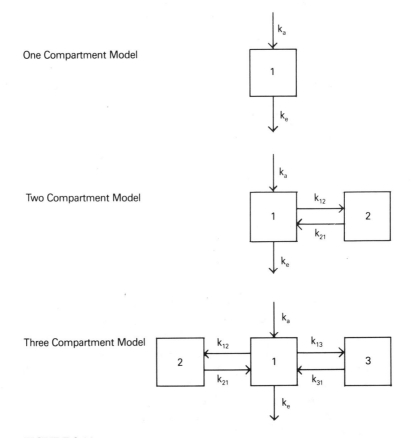

One Compartment Model

Two Compartment Model

Three Compartment Model

FIGURE 2.11.
Open-compartment toxicokinetic models: k_a is the absorption rate constant and k_e is the excretion rate constant. The other rate constants are for transfers between compartments, eg, k_{12} is the rate constant for transfer from compartment 1 to compartment 2, and k_{21} is the constant for transfer from compartment 2 to compartment 1.

physicochemical properties of the contaminant suggest that prolonged exposure to small amounts may lead to toxicity. Whereas a single dose of 1 μg/kg/ TCDD in rats decreased at an apparent first-order rate ($t_{0.5} = 21 - 39$ days, elimination through feces), when rats were given 1.0 or 0.1 μg/kg/day for 5 days a week for 7 weeks, the amount of TCDD in the body increased but the rates of increase decreased with time. A plateau effect was noted despite continued exposure (Figure 2.12). The rate constant for excretion was determined to be 0.0293 day^{-1} (half-life of 23.7 days), and the fraction of each dose absorbed was 0.861. From these values, it was calculated that if a given dose (D) were administered every day for an indefinite time, the steady-state body burden would be 29 times that dose (D $\times$ 29).

The calculations show that in the rat, small amounts of TCDD will not accumulate in the body; this was tested experimentally. Whereas 1.0 or 0.1 μg/

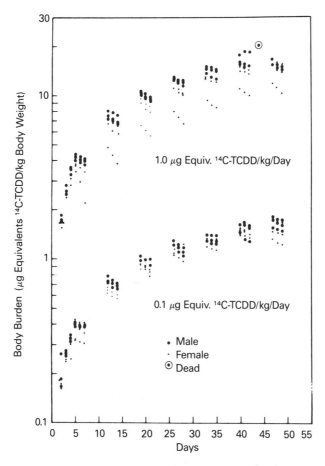

FIGURE 2.12.
Concentration of microgram equivalents of 2,3,7,8-tetrachlorodibenzo-*p*-dioxin (TCDD) in rats given 0.1 or 1.0 μg/kg/day, 5 days per week for 7 weeks. Source: Gehring et al., Ch. 8 in Mehlman, Shapiro, Blumenthal (eds.). New Concepts in Safety Evaluation, Pt. 1. Washington, D.C.: Halsted Press, 1976. Used by permission.

kg/day caused toxic manifestations (hepatic pathology and functional changes), longer exposure at lower rates (0.01 μg/kg/day) did not cause accumulation. Because TCDD in the tissues reached a plateau within 90 days, more prolonged exposure of amounts <0.1 μg/kg/day would not be expected to cause toxic levels of TCDD in body tissues.

The compartmental-model approach is being challenged by a more dynamic systems approach as discussed by Van Rossum et al (see Selected Reading). The systems-dynamics approach offers a new and stimulating viewpoint to study the relationship between kinetics and pharmacological effects.

2.10 SUGGESTED FURTHER READING

GENERAL

Doull, J., Klaasson, C.D., Amdur, M.D. Toxicology: The Basic Science of Poisons. New York: Macmillan, 1980, p. 778.

Goldstein, A., Aranow, L., Kalman, S.M. Principles of Drug Action. New York: Wiley-Heath, 1974.

Mehlman, M.H., et al. Advances in Modern Toxicology. 1976. Washington, D.C.: Hemisphere.

ABSORPTION

Lee, D.H.K., Falk, H.L., Murphy, S.D. (eds.). Handbook of Physiology, Section 9., Reaction to Environmental Agents. Bethesda, Md.: American Physiology Society, 1977. See especially chapters on skin (p. 299), gastrointestinal tract (p. 349), and respiratory system (p. 213).

Marzulli, F.M., Maibach, H.I. (eds.). Dermatotoxicology, New York: Hemisphere, 1983, 693 pp.

Mullins, L.J. (ed.). Annual Reviews Reprints: Cell Membranes. Palo Alto, Calif.: Annual Reviews, 1981, p. 889.

TRANSPORT

Steinhardt, J., Reynolds, J.A. Multiple Equilibria in Proteins. New York: Academic Press, 1969, p. 391.

Westphal, U. Steroid–Protein Interactions. New York: Springer, 1971.

TOXICOKINETICS

Boxenbaum, H., Pivinski, F. Frequently cited references in contemporary pharmacokinetics. Drug Metab. Rev. 1984–1985; 15:1385–1402.

Plaa, G.L., Duncan, W.A.M. (eds.). Proceedings of the 1st International Congress of Toxicology. New York: Academic Press, 670 pp.

Ramsey, J.C., Reitz, R.H. Pharmacokinetics and threshold concepts. Chapter 15. In Bandal, S.K., Marco, G.J., Goldberg, M., Leng, M.L. (eds.). The Pesticide Chemist and Modern Toxicology. ACS Symposium No. 160, 1981. Washington, D.C.

Tuey, D.B. Toxicokinetics. In Hodgson, E., Guthrie, F.E. (eds.). Introduction to Biochemical Toxicology. New York: Elsevier, 1980, 437 pp.

Van Rossum, J.M., Burgers, J., Van Lingen, G., de Bie, J. Pharmacokinetics: A dynamic systems approach. Trends Pharm. Sci. 1983; 4:27.

Withey, J.R. Pharmacokinetic principles; and Gehring, P.J., Young, J.D. Application of Pharmacokinetic principles in practice. In Plaa, G.L., Duncan, W.A.M. (eds.). Proceedings of the 1st International Congress of Toxicology. New York: Academic Press, 1978, 670 pp.

chapter three

METABOLISM OF TOXICANTS

Ernest Hodgson

3.1 INTRODUCTION

Metabolism by a wide array of enzymes that are capable of using xenobiotics as substrates is the principle means by which the toxicity of endogenous chemicals is modified in vivo, either increased or decreased. This chapter and the next are based on chapters 4–8 in Hodgson and Guthrie (1980). They are, however, both considerably condensed and revised in the light of more recent findings.

Most xenobiotics that enter the body are lipophilic, a property that enables them to penetrate lipid membranes and to be transported by lipoproteins in the blood. Xenobiotic metabolism consists of two phases. In phase one, a polar reactive group is introduced into the molecule, rendering it a suitable substrate for phase-two enzymes. These latter enzymes bring about conjugations to various endogenous substrates such as sugars, amino acids, etc., forming exceedingly water-soluble products that are readily excreted. Although this process is generally a detoxication sequence, reactive intermediates may be formed that are much more toxic than the parent compound. It is, however, usually a sequence that increases water solubility and hence decreases $t_{0.5}$ in vivo.

Formation of reactive intermediates is more frequently the case with phase-one monooxygenations since the products are often potent electrophiles capable of reacting with nucleophilic substituents on macromolecules, unless detoxified by some subsequent reaction. In the following discussion, examples of both detoxication and intoxication reactions are given.

3.2 PHASE-ONE REACTIONS

Phase-one reactions include microsomal monooxygenations, cytosolic and mitochondrial oxidations, cooxidations in the prostaglandin synthetase reaction, reductions, hydrolyses, and epoxide hydration. All of these reactions introduce

51

a polar group which, in most cases, can be conjugated during phase-two metabolism.

3.2.1 The Endoplasmic Reticulum, Microsomes, and Monooxygenations

Monooxygenations of xenobiotics are catalyzed either by the cytochrome P-450–dependent monoxygenase system or by the FAD-containing monooxygenase. Both are located in the endoplasmic reticulum of the cell and have been studied in many tissues and organisms. This is particularly true of cytochrome P-450, probably the most studied of all enzymes.

Microsomes are derived from the endoplasmic reticulum as a result of homogenization and are isolated by ultracentrifugation of the postmitochondrial supernatant fraction. The endoplasmic reticulum is an anastomosing network of lipoprotein membranes extending from the plasma membrane to the nucleus and mitochondria, whereas the microsomal fraction derived from it consists of membranous vesicles contaminated with free ribosomes, glycogen granules, and fragments of other subcellular structures such as mitochondria and Golgi apparatus. The endoplasmic reticulum, and consequently the microsomes derived from it, consists of two types, rough and smooth, the former having the outer membrane studded with ribosomes, which the latter characteristically lack. Although both rough and smooth microsomes have all the components of the cytochrome P-450-dependent monooxygenase system, the specific activity of the smooth type is usually higher.

Monooxygenations, also known as mixed-function oxidations, are those oxidations in which one atom of a molecule of oxygen is incorporated into the substrate while the other is reduced to water. Because the electrons involved in the reduction of cytochrome P-450 or FAD are derived from NADPH, the overall reaction can be written as follows (where RH is the substrate):

$$RH + O_2 \xrightarrow[\quad\quad\quad\quad\quad\quad]{NADPH + H^+ \quad\quad NADP^+} ROH + H_2O.$$

3.2.2 The Cytochrome P-450–Dependent Monooxygenase System

Cytochrome P-450s, the carbon monoxide-binding pigments of microsomes, are hemoproteins of the b cytochrome type. Unlike most cytochromes, they are named, not from the absorption maximum of the reduced form in the visible region but from the unique wavelength of the absorption maximum of the carbon monoxide derivative of the reduced form, namely 450 nm.

The role of cytochrome P-450 as the terminal oxidase in monooxygenase reactions is supported by considerable evidence. The initial proof was derived from the demonstration of the concomitant light reversibility of the CO complex of cytochrome P-450 and the inhibition, by CO, of the C-21 hydroxylation of $17\,\alpha$-hydroxy-progesterone by adrenal gland microsomes. This was followed by a number of indirect but nevertheless convincing proofs involving the effects on both cytochrome P-450 and monooxygenase activity of CO, inducing agents, spectra resulting from ligand binding, and the loss of activity on degradation of cytochrome P-450 to cytochrome P-420. Direct proof was subsequently provided by the demonstration that monooxygenase systems, reconstituted from apparently homogenous cytochrome P-450, NADPH-cytochrome P-450 reductase, and phosphatidylcholine, can catalyze many monooxygenase reactions.

Cytochrome P-450, like other hemoproteins, has a characteristic absorption in the visible region. The addition of many organic, and some inorganic, ligands results in perturbations of this spectrum. Although their detection and measurement requires a high-resolution instrument that must be used with considerable care, these perturbations, measured as optical difference spectra, have been of tremendous use in the characterization of cytochrome P-450.

The most important difference spectra of oxidized cytochrome P-450 are type I, with an absorption maximum at 385–390 nm and a minimium near 420 nm, and type II, with a peak at 420–435 nm and a trough at 390–410 nm. Type I ligands are found in many different chemical classes and include drugs, environmental contaminants, insecticides, etc. They appear to be generally unsuitable, on chemical grounds, as ligands for the heme iron and are believed to bind to a hydrophobic site in the protein that is close enough to the heme to allow both spectral perturbation and interaction with the activated oxygen. Although most type I ligands are substrates, it has not been possible to demonstrate a quantitative relationship between K_s (concentration required for half-maximal spectral development) and K_m (Michaelis constant).

Type II ligands, on the other hand, interact directly with the heme iron of cytochrome P-450 and are associated with organic compounds having nitrogen atoms with sp^2 or sp^3 nonbonded electrons that are sterically accessible. Such ligands are frequently inhibitors of cytochrome P-450-dependent monooxygenase activity.

The two most important difference spectra of reduced cytochrome P-450 are the well-known CO spectrum, with its maximum at or about 450 nm and the type III spectrum, with two pH-dependent peaks at approximately 430 and 455 nm. The CO spectrum forms the basis for the quantitative estimation of cytochrome P-450. The best known type III ligands for cytochrome P-450 are ethyl isocyanide and compounds such as the methylenedioxyphenyl synergists and SKF-525A, the last two forming stable type III complexes that appear to be related to the mechanism by which they inhibit monooxygenations.

Reducing equivalents are transferred from NADPH to cytochrome P-450 by a flavoprotein enzyme known as NADPH-cytochrome P-450 reductase. The evidence that this enzyme is involved in cytochrome P-450–dependent monooxygenations was originally derived from the observation that cytochrome c, which can function as an artificial electron acceptor for the enzyme, is an inhibitor of such oxidations. More recently, this reductase was shown to be an essential component in cytochrome P-450–dependent monooxygenase systems reconstituted from purified components. Antibodies prepared from purified reductase are inhibitors of microsomal monooxygenase reactions. The reductase is a flavoprotein of approximately 80,000 daltons that contains 1 mole each of flavin mononucleotide (FMN) and FAD per mole of enzyme.

The only other component necessary for activity in the reconstituted system is a phospholipid, phosphatidylcholine. This is not involved directly in electron transfer but appears to be involved in the coupling of the reductase to the cytochrome and in the binding of the substrate to the cytochrome.

The mechanism of cytochrome P-450 function has not been established unequivocally; however, the generally recognized steps are shown in Figure 3.1. The initial step consists of the binding of substrate to oxidized cytochrome P-450 followed by a one-electron reduction catalyzed by NADPH-cytochrome P-450 reductase to form a reduced cytochrome–substrate complex. This complex can interact with CO to form the CO-complex, which gives rise to the well-known difference spectrum with a peak at 450 nm and also inhibits monooxygenase activity.

The next several steps are less well understood. They involve an initial interaction with molecular oxygen to form a ternary oxygenated complex. This ternary complex accepts a second electron, resulting in the further formation of one or more poorly understood complexes. One of these, however, is probably the equivalent of the peroxide anion derivative of the substrate-bound hemoprotein. Under some conditions, this complex may break down to yield hydrogen peroxide and the oxidized cytochrome–substrate complex. Normally, however, one atom of molecular oxygen is transferred to the substrate and the other is reduced to water, followed by dismutation reactions leading to the formation of the oxygenated product, water, and the oxidized cytochrome.

The possibility that the second electron is derived from NADH through cytochrome b_5 has been the subject of argument for some time and has yet to be resolved. Cytochrome b_5 is a widely distributed microsomal heme protein that is involved in metabolic reactions such as fatty acid desaturation that involve endogenous substrates. It is clear, however, that this pathway is not essential for all cytochrome P-450-dependent monooxygenations since many occur in systems reconstituted from NADPH, O_2, phosphatidylcholine and highly purified NADPH-cytochrome P-450 reductase, and cytochrome P-450. Nevertheless, cytochrome b_5 is stimulatory in some cases and thus may facilitate oxidative activity in the intact endoplasmic reticulum. The recent isolation of forms of cytochrome P-450 that bind avidly to cytochrome b_5 also tends to support this idea.

3.2.2.1 Distribution of Cytochrome P-450

In vertebrates, the liver is the richest source of cytochrome P-450 and is most active in the monooxygenation of xenobiotics. Cytochrome P-450 and other components of the monooxygenase system dependent on it are also found in skin, nasal mucosa, lung, and GI tract, presumably reflecting the evolution of defense mechanisms at portals of entry. In addition to these organs, cytochrome P-450 has been demonstrated in kidney, adrenal cortex and medulla, placenta, testes, ovaries, fetal and embryonic liver, corpus luteum, aorta, blood platelets, and the nervous system. In humans, cytochrome P-450 has been demonstrated in fetal and adult liver, placenta, kidney, testes, fetal and adult adrenal gland, skin, blood platelets, and lymphocytes.

Although cytochrome P-450 is found in many tissues, its function does not appear to be the same in all cases. In the liver, cytochrome P-450 oxidizes a number of xenobiotics as well as some endogenous steroids and bile pigments. The cytochrome P-450 of the lung also appears to be concerned primarily with xenobiotic oxidation, although the range of substrates is more limited than that of the liver. Skin and small intestine also carry out xenobiotic oxidations, but

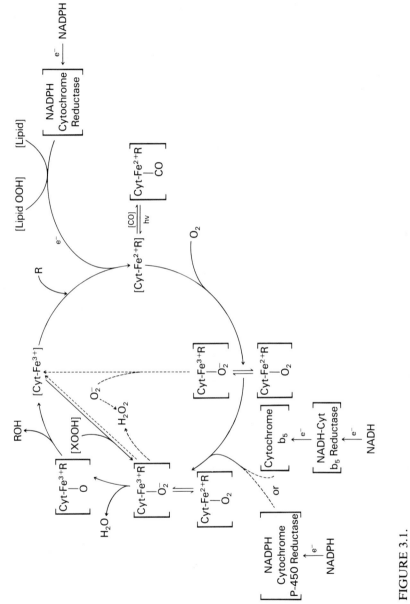

FIGURE 3.1.
Generalized scheme showing the sequence of events for cytochrome P-450 monooxygenations.

only aryl hydrocarbon hydroxylase activity has been investigated to any extent. In the uninduced pregnant female, the placental microsomes display little or no ability to oxidize foreign compounds, appearing to function as a steroid hormone metabolizing system. On induction, however, such as occurs in pregnant women who smoke, aryl hydrocarbon hydroxylase activity is readily apparent.

The cytochrome P-450 of the kidney is active in the ω-oxidation of fatty acids, such as lauric acid, but is relatively inactive in xenobiotic oxidation. Mitochondrial cytochromes P-450, such as those of the placenta and adrenal cortex, are active in the oxidation of steroid hormones rather than xenobiotics.

Distribution of cytochrome P-450 within the cell has been studied primarily in the mammalian liver, where it is present in greatest quantity in the smooth endoplasmic reticulum and in smaller but appreciable quantities in the rough endoplasmic reticulum. The nuclear membrane has also been reported to contain cytochrome P-450 and to have detectable aryl hydrocarbon hydroxylase activity, an observation that may be of considerable importance in studies of the metabolic activation of carcinogens.

3.2.2.2 Multiplicity of Cytochrome P-450 and Purification and Reconstitution of Cytochrome P-450 – Dependent Monooxygenase Systems

Even before appreciable purification of cytochrome P-450 had been accomplished, it was already apparent from indirect evidence that mammalian liver cells contained more than one cytochrome P-450. The more recent direct evidence on the multiplicity of cytochrome P-450 is of two types: (1) the separation and purification of cytochrome P-450 isozymes, which can be distinguished from each other by chromatographic behavior, immunological specificity, and/or substrate specificity after reconstitution; and (2) separation of distinct polypeptides by polyacrylamide gel electrophoresis (PAGE) in the presence of sodium dodecyl sulfate (SDS), which can be related to distinct cytochromes P-450 present in the original microsomes.

Recent studies have raised the possibility that these different cytochromes P-450 may have specific locations within the cell since microsomal fractions of different densities show qualitative differences in spectral characteristics related to cytochrome P-450.

Considerations of multiplicity may be of considerable importance in several areas of toxicology, including developmental changes, sex differences, inhibition, induction, and comparative toxicology. Any of these effects on cytochrome P-450 or monooxygenase could involve either specificity differences between different cytochromes or different proportions of cytochromes. Multiplicity of cytochrome P-450 is known or inferred in many tissues and organisms and may be considered the usual state of affairs rather than the exception.

Purification of cytochrome P-450 was, for many years, an elusive goal; however, during the past decade considerable progress has been made. The problem of instability on solubilization, which led to the formation of the inactive form, cytochrome P-420, was solved by the use of glycerol and dithiothreitol as protectants. Subsequent to solubilization, the hydrophobicity of the protein causes reaggregation, a problem that can be overcome by maintaining a low concentration of a suitable detergent, such as Emulgen 911 (Kas-Atlas,

Tokyo), throughout the procedure. Multiple forms, as discussed previously, must be separated from each other and purified as separate entities. The final problem involves the removal of detergent, which is necessary before reconstitution experiments can be carried out.

Using the above precautions and by a judicious selection of traditional and recent methods for protein purification, it has been possible to purify cytochrome P-450 as well as NADPH-cytochrome P-450 reductase from both mammalian liver and lung. These methods include the following:

1. Solubilization. Various detergents have been used, but sodium cholate is by far the most commonly used.
2. Protein precipitation. The two reagents commonly used are ammonium sulfate and polyethylene glycol.
3. Column chromatography. The materials commonly used are DEAE-cellulose, CM-cellulose, hydroxylapatite, and "affinity" columns based on *n*-octylamine or *n*-hexylamine, although the latter may act as hydrophobic columns rather than as true affinity columns.

A typical protocol and the substrate specificity of the purified cytochromes is shown in Figure 3.2. As a result of these and similar methods, highly purified preparations that appear homogeneous on PAGE can now be prepared. These cytochromes have a molecular mass of about 50,000 daltons. It is also true, however, that most of these cytochromes are purified from animals treated with a variety of inducing agents and they may, in the uninduced animal, represent a very small proportion of the total cytochrome P-450. Progress in purification of cytochrome P-450 from uninduced animals has been much less dramatic.

Systems reconstituted from purified cytochrome P-450, NADPH-cytochrome P-450 reductase, and phosphatidylcholine will, in the presence of NADPH and O_2, oxidize xenobiotics such as benzphetamine, often at rates comparable with those of microsomes. Although systems reconstituted from this minimal number of components are enzymatically active, other microsomal components, such as cytochrome b_5, may facilitate activity either in vivo or in vitro or may even be essential for the oxidation of certain substrates.

One important finding from purification studies (see Figure 3.2) is that the lack of substrate specificity of microsomes for monooxygenase activity is not an artifact caused by the presence of several specific cytochromes since it appears that all of the cytochromes isolated are relatively nonspecific. The relative activity toward different substrates does, however, vary greatly from one to another.

3.2.2.3 Microsomal Cytochrome P-450 – Dependent Monooxygenase Reactions

Although microsomal monooxygenase reactions are basically similar in the role played by molecular oxygen and in the supply of electrons, the enzymes are nonspecific, both substrates and products falling into many different chemical classes. In the following sections, therefore, these activities are classified on the basis of the overall chemical reaction catalyzed; one should bear in mind, however, that not only do these classes often overlap but that a substrate may undergo more than one reaction.

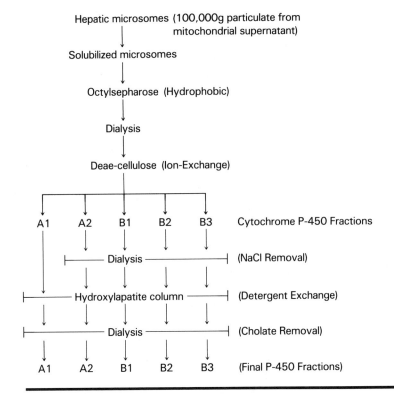

	Cytochrome P-450 Fractions					
Assay	A1	A2	B1	B2	B3	Microsomes
CO-Spectrum (λMax-nm)	452	449.5	450	451	450	
Molecular Mass (Daltons)	53,000 56,000	48,000 53,000 56,000	53,000	53,000	54,500	
Benzphetamine N-Demethylation	26	15	ND[1]	184	ND	ND
Ethoxyresorufin O-Deethylation	0.7	0.7	8.1	1.8	9.9	0.5
Benzo(a)pyrene Hydroxylation	3.8	11.4	0.6	1.5	1.4	12.1
Ethoxycoumarin O-Deethylation	20.2	1.1	0.2	0.4	0.2	4.6
Biphenyl 4-Hydroxylation	1.1	1.3	23.6	5.3	20.8	11.1
Biphenyl 2-Hydroxylation	0.08	ND	ND	ND	ND	1.6

Rates of product formation were determined in reaction mixtures in which cytochrome P-450 was the rate limiting component.

(1)ND, no product was detected under conditions of the assay.

FIGURE 3.2.
Purification and properties of multiple forms of cytochrome P-450 isozymes from uninduced mouse liver. Source: Levi and Hodgson. Int. J. Biochem. 1983; 15:349.

3.2.2.3a Epoxidation and Aromatic Hydroxylation

Epoxidation is an extremely important microsomal reaction; not only can stable and environmentally persistent epoxides be formed (see 3.2.2.3c), but also highly reactive intermediates of aromatic hydroxylations, such as arene oxides, are produced. These highly reactive intermediates are known to be involved in chemical carcinogenesis.

The oxidation of naphthalene was one of the earliest examples of an epoxide as an intermediate in aromatic hydroxylations. As shown in Figure 3.3, the

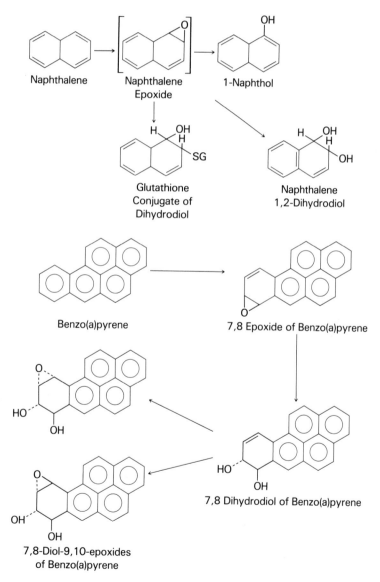

FIGURE 3.3.
Examples of epoxidation and aromatic hydroxylation.

epoxide can rearrange nonenzymatically to yield predominantly 1-naphthol, can interact with the enzyme epoxide hydrolase to yield the dihydrodiol, or can interact with glutathione S-transferase to yield the glutathione conjugate, which is ultimately metabolized to a mercapturic acid. These reactions are also of importance in the metabolism of the insecticide carbaryl, which contains the naphthalene nucleus.

The ultimate carcinogens arising from the metabolic activation of benzo(a)pyrene are stereoisomers of benzo(a)pyrene 7,8-diol-9,10-epoxide (Figure 3.3). These metabolites arise by prior formation of the 7,8-epoxide, which gives rise to the 7,8-dihydrodiol through the action of epoxide hydrolase. This is further metabolized by the cytochrome P-450–dependent monooxygenase system to the 7,8-diol-9,10-epoxides, which are both potent mutagens and unsuitable substrates for the further action of epoxide hydrolase. Stereochemistry is important in the toxicity of the final product. Of the four possible isomers of the diol epoxide, one, the +-benzo(a)pyrene diol epoxide-2 is much more toxic.

3.2.2.3b Aliphatic Hydroxylation

Although simple aliphatic molecules such as *n*-butane, *n*-pentane, *n*-hexane, etc., as well as alicyclic compounds such as cyclohexane, are known to be oxidized to alcohols, alkyl side chains of aromatic compounds are more readily oxidized, often at more than one position, and provide good examples of this type of oxidation. The *n*-propyl side chain of *n*-propyl benzene can be oxidized, in the rabbit, at any one of the three carbons to yield 3-phenylpropan-1-ol ($C_6H_5CH_2CH_2CH_2OH$) by ω-oxidation, benzylmethyl carbinol ($C_6H_5CH_2CHOHCH_3$) by ω-1 oxidation, and ethylphenylcarbinol ($C_6H_5CHOHCH_2CH_3$) by α-oxidation. Further oxidation of these alcohols is also possible.

3.2.2.3c Aliphatic Epoxidation

Many aliphatic and alicyclic compounds containing unsaturated carbon atoms are thought to be metabolized to epoxide intermediates (Figure 3.4). In the case of aldrin, the product, dieldrin, is an extremely stable epoxide and represents the principal residue found in animals exposed to aldrin. Epoxide formation in the case of aflatoxin is believed to be the final step in the expression of carcinogenicity and is, therefore, an activation reaction.

3.2.2.3d Dealkylation: *O*-, *N*-, and *S*-Dealkylation

Probably the best known example of *O*-dealkylation is the demethylation of *p*-nitroanisole. Due to the ease with which the product, *p*-nitrophenol, can be measured, it is a frequently used substrate for the demonstration of cytochrome P-450–dependent monooxygenase activity. The reaction is believed to proceed by an unstable methylol intermediate (Figure 3.5).

The *O*-dealkylation of organophosphorus triesters differs from that of *p*-nitroanisole in that it involves the dealkylation of an ester rather than an ether. The reaction was first described for the insecticide chlorfenvinphos and is known to occur with a wide variety of vinyl, phenyl, phenylvinyl, and naphthyl phosphate and thionophosphate triesters (Figure 3.5).

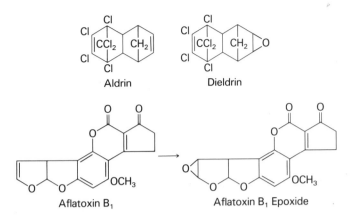

FIGURE 3.4.
Examples of aliphatic epoxidation.

N-Dealkylation is a common reaction in the metabolism of drugs, insecticides, and other xenobiotics. Both the *N*-alkyl and the *N,N*-dialkyl carbamates are readily dealkylated; in some cases, the methylol intermediates are stable enough to be isolated. *N,N*-Dimethyl-*p*-nitrophenyl carbamate is a useful model compound for this reaction (Figure 3.5). The insecticide carbaryl undergoes several monooxygenations, including attack on the *N*-methyl group. In this case the methylol derivative is stable enough to be isolated or to be conjugated in vivo.

S-Dealkylation is believed to occur with a number of thioethers, including methylmercaptan and 6-methylthiopurine, although with newer knowledge of the specificity of the FAD-containing monooxygenase (see Section 3.2.2.4) it is possible that the initial attack is through sulfoxidation mediated by the latter enzyme rather than cytochrome P-450.

3.2.2.3e *N*-Oxidation

N-Oxidation can occur in a number of ways, including hydroxylamine formation, oxime formation, and *N*-oxide formation, although the latter is primarily dependent on the FAD-containing monooxygenase also found in microsomes. Hydroxylamine formation occurs with a number of amines such as aniline and many of its substituted derivatives. In the case of 2-acetylaminofluorene, the product is a potent carcinogen and thus the reaction is an activation reaction (Figure 3.6).

Oximes can be formed by the *N*-hydroxylation of imines and primary amines. Imines have been suggested as intermediates in the formation of oximes from primary amines (Figure 3.6).

3.2.2.3f Oxidative Deamination

Oxidative deamination of amphetamine occurs in rabbit liver but not to any extent in liver of either dog or rat, which tend to hydroxylate the aromatic ring. A close examination of the reaction indicates that it is probably not an attack on

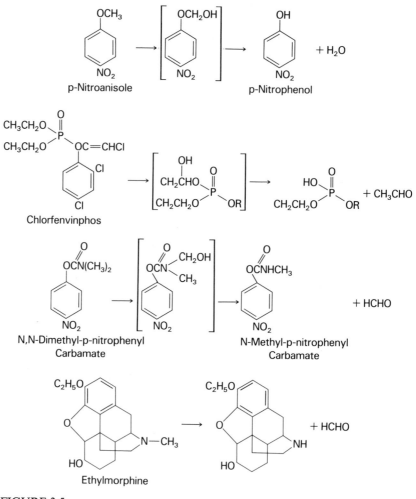

FIGURE 3.5.
Examples of dealkylation.

the nitrogen but rather on the adjacent carbon atom, giving rise to a carbinol amine, which eliminates ammonia, producing a ketone.

$$R_2CHNH_2 \xrightarrow{\text{O}} R_2C(OH)NH_2 \xrightarrow{-NH_3} R_2C=O.$$

The carbinol, by another reaction sequence, can also give rise to an oxime, which can be hydrolyzed to yield the ketone, which is thus formed by two different routes.

$$R_2C(OH)NH_2 \xrightarrow{-H_2O} R_2C=NH \xrightarrow{+O} R_2CNOH \xrightarrow{+H_2O} R_2C=O.$$

3.2.2.3g *S*-Oxidation

Thioethers in general are oxidized by microsomal monooxygenases to sulfoxides, some of which are further oxidized to sulfones. This reaction is very

a. Hydroxylamine formation

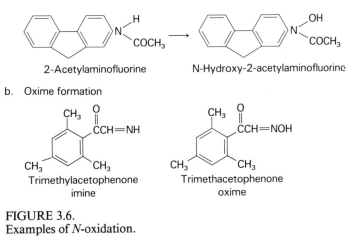

2-Acetylaminofluorine   N-Hydroxy-2-acetylaminofluorine

b. Oxime formation

Trimethylacetophenone   Trimethacetophenone
imine   oxime

FIGURE 3.6.
Examples of *N*-oxidation.

common among insecticides of several different chemical classes, including carbamates, organophosphates, and chlorinated hydrocarbons. The organophosphates include phorate, demeton, and others, whereas among the chlorinated hydrocarbons, endosulfan is oxidized to endosulfan sulfate and methiochlor to a series of sulfoxides and sulfones, eventually yielding the *bis*-sulfone. Among carbamates, methiocarb yields the sulfoxide and sulfone, and drugs such as chloropromazine and solvents such as dimethyl sulfoxide are also subject to *S*-oxidation. The current knowledge that the FAD-containing monooxygenase, formerly known as an amine oxidase, is actually a versatile sulfur oxidase carrying out many of the above reactions raises important questions as to the relative role of this enzyme *v* that of cytochrome P-450. Thus, a reexamination of earlier work in which many of these reactions were ascribed to cytochrome P-450 is required.

3.2.2.3h *P*-Oxidation
P-Oxidation, a little known reaction, involves the conversion of trisubstituted phosphines to phosphine oxides, eg, diphenylmethylphosphine to diphenylmethylphosphine oxide. Although described as a typical cytochrome P-450–dependent monooxygenation, it too is now known to be catalyzed by the FAD-containing monooxygenase as well.

3.2.2.3i Desulfuration and Ester Cleavage
The insecticides phosphorothionate $[(R^1O)_2P(S)OR^2]$ and phosphorodithioate $[(R^1O)_2P(S)SR^2]$ owe their insecticidal activity and their mammalian toxicity to an oxidative reaction in which the P=S group is converted to P=O, thereby converting them from compounds relatively inactive toward cholinesterases into potent cholinesterase inhibitors. This reaction is known for many organophosphorus compounds but has been studied most intensively in the case of parathion. Much of the splitting of the phosphorus ester bonds in organophosphorus insecticides, formerly believed to be due to hydrolysis, is now known to be due to oxidative dearylation. This is a typical cytochrome P-450–dependent

monooxygenation, requiring NADPH and O_2 and being inhibited by CO, and persuasive evidence supports the hypothesis that this reaction and oxidative desulfuration involve a common intermediate of the "phosphooxithirane" type (Figure 3.7).

Some organophosphorus insecticides, all phosphonates, are activated by the FAD-containing monooxygenase as well as by cytochrome P-450 (see Figure 6.1).

3.2.2.3j Methylenedioxy (Benzodioxole) Ring Cleavage

Methylenedioxyphenyl compounds, such as safrole or the insecticide synergist, piperonyl butoxide, many of which are effective inhibitors of cytochrome P-450–dependent monooxygenations, are themselves metabolized to catechols. The most probable mechanism appears to be an attack on the methylene carbon, followed by elimination of water to yield a carbene. The highly reactive carbene either reacts with the heme iron to form a cytochrome P-450–inhibitory complex or breaks down to yield the catechol (Figure 3.8).

3.2.3 The Microsomal FAD-Containing Monooxygenase

Tertiary amines such as trimethylamine and dimethylaniline have long been known to be metabolized to *N*-oxides by an amine oxidase which is microsomal, but not dependent on cytochrome P-450. This enzyme, now known as the microsomal FAD-containing monooxygenase, is also dependent on NADPH and O_2, and has been purified to homogeneity from pig and mouse liver microsomes. It has a monomeric molecular mass of about 56,000/mol of FAD.

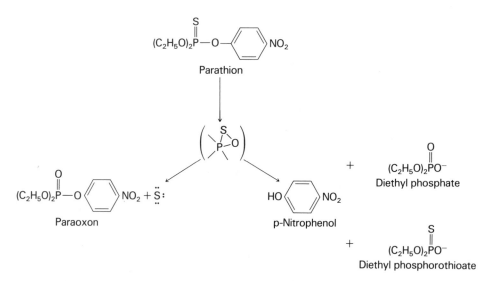

FIGURE 3.7.
Desulfuration and oxidative dearylation.

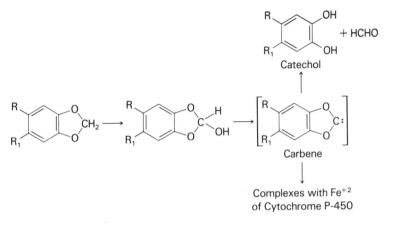

FIGURE 3.8.
Monooxygenation of methylenedioxyphenyl compounds.

The FAD-contaning monooxygenase is now known to have a much wider substrate specificity than formerly supposed. It includes tertiary and secondary amines as well as a number of different types of sulfur compounds such as sulfides, thioethers, thiols, and thiocarbamates. More recently still, this enzyme has been shown to attack organophosphorus compounds in the case of phosphines and in the activation of phosphonates to their oxons (Figure 3.9).

Many of these compounds are also known to be substrates for cytochrome P-450, and current research is being directed toward an assessment of their relative importance in both detoxication and activation reactions.

Toxicologically, it is of interest that this enzyme is responsible for the oxidation of nicotine to nicotine-1'-N-oxide, whereas the oxidation of nicotine to cotinine is catalyzed by two enzymes acting in sequence: cytochrome P-450 and a soluble aldehyde dehydrogenase. Thus, nicotine is metabolized by two different routes, the relative contributions of which may vary with both the extrinsic and intrinsic factors outlined in Chapter 4.

3.2.4 Nonmicrosomal Oxidations

In addition to the microsomal monooxygenases, other enzymes are involved in the oxidation of xenobiotics. These enzymes are located in the mitochondria or in the soluble cytoplasm of the cell.

3.2.4.1 Alcohol Dehydrogenases

Alcohol dehydrogenases catalyze the conversion of alcohols to aldehydes or ketones:

$$RCH_2OH + NAD^+ \rightleftharpoons RCHO + NADH + H^+.$$

This reaction should not be confused with the monooxygenation of ethanol that occurs in the microsomes. The alcohol dehydrogenase reaction is reversible, with the carbonyl compounds being reduced to alcohols.

This enzyme is found in the soluble fraction of the liver, kidney, and lung

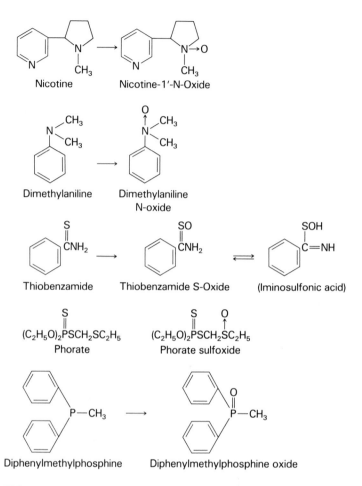

FIGURE 3.9.
Examples of oxidations catalyzed by the microsomal FAD-containing monooxygenase.

and is probably the most important enzyme involved in the metabolism of foreign alcohols. Alcohol dehydrogenase is a dimer, the subunits of which can occur in several forms that are under genetic control, thus giving rise to a large number of variants of the enzyme. It can use either NAD or NADP as a co-enzyme, but the reaction proceeds at a much slower rate with NADP. In the intact organism, the reaction proceeds in the direction of alcohol consumption, since aldehydes are further oxidized to acids. Because aldehydes are toxic and are not readily excreted because of their lipophilicity, alcohol oxidation may be considered an activation reaction, the further oxidation of the aldehyde being detoxication step.

Primary alcohols are oxidized to aldehydes, n-butanol being the substrate oxidized at the highest rate. Although secondary alcohols are oxidized to ketones, the rate is less than that for primary alcohols, and tertiary alcohols are not readily oxidized. Alcohol dehydrogenase is inhibited by a number of heterocyclic compounds such as pyrazole, imidazole, and their derivatives.

3.2.4.2 Aldehyde Dehydrogenase

This enzyme catalyzes the formation of acids from aliphatic and aromatic aldehydes; the acids are then available as substrates for conjugating enzymes:

$$RCHO + NAD^+ \longrightarrow RCOOH + NADH + H^+.$$

The enzyme from mammalian liver has been isolated, and many aldehydes can serve as substrates. Other enzymes in the soluble fraction of liver that oxidize aldehydes are aldehyde oxidase and xanthine oxidase, both flavoproteins that contain molybdenum; however, their primary role seems to be the oxidation of endogenous aldehydes formed as a result of deamination reactions.

3.2.4.3 Amine Oxidases

The most important function of amine oxidases appears to be the oxidation of amines formed during normal processes. Two types of amine oxidases are concerned with the oxidative deamination of both endogenous and exogenous amines. Typical substrates are shown in Figure 3.10.

3.2.4.3a Monoamine Oxidases

The monoamine oxidases are a family of flavoproteins found in the mitochondria of a wide variety of tissues: liver, kidney, brain, intestine, and blood platelets. They are a group of similar enzymes with overlapping substrate specificities and inhibition. Although the number is difficult to estimate, two forms from rat liver have been characterized in some detail. Although the enzyme in the central nervous system is concerned primarily with neurotransmitter turnover, that in the liver will deaminate primary, secondary, and tertiary aliphatic amines, reaction rates with the primary amines being faster. Electron-withdrawing substitutions on an aromatic ring increase the reaction rate, whereas compounds with a methyl group on the α-carbon such as amphetamine and ephedrine are not metabolized.

3.2.4.3b Diamine Oxidases

Diamine oxidases are enzymes that also oxidize amines to aldehydes. The preferred substrates are aliphatic diamines in which the chain length is four (putrescine) or five (cadaverine) carbon atoms. Diamines with carbon chains longer than nine will not serve as substrates but can be oxidized by monoamine

a. Monoamine oxidase

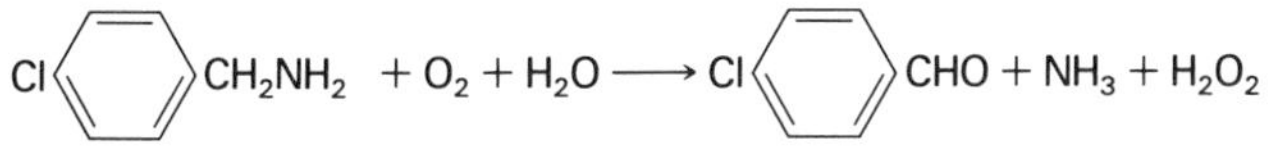

$$Cl \langle \rangle CH_2NH_2 + O_2 + H_2O \longrightarrow Cl \langle \rangle CHO + NH_3 + H_2O_2$$

p-Chlorobenzylamine

b. Diamine oxidase

$$H_2N(CH_2)_5NH_2 + O_2 + H_2O \longrightarrow H_2N(CH_2)_4CHO + NH_3 + H_2O_2$$
Cadaverine

FIGURE 3.10.
Examples of oxidations catalyzed by amine oxidases.

oxidases. Secondary and tertiary amines are not metabolized. Diamine oxidases are typically soluble pyridoxal phosphate-containing proteins that also contain copper. They have been found in a number of tissues, including liver, intestine, kidney, and placenta.

3.2.5 Cooxidation During Prostaglandin Biosynthesis

During the biosynthesis of prostaglandins, a polyunsaturated fatty acid, such as arachidonic acid, is first oxygenated to yield a hydroperoxy endoperoxide, prostaglandin G. This is then further metabolized to prostaglandin H_2, both reactions being catalyzed by the same enzyme, prostaglandin synthase (Figure 3.11). This enzyme is located in the microsomal membrane and is found in high levels in such tissues as seminal vesicle. It is a glycoprotein with a subunit molecular mass of about 70,000 daltons, containing one heme per subunit. During the second step of the above sequence (peroxidase), many xenobiotics can be cooxidized, and investigations of the mechanism have shown that the reactions are hydroperoxide-dependent reactions catalyzed by a peroxidase that uses prostaglandin G as a substrate. In at least some of these cases, the identity of this peroxidase has been established as prostaglandin synthase. Many of the reactions are similar or identical to those catalyzed by other peroxidases and also by microsomal monooxygenases; they include both detoxication and activation reactions (Figure 3.11). This mechanism has been discovered relatively recently. Further studies are likely to demonstrate that it is important in xenobiotic metabolism, particularly in tissues that are low in cytochrome P-450 and/or the FAD-containing monooxygenase but high in prostaglandin synthase.

a. PROSTAGLANDIN SYNTHASE REACTION

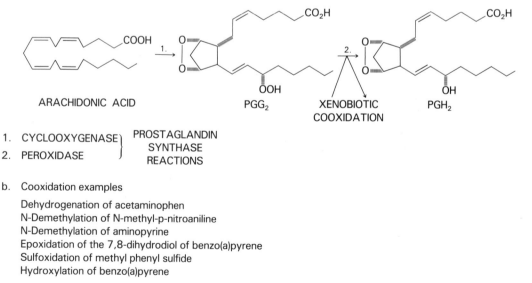

1. CYCLOOXYGENASE ⎫ PROSTAGLANDIN
2. PEROXIDASE ⎬ SYNTHASE
          ⎭ REACTIONS

b. Cooxidation examples

Dehydrogenation of acetaminophen
N-Demethylation of N-methyl-p-nitroaniline
N-Demethylation of aminopyrine
Epoxidation of the 7,8-dihydrodiol of benzo(a)pyrene
Sulfoxidation of methyl phenyl sulfide
Hydroxylation of benzo(a)pyrene

FIGURE 3.11.
Cooxidation during prostaglandin biosynthesis.

3.2.6 Reduction Reactions

A number of functional groups, such as nitro, diazo, carbonyl, disulfide sulfoxide, alkene, pentavalent arsenic, etc., are susceptible to reduction, although in many cases it is difficult to tell whether the reaction proceeds enzymatically or nonenzymatically by the action of such biological reducing agents as reduced flavins or reduced pyridine nucleotides. In some cases, such as the reduction of the double bond in cinnamic acid ($C_6H_5CH{=}CHCOOH$), the reaction has been attributed to the intestinal microflora. Examples of reduction reactions are shown in Figure 3.12.

3.2.6.1 Nitro Reduction

Aromatic amines are susceptible to reduction by both bacterial and mammalian nitroreductase systems. Convincing evidence has been presented that this

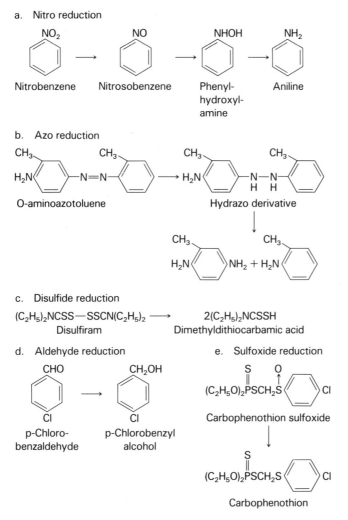

a. Nitro reduction

Nitrobenzene   Nitrosobenzene   Phenyl-hydroxyl-amine   Aniline

b. Azo reduction

O-aminoazotoluene   Hydrazo derivative

c. Disulfide reduction

$(C_2H_5)_2NCSS{-}SSCN(C_2H_5)_2 \longrightarrow 2(C_2H_5)_2NCSSH$
Disulfiram   Dimethyldithiocarbamic acid

d. Aldehyde reduction

p-Chloro-benzaldehyde   p-Chlorobenzyl alcohol

e. Sulfoxide reduction

$(C_2H_5O)_2PSCH_2S$ ... Cl
Carbophenothion sulfoxide

$(C_2H_5O)_2PSCH_2S$ ... Cl
Carbophenothion

FIGURE 3.12.
Examples of metabolic reduction reactions.

reaction sequence is catalyzed by cytochrome P-450. It is inhibited by oxygen, although NADPH is still consumed. Earlier workers had suggested a flavoprotein reductase was involved, and it is not clear whether this is incorrect or whether both mechanisms occur. It is true, however, that high concentrations of FAD or FMN will catalyze the nonenzymatic reduction of nitro groups.

3.2.6.2 Azo Reduction

Requirements for azoreduction are similar to those for nitroreduction, namely, anaerobic conditions and NADPH. They are also inhibited by CO, and presumably they involve cytochrome P-450. The ability of mammalian cells to reduce azo bonds is rather poor, and intestinal microflora may play a role.

3.2.6.3 Disulfide Reduction

Some disulfides, such as the drug disulfiram (Antabuse), are reduced to their sulfhydryl constituents. Many of these reactions are three-step sequences, the last reaction of which is catalyzed by glutathione reductase.

$$XSSX + GSH \longrightarrow XSSG + XSH$$

$$XSSG + GSH \longrightarrow GSSG + XSH$$

$$GSSG + NADPH + H^+ \longrightarrow 2GSH + NADP^+.$$

3.2.6.4 Ketone and Aldehyde Reduction

In addition to the reduction of aldehyde and ketones through the reverse reaction of alcohol dehydrogenase (Section 3.2.4.1) a family of aldehyde reductases also reduces these compounds. These reductases are NADPH-dependent, cytoplasmic enzymes of low mol wt and have been found in liver, brain, kidney, and other tissues.

3.2.6.5 Sulfoxide Reduction

The reduction of sulfoxides has been reported to occur in mammalian tissues. Soluble thioredoxin-dependent enzymes in the liver are known to be responsible in some cases. It has been suggested that oxidation in the endoplasmic reticulum followed by reduction in the cytoplasm may be a form of recyling that could extend the in vivo half-life of certain toxicants.

3.2.7 Hydrolysis

Enzymes with carboxylesterase and amidase activity are widely distributed in the body, occurring in many tissues and in both microsomal and soluble fractions. They catalyze the following general reactions:

$$RC(O)OR' + H_2O = RCOOH + HOR' \text{—Carboxylester hydrolysis}$$

$$RC(O)NR'R'' + H_2O = RCOOH + HNR'R'' \text{—Carboxyamide hydrolysis}$$

$$RC(O)SR' + H_2O = RCOOH + HSR' \text{—Carboxythioester hydrolysis.}$$

Although carboxylesterases and amidases were thought to be different, no purified carboxylesterase has been found that does not have amidase activity toward the corresponding amide. Similarly, enzymes purified on the basis of their amidase activity have been found to have esterase activity. Thus, these two activities are now regarded as different manifestations of the same activity, specificity depending on the nature of R, R', and R" groups and, to a lesser extent, on the atom (O, S, or N) adjacent to the carboxyl group.

In view of the large number of esterases in many tissues and subcellular fractions, as well as the large number of substrates hydrolyzed by them, it is difficult to derive a meaningful classification scheme. The division into A-, B-, and C-esterases on the basis of their behavior toward such phosphate triesters are paraoxon, first devised by Aldridge, is still of some value, although not entirely satisfactory.

B-Esterases, the most important group, are all inhibited by paraoxon, and all have a serine residue in their active site that is phosphorylated by this inhibitor. This group includes a number of different enzymes and their isozymes, many of which have quite different substrate specificities. For example, the group contains carboxylesterase/amidases, cholinesterases, monoacylglycerol lipases, and arylamidases. Many of these enzymes hydrolyze physiological (endogenous) substrates as well as xenobiotics. Several examples of their activity toward xenobiotic substrates are shown in Figure 3.13.

a. Esterase

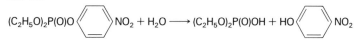

b. Esterase

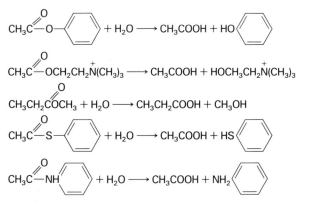

c. Esterase

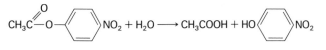

FIGURE 3.13.
Examples of esterase/amidase reactions involving xenobiotics.

A-Esterases, often referred to as arylesterases, are not inhibited by phosphotriesters such as paraoxon, but hydrolyze them instead.

C-Esterases, or acetylesterases, are defined as those esterases that prefer acetyl esters as substrates, and for which paraoxon serves as neither substrate nor inhibitor.

3.2.8 Epoxide Hydration

Epoxide rings of alkene and arene compounds are hydrated by enzymes known as epoxide hydrolases, the animal enzyme forming the corresponding *trans* diols, although bacterial hydrolases are known that form *cis* diols. In some cases, such as benzo(a)pyrene, the hydration of an epoxide is the first step in an activation sequence that ultimately yields highly toxic *trans*-dihydrodiol intermediates. In others, reactive epoxides are detoxified by both glutathione transferase and epoxide hydrolase. The reaction probably involves a nucleophilic attack by –OH on the oxirane carbon. The most studied epoxide hydrolase is microsomal, and the enzyme has been purified from hepatic microsomes of several species. Although less well known, soluble epoxide hydrolases with different substrate specificities have also been described. Examples of epoxide hydrolase reactions are shown in Figure 3.14.

3.2.9 DDT-Dehydrochlorinase

DDT-Dehydrochlorinase is an enzyme that occurs in both mammals and insects but has been studied most intensively in DDT-resistant houseflies. It catalyzes the dehydrochlorination of DDT to DDE and occurs in the soluble fraction of homogenates. Although the reaction requires glutathione, it apparently serves in a catalytic role since it does not appear to be consumed during the reaction. The K_m for DDT is 5×10^{-7} mol/L with optimum activity at pH 7.4. The monomeric form of the enzyme has a molecular mass of about 36,000 daltons, but the enzyme normally exists as a tetramer. In addition to catalyzing the dehydrochlorination of DDT to DDE and DDD (2,2-*bis*(*p*-chlorophenyl)-1,1-dichloroethane) to TDE (2,2-*bis*-(*p*-chlorophenyl)-1-chlorothylene), DDT dehydrochlorinase catalyzes the dehydrohalogenation of a number of other

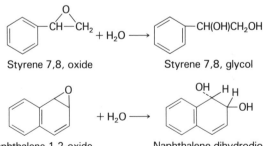

Styrene 7,8, oxide   Styrene 7,8, glycol

Naphthalene 1,2-oxide   Naphthalene dihydrodiol

FIGURE 3.14.
Examples of epoxide hydrolase reactions.

DDT analogs. In all cases, the *p,p* configuration is required, *o,p* and other analogs are not utilized as substrates. The reaction is illustrated in Figure 3.15.

3.3 PHASE-TWO REACTIONS

Metabolism of phase-one products and other xenobiotics containing functional groups such as hydroxyl, amino, carboxyl, epoxide, or halogen can undergo conjugation reactions with endogenous metabolites, these conjugations being collectively termed phase-two reactions. The endogenous metabolites in question include sugars, amino acids, glutathione, sulfate, etc. Conjugation products, with only rare exceptions, are more polar, less toxic, and more readily excreted than are their parent compounds.

Conjugation reactions usually involve activation by some high energy intermediate and have been classified into two general types: type I, in which an activated conjugating agent combines with the substrate to yield the conjugated product, and type II, in which the substrate is activated and then combines with an amino acid to yield a conjugated product. The formation of sulfates and glycosides are examples of type I, where type II consists primarily of amino acid conjugations.

3.3.1 Glycoside Conjugation

The formation of an activated intermediate, either uridine diphosphate glucose (UDPG) or uridine diphosphate glucuronic acid (UDPGA), is required for glycoside formation. The enzymes involved occur in the soluble fraction of the liver and other organs. The activation sequence and examples of the various types of glycosides described in the following section are shown in Figure 3.16.

3.3.1.1 Glucuronides

The final step of glucuronide formation involves the reaction of UDPGA with the aglycone, the latter being, in many cases, a xenobiotic. The reaction involves a nucleophilic displacement (SN₂ reaction) of the functional group of the substrate with Walden inversion. UDPGA is in the α-configuration whereas, due to the inversion, the glucuronide formed is in the β-configuration. The enzyme involved, glucuronosyl transferase, is found in the microsomal fraction of liver, kidney, and other tissues.

Whether this is one enzyme or a family of closely related enzymes is not entirely clear, although the latter is indicated from both purification and induc-

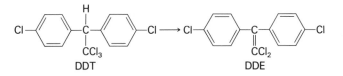

FIGURE 3.15.
DDT-dehydrochlorinase.

Reaction sequence

1. Uridine triphosphate (UTP) + Glucose-1-phosphate $\xrightarrow[\text{Pyrophosphorylase}]{\text{UDPG}}$
    Uridine diphosphate glucose (UDPG) + Pyrophosphate

2. UDPG + 2NAD + H_2O $\xrightarrow[\text{Dehydrogenase}]{\text{UDPG}}$
    Uridine diphosphate glucuronic acid (UDPGA) + 2NADH$_2$

3. a. O-Glucuronide formation

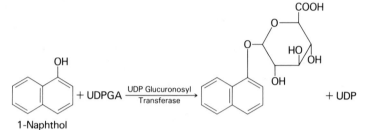

1-Naphthol

    b. N-Glucuronide formation

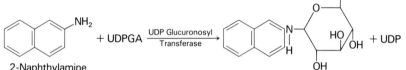

2-Naphthylamine

    c. S-Glucuronide formation

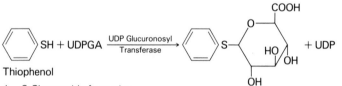

Thiophenol

    d. C-Glucuronide formation

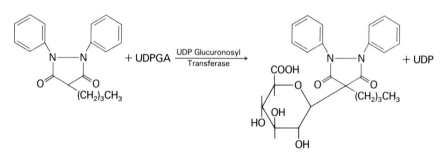

    e. O-Glucoside formation

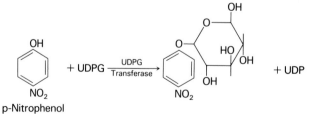

p-Nitrophenol

FIGURE 3.16.
Glycoside formation.

tion studies. Homogeneous glucuronosyl transferase has been isolated as a single polypeptide chain of about 59,000 daltons, apparently containing carbohydrate, the activity of which appears to be dependent on reconstitution with microsomal lipid. There appears to be an absolute requirement for UDPGA; related UDP-sugars will not suffice. This enzyme, as it exists in the microsomal membrane, does not exhibit its maximal capacity for conjugation; activation by some means (detergents, for example) is required.

A wide variety of reactions are mediated by glucuronosyltransferases. *O*-Glucuronides, *N*-glucuronides and *S*-glucuronides have all been identified.

3.3.1.2 Glucosides

Although rare in vertebrates, glucosides formed from xenobiotics are common in insects and plants. Formed from UDP-glucose, they appear to fall into the same classes as the glucuronides.

3.3.2 Sulfate Conjugation

Sulfate esters, which are water soluble and readily eliminated from the organism, are formed with xenobiotics such as alcohols, arylamines, and phenols. This process requires the prior activation of sulfate ions to 3'-phospho-adenosine-5'-phosphosulfate (PAPS), a reaction sequence (Figure 3.17) requiring the consumption of ATP and hence using a considerable amount of energy.

In addition to inorganic sulfate and adenosine triphosphate (ATP), the formation of PAPS requires the sequential action of ATP sulfurylase and adenosine 5'-phosphosulfate kinase. ATP sulfurylase from rat liver is a large molecule of about 500,000 daltons. Several group VI anions other than sulfate can also serve as substrates, although the resultant anhydrides are unstable. Because this instability would lead to the overall consumption of ATP, these other anions can exert a toxic effect by depleting the cell of ATP. The second enzyme, the kinase, is not well known from mammalian tissues, but that from yeast shows a high affinity for APS and the reaction is essentially irreversible.

The final step is catalyzed by a family of related sulfotransferases that have been classified as follows: aryl sulfotransferase; hydroxysteroid sulfotransferase; estrone sulfotransferase; and bile salt sulfotransferase. Aryl sulfotransferases from rat liver have been separated into four distinct forms, each of which catalyzes the sulfation of various phenols and catecholamines. They differ, however, in pH optimum, relative substrate specificity, and immunological properties. The molecules of all of them are in the range of 61,000–64,000 daltons.

Hydroxysteroid sulfotransferase also appears to exist in several forms. This reaction is now known to be important, not only as a detoxication mechanism, but also in the synthesis and possibly the transport of steroids. Hydroxysteroid sulfotransferase will react with hydroxysterols and primary and secondary alcohols but not with hydroxy groups on the aromatic rings of steroids.

The third sulfotransferase, estrone sulfotransferase, has been purified from bovine adrenal gland. This enzyme will conjugate hydroxyl groups on the A ring of sterols.

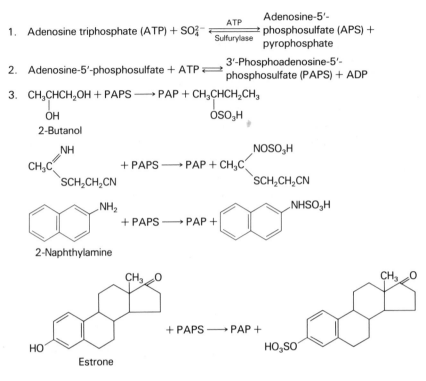

1. Adenosine triphosphate (ATP) + SO_4^{2-} $\underset{\text{Sulfurylase}}{\overset{\text{ATP}}{\rightleftharpoons}}$ Adenosine-5'-phosphosulfate (APS) + pyrophosphate

2. Adenosine-5'-phosphosulfate + ATP $\rightleftharpoons$ 3'-Phosphoadenosine-5'-phosphosulfate (PAPS) + ADP

3. CH_3CHCH_2OH + PAPS $\longrightarrow$ PAP + $CH_3CHCH_2CH_3$

FIGURE 3.17.
Sulfate ester formation.

Bile salt sulfotransferase appears to have the function of detoxifying bile salts, the toxic properties of which are well documented. This enzyme has been purified from both liver and kidney, the two forms appearing to be distinct entities.

3.3.3 Methyltransferases

A large number of both endogenous and exogenous compounds can be methylated by several *N*-, *O*-, and *S*-methyl transferases. The most common methyl donor is *S*-adenosyl methionine (SAM), formed from methionine and ATP. Even though these reactions may involve a decrease in water solubility, they are generally detoxication reactions. Examples of biological methylation reactions are seen in Figure 3.18.

3.3.3.1 *N*-Methylation

Several enzymes are known that catalyze *N*-methylation reactions. They include histamine *N*-methyltransferase, a highly specific enzyme that occurs in the soluble fraction of the cell, phenylethanolamine *N*-methyltransferase, which catalyzes the methylation of noradrenaline to adrenaline as well as the methylation of other phenylethanolamine derivatives. A third *N*-methyltrans-

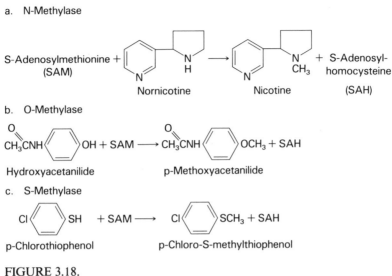

FIGURE 3.18.
Examples of methyl transferase reactions.

ferase is the indoethylamine N-methyltransferase, or nonspecific N-methyltransferase. This enzyme has been isolated from rabbit lung and is known to occur in various tissues. It methylates endogenous compounds such as serotonin and tryptamine and exogenous compounds such as nornicotine and norcodeine. The relationship between this enzyme and phenylethanolamine N-methyltransferase is not yet entirely clear.

3.3.3.2 O-Methylation

Catechol O-methyltransferase occurs in the soluble fraction of several tissues and has been purified from rat liver. The purified form has a molecular weight of 23,000 daltons, requires S-adenosylmethionine and Mg^+, and catalyzes the methylation of epinephrine, norepinephrine, and other catechol derivatives. There is evidence that this enzyme exists in multiple forms.

A microsomal O-methyltransferase that methylates a number of alkyl-, methoxy-, and halophenols has been described from rabbit liver and lungs. These methylations are inhibited by SKF-525A, N-ethyl-maleimide and p-chloromercuribenzoate.

A hydroxyindole O-methyltransferase, which methylates N-acteyl-serotonin to melatonin and, to a lesser extent, other 5-hydroxyindoles and 5,6-dihydroxyindoles, has been described from the pineal gland of mammals, birds, reptiles, amphibians, and fish.

3.3.3.3 S-Methylation

Thiol groups of some foreign compounds are also methylated, the reaction being catalyzed by the enzyme, thiol S-methyltransferase. This enzyme is microsomal and, as with most methyl transferases, utilizes S-adenosylmethionine. It has been purified from rat liver and is a monomer of about 28,000 daltons. A wide variety of substrates are methylated, including thioacetanilide, mercaptoethanol, and phenylsulfide. This enzyme may also be important in the detoxication of hydrogen sulfide, which is methylated in two steps, first to the highly toxic methanethiol and then to dimethylsulfide.

Methylthiolation, or the transfer of a methylthio (CH_3S-) group to a foreign compound may occur through the action of another recently discovered enzyme, cysteine conjugate β-lyase. This enzyme acts on cytsteine conjugates of foreign compounds as follows:

$$RSCH_2CH(NH_2)COOH \longrightarrow RSH + NH_3 + CH_3C(O)COOH.$$

The thiol group can then be methylated to yield the methylthio derivative of the original xenobiotic.

3.3.3.4 Biomethylation of Elements

The biomethylation of elements is primarily carried out by microorganisms but is important in environmental toxicology, particularly in the case of heavy metals, since the products are absorbed through the membranes of the gut, the blood-brain barrier, and the placenta more readily than are the inorganic forms. For example, inorganic mercury can be methylated first to monomethylmercury and subsequently to dimethylmercury:

$$Hg^{2+} \longrightarrow CH_3Hg^+ \longrightarrow (CH_3)_2Hg.$$

The enzymes involved are reported to use either S-adenosylmethionine or vitamin B_{12} derivatives as methyl donors and, in addition to mercury; the metals, lead, tin, and thallium, as well as the metalloids, arsenic, selenium, tellurium, and sulfur are methylated. Even the unreactive metals, gold and platinum, are reported as substrates for these reactions.

3.3.4 Glutathione Transferases and Mercapturic Acid Formation

Although mercapturic acids, the N-acetylcysteine conjugates of xenobiotics, have been known for > 75 years, only in the last 25 years have the source of the cysteine moiety (glutathione) and the enzymes required for the formation of these acids been identified and characterized. The overall pathway and examples of reactions that are mentioned in this section are shown in Figure 3.19.

The initial reaction is the conjugation of xenobiotics having electrophilic substituents with glutathione, a reaction catalyzed by one of the various forms of glutathione transferase. This is followed by transfer of the glutamate by γ-glutamyltranspeptidase, by loss of glycine through cysteinyl glycinase, and finally by acetylation of the cysteine amino group. The overall sequence, but particularly the initial reaction, is extremely important in toxicology since, by removing reactive electrophiles, it protects vital nucleophilic groups in macromolecules such as proteins and nucleic acids. The mercapturic acids formed can be excreted either in the bile or in the urine.

The glutathione transferases, the family of enzymes that catalyzes the initial step, are widely distributed, being found in essentially all groups of living organisms. Although the best known examples have been described from the

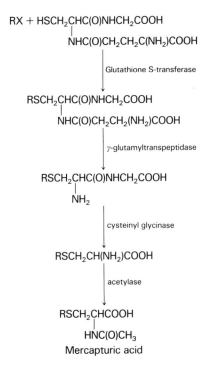

FIGURE 3.19.
Glutathione transferase reaction and formation of mercapturic acids.

soluble fraction of mammalian liver, these enzymes have also been demonstrated in microsomes. All forms appear to be highly specific with respect to glutathione but nonspecific with respect to the xenobiotic substrate, although the relative rates for different substrates can vary widely from one form to another.

The types of reactions catalyzed include the following: alkyltransferase; aryltransferase; aralkyltransferase; alkenetransferase; epoxidetransferase. Examples are shown in Figure 3.20.

The presence of multiple forms of glutathione transferase has been demonstrated in the liver of rat, mouse, and humans; multiple forms also occur in insects. Seven forms have been purified from rat liver and five from human liver. These enzymes have molecular weights in the range of 45,000–50,000 daltons and consist of two subunits. All forms appear to be nonspecific with respect to the reaction types described, although the kinetic constants for particular substrates vary from one form to another. They are usually identified and named from their chromatographic behavior. One of them, form B, appears to be identical to the binding protein, ligandin.

γ-Glutamyltranspeptidase is a membrane-bound glycoprotein that has been purified from the kidney of several other species as well as from human and rat liver. Molecular weights for the kidney enzyme are in the range of 68,000–90,000 daltons, and the enzyme appears to consist of two unequal subunits; the different forms appear to differ in the degree of sialalylation. This enzyme,

a. Aryl transferase

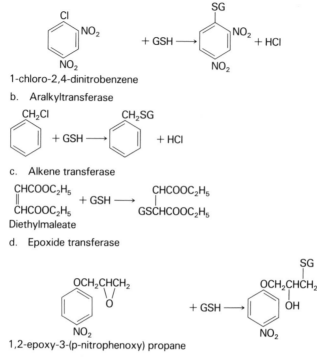

1-chloro-2,4-dinitrobenzene

b. Aralkyltransferase

c. Alkene transferase

Diethylmaleate

d. Epoxide transferase

1,2-epoxy-3-(p-nitrophenoxy) propane

e. Sulfate ester transferase

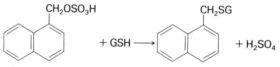

Menaphthyl sulfate

FIGURE 3.20.
Examples of glutathione transferase reactions.

which exhibits wide specificity toward γ-glutamyl peptides and has a number of acceptor amino acids, catalyzes three types of reaction.

Hydrolysis. γ-Glu-X + H$_2$O $\longrightarrow$ Glu + HX

Transpeptidation. γ-Glu-X + Acceptor $\longrightarrow$ γ-Glu-Acceptor + HX

γ-Glu-X + γ-Glu-X $\longrightarrow$ γ-Glu-γ-Glu-X + HX

Aminopeptidases that catalyze the hydrolysis of cysteinyl peptides are known. The membrane-bound aminopeptidases are glycoproteins, usually with molecular weights of about 100,000 daltons. They appear to be metalloproteins, one of the better known being a zinc-containing enzyme. Other enzymes, such as the leucine aminopeptidase, are cytosolic but, at least in this case, are also zinc-containing. The substrate specificity of these enzymes varies, but most are relatively nonspecific.

Little is known of the *N*-acetyltransferase(s) responsible for the acetylation of *S*-substituted cysteine. It is found in the microsomes of kidney and liver, however, and is specific for acetyl CoA as the acetyl donor. It is distinguished from other *N*-acetyltransferases by its substrate specificity and subcellular location.

3.3.5 Cysteine Conjugate *β*-Lyase

As indicated in Section 3.3.3.3, this enzyme uses cysteine conjugates as substrates, releasing the thiol of the xenobiotic, pyruvic acid, and ammonia, with subsequent methylation giving rise to the methylthio derivative. The enzyme from the cytosolic fraction of rat liver is a pyridoxal phosphate requiring protein of about 175,000 daltons. Cysteine conjugates of aromatic compounds are the best substrates and it is necessary for the cysteine amino and carboxyl groups to be unsubstituted for enzyme activity.

3.3.6 Acylation

Acylation reactions are of two general types, the first involving an activated conjugation agent, CoA, and the second involving activation of the foreign compounds and subsequent acylation of an amino acid. This type of conjugation is commonly undergone by exogenous carboxylic acids and amides and, although the products are often less water soluble than the parent compound, they are usually less toxic.

Examples of the reactions mentioned in Section 3.3.6 are shown in Figure 3.21.

a.   Acetylation

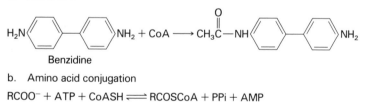

Benzidine

b.   Amino acid conjugation

$$RCOO^- + ATP + CoASH \rightleftharpoons RCOSCoA + PPi + AMP$$

$$RCOSCoA + R^1NH_2 \xrightarrow{CoA} CoASH + RCONHR^1$$

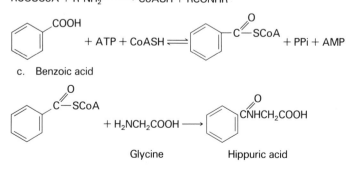

c.   Benzoic acid

Glycine   Hippuric acid

FIGURE 3.21.
Examples of acylation reactions.

3.3.6.1 Acetylation

Acetylated derivatives of foreign exogenous amines are acetylated by *N*-acetyl transferase, the acetyl donor being CoA. This enzyme is cytosolic, has been purified from rat liver, and is known to occur in several other organs. Evidence exists for the existence of multiple forms of the enzyme. Although endogenous amino, hydroxy, and thiol compounds are acetylated in vivo, the acetylation of exogenous hydroxy and thiol groups is presently unknown.

Acetylation of foreign compounds is influenced by both development and genetics. Newborn mammals generally have a low level of the transferase whereas, due to the different genes involved, fast and slow acetylators can be identified in both rabbit and human populations. Slow acetylators are more susceptible to the effects of compounds detoxified by acetylation.

3.3.6.2 *N,O*-Acyltransferase

This enzyme is believed to be involved in the carcinogenicity of arylamines. These compounds are first *N*-oxidized and then, in species capable of their *N*-acetylation, acetylated to arylhydroxamic acids. The effect of *N,O*-transacetylation is shown in Figure 3.22. The *N*-acyl group of the hydroxamic acid is first removed and is then transferred, either to an amine to yield a stable amide, or to the oxygen of the hydroxylamine to yield a reactive *N*-acyloxyarylamine. These compounds are highly reactive in the formation of adducts with both proteins and nucleic acids, and *N,O*-acyltransferase, added to the medium in the Ames test, increases the mutagenicity of compounds such as *N*-hydroxy-2-acetylaminofluorene. Despite its great instability, this enzyme has been purified from the cytosolic fraction of rat liver.

3.3.6.3 Amino Acid Conjugation

In the second type of acylation reaction, exogenous carboxylic acids are activated to form *S*-CoA derivatives in a reaction involving ATP and CoA. These CoA derivatives then acylate the amino group of a variety of amino acids.

Glycine and glutamate appear to be the most common acceptor of amino acids in mammals; in other organisms, other amino acids are involved. These include ornithine in reptiles and birds and taurine in fish.

The activating enzyme occurs in the mitochondria and belongs to a class of

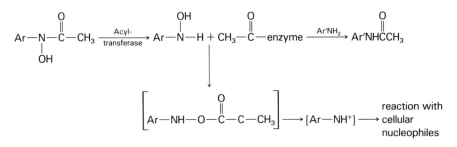

FIGURE 3.22.
N,O-Acyltransferase, reactions of arylhydroxamic acid. Ar, aryl group.

enzymes known as the ATP-dependent acid:CoA ligases (AMP), but has also been known as acyl CoA synthetase and acid-activating enzyme. It appears to be identical to the intermediate chain length fatty acyl-CoA synthetase.

Two acyl-CoA:amino acid N-acyltransferases have been purified from liver mitochondria of cattle, Rhesus monkey, and humans. One is a benzoyltransferase that utilizes benzoyl-CoA, isovaleryl-CoA, and tiglyl-CoA, but not phenylacetyl-CoA, malonyl-CoA, or indoleacetyl CoA. The other is a phenylacetyl transferase that utilizes phenylacetyl-CoA and indoleacetyl-CoA but is inactive toward benzoyl CoA. Neither is specific for glycine, as had been supposed from studies using less defined systems; both also utilize asparagine and glutamine, although at lower rates than glycine.

Bile acids are also conjugated by a similar sequence of reactions involving a microsomal bile acid:CoA ligase and a soluble bile acid-CoA amino acid N-acyltransferase. The latter has been extensively purified, and differences in acceptor amino acids, of which taurine is the most common, have been related to the evolutionary history of the species.

3.3.6.4 Deacetylation

Deacetylation occurs in a number of species, but there is a large difference between species, strains, and individuals in the extent to which the reaction occurs. Because acetylation and deacetylation are catalyzed by different enzymes, the levels of which vary independently in different species, the importance of acetylation as a xenobiotic metabolizing mechanism also varies between species. This can be seen in a comparison of the rabbit and the dog. The former, which has high acetyltransferase activity and low deacetylase, excretes significant amounts of acetylated amines. The dog, in which the opposite situation obtains, does not.

A typical substrate for the aromatic deacetylase of the liver and kidney is acetanilide, which is deacetylated to yield aniline.

3.3.7 Phosphate Conjugation

Phosphorylation of xenobiotics is not a widely distributed conjugation reaction, insects being the only major group of animals in which it is found. The enzyme from the gut of cockroaches utilizes ATP, requires Mg^+, and is active in the phosphorylation of 1-naphthol and p-nitrophenol.

3.4 SUGGESTED FURTHER READING

Arias, I.M., Jakoby, W.B. (eds.) Glutathione: Metabolism and Function. New York: Raven Press, 1976.

Bend, J.R., Hook, G.E.R. Hepatic and extrahepatic mixed function oxidases. In Lee, D.H.K., Falk, H.L., Murphy, S.D. (eds.). Handbook of Physiology, Section 9, Reactions to Environmental Agents. Bethesda, Md.: American Physiological Society, 1977.

Brodie, B.B., Gillette, J.R., Ackerman, H.S. (eds.). Handbook of Experimental Pharmacology, Vol. 28, Part 2, Concepts in Biochemical Pharmacology. Berlin: Springer, 1971.

Coon, M.J., Conney, A.H., Estabrook, R.W., Gelboin, H.V., Gillette, J.R., O'Brien, P.J. (eds.). Microsomes, Drug Oxidations and Chemical Carcinogenesis. 2 vols. New York: Academic Press, 1980.

Estabrook, R.W., Gillette, J.R., Leibman, K.C. (eds.). Microsomes and Drug Oxidations (Proceedings of the Second International Symposium). Baltimore: Williams & Wilkins, 1972.

Eling, T., Boyd, J., Reed, G., Mason, R., Sivarajoh, K. Xenobiotic metabolism by prostaglandin endoperoxide synthetase. Drug Metab. Rev. 1983; 14:1023.

Goldstein, A., Aronow, L., Kalman, S.M. Principles of Drug Action: The Basis of Pharmacology, Second Edition. New York: Wiley, 1974.

Hodgson, E., Guthrie, F.E. (eds.). Introduction to Biochemical Toxicology. New York: Elsevier, 1980.

Jakoby, W.B. (ed.). Enzymatic Basis of Detoxication, 2 vols. New York: Academic Press, 1980. These volumes contain many chapters of particular importance to this chapter.

Jakoby, W.B., Bend, J.R., Caldwell, J. Metabolic Basis of Detoxication. New York: Academic Press, 1980.

Jallow, D.R., Locsis, J.J., Snyder, R., Vainio, H. (eds.). Biological Reactive Intermediates: Formation, Toxicity and Inactivation. New York: Plenum Press, 1977.

Jenner, P., Testa, B. Novel pathways in drug metabolism. Xenobiotica, 1978; 8:1.

Jerina, D.M. (ed.). Drug Metabolism Concepts. New York: American Chemical Society Symposium Series 44, 1977. This symposium contains the following articles of particular relevance to this chapter.

Coon, M.J., Vermilion, J.L., Vatsii, K.P., et al. Biochemical studies on drug metabolism: Isolation of multiple forms of liver microsomal cytochrome P-450, p. 46.

Estabrook, R.W., Werringloer, J. Cytochrome P-450—Its role in oxygen activation for drug metabolism, p. 1.

Johnson, E.J., Muller-Eberhard, U. Resolution of multiple forms of rabbit liver cytochrome P-450, p. 72.

Moore, P.D., Koreeda, M., Wislocki, P.G. *In vitro* reactions of the diastereomeric 9,10-epoxides of (+) and (−)-trans-7,8-dihydroxy-7,8 dihydrobenzo(a)pyrene with polyguanylic acid and evidence for formation of an enantiomer of each diastereomeric 9,10-epoxide from benzo(a)pyrene in mouse skin, p. 127.

Kulkarni, A.P., Hodgson, E. Metabolism of insecticides by mixed function oxidase systems. Pharmacol. Ther. 1980; 8:379.

Lee, A.Y.H., Levin, W. The resolution and reconstitution of the liver microsomal hydroxylation system. Biochem. Biophys. Acta 1974; 344:205.

Lu, A.Y.H., West, S.B. Multiplicity of mammalian microsomal cytochrome P-450. Pharmacol. Rev. 1980; 31:277.

Parke, D.V. The Biochemistry of Foreign Compounds. London: Pergamon Press, 1968.

Snyder, R., Parke, D.V., Kocsis, J.J., Jallow, D.J., Gibson, C.G. and Witner, C.M. (eds.). Biological Reactive Intermediate II, Parts A & B. New York: Plenum Press, 1982.

Timbrell, J.A. Principles of Biochemical Toxicology. London: Taylor & Francis, 1982.

Wilkinson, C.F. (ed.). Insecticide Biochemistry and Physiology. Chapter 15. New York: Plenum Press, 1976.

Williams, R.T. Interspecies variations in the metabolism of xenobiotics. Biochem. Soc. Trans. 1974; 2:359.

chapter four

MODIFICATION OF METABOLISM

Ernest Hodgson

4.1 INTRODUCTION

Both the metabolism of toxicants and overall toxicity can be modified by many factors, both extrinsic and intrinsic to the normal functioning of the organism. It is entirely possible that many changes in toxicity are due to changes in metabolism, since most sequences of events that lead to overt toxicity involve activation and/or detoxication of the parent compound. In many cases, the chain of cause and effect is not entirely clear, due to the difficulty of relating single events, measured in vitro, to the complex and interrelated effects that occur in vivo. This relationship between in vitro and in vivo studies is important and is discussed in connection with enzymatic inhibition and induction (see Section 4.5). It is important to note that the chemical, nutritional, physiological, and other effects noted herein have been described primarily from experiments carried out on experimental animals. They indicate that similar effects may occur in humans or other animals, but not that they must occur, or that they occur at the same magnitude if they do.

4.2 NUTRITIONAL EFFECTS

Many nutritional effects on xenobiotic metabolism have been noted, but the information is scattered and often appears contradictory. This is one of the most important of several neglected areas of toxicology. This section is concerned only with the effects of nutritional constituents of the diet; the effects of other xenobiotics in the diet are discussed under chemical effects (see Section 3.4.4).

4.2.1 Protein

Low protein diets generally decrease monooxygenase activity in rat liver microsomes, and sex and substrate differences may be seen in the effect. For example, aminopyrine N-demethylation, hexobarbital hydroxylation, and aniline hydroxylation are all decreased, but the effect on the first two is greater in males than in females. In the third case, aniline hydroxylation, the reduction in males is equal to that in females. Tissue differences may also be seen. These changes are presumably related to the reductions in the levels of cytochrome P-450 and NADPH-cytochrome P-450 reductase that are also noted. One might speculate that the sex and other variations are due to differential effects on cytochrome P-450 isozymes. Even though enzyme levels are reduced by low protein diets, they can still be induced to some extent by compounds such as phenobarbital.

Such changes may also be reflected in changes in toxicity. Changes in the level of azoreductase activity in rat liver brought about by a low protein diet is reflected in an increased severity in the carcinogenic effect of dimethylaminoazobenzene. The liver carcinogen, dimethylnitrosamine, which must be activated metabolically, is almost without effect in protein-deficient rats. Strychnine, which is detoxified by microsomal monooxygenase action, is more toxic to animals on low protein diets, whereas octamethylpyrophosphoramide, carbon tetrachloride, and heptachlor, which are activated, are less toxic.

Phase-two reactions may also be affected by dietary protein levels. Chloramphenicol glucuronidation is reduced in protein-deficient guinea pigs, although no effect is seen on sulfotransferase activity in protein-deficient rats.

4.2.2 Carbohydrates

High dietary carbohydrate levels in the rat tend to have much the same effect as low dietary protein, decreasing such activities as aminopyrine N-demethylase, pentobarbital hydroxylation, and p-nitrobenzoic acid reduction along with a concomitant decrease in the enzymes of the cytochrome P-450-dependent monooxygenase system. Because rats tend to regulate total caloric intake, this may actually reflect low protein intake.

4.2.3 Lipids

Dietary deficiencies in linoleic or in other unsaturated fats generally bring about a reduction in cytochrome P-450 and related monooxygenase activities in the rat. The increase in effectiveness of breast and colon carcinogens brought about in animals on high fat diets, however, appears to be related to events during the promotion phase rather than the activation of the causative chemical. Lipids also appear to be necessary for the effect of inducers, such as phenobarbital, to be fully expressed.

4.2.4 Micronutrients

Vitamin deficiencies in general bring about a reduction in monooxygenase activity, although exceptions can be noted. Riboflavin deficiency causes an increase in cytochrome P-450 and aniline hydroxylation, although at the same time it causes a decrease in NADPH-cytochrome P-450 reductase and benzo(a)pyrene hydroxylation. Ascorbic acid deficiency in the guinea pig not only causes a decrease in cytochrome P-450 and monooxygenase activity but also causes a reduction in microsomal hydrolysis of procaine. Deficiencies in vitamins A and E cause a decrease in monooxygenase activity, whereas thiamine deficiency causes an increase. The effect of these vitamins on different cytochrome P-450 isozymes has not been investigated.

Changes in mineral nutrition have also been observed to affect monooxygenase activity. In the immature rat, calcium or magnesium deficiency causes a decrease whereas, quite unexpectedly, iron deficiency causes an increase. This increase is not accompanied by a concomitant increase in cytochrome P-450, however. An excess of dietary cobalt, cadmium, manganese, and lead all cause an increase in hepatic glutathione levels and a decrease in cytochrome P-450 content.

4.2.5 Starvation and Dehydration

Although in some animals starvation appears to have effects similar to those of protein deficiency, this is not necessarily the case. For example, in the mouse, monooxygenation is decreased but reduction of p-nitrobenzoic acid is unaffected. In male rats, hexobarbital and pentabarbital hydroxylation as well as aminopyrine N-demethylation are decreased, but aniline hydroxylation is increased. All of these activities are stimulated in the female. Water deprivation in gerbils causes an increase in cytochrome P-450 and a concomitant increase in hexobarbital metabolism, which is reflected in a shorter sleeping time.

4.3 PHYSIOLOGICAL EFFECTS

4.3.1 Development

Birth, in mammals, initiates an increase in the activity of many hepatic enzymes, including those involved in xenobiotic metabolism. The ability of the liver to carry out monooxygenation reactions appears to be very low during gestation and to increase after birth, with no obvious differences being seen between immature males and females. This general trend has been observed in many species, although the developmental pattern may vary according to the sex and genetic strain involved. The component enzymes of the cytochrome P-450–dependent monooxygenase system both follow the same general trend although there may be differences in the rate of increase. In the rabbit, the postnatal increase in cytochrome P-450 and its reductase is parallel; in the rat, the increase in the reductase is slower than that of the cytochrome.

Phase-two reactions may also be age dependent. Glucuronidation of many substrates is low or undetectable in fetal tissues but increases with age. The inability of newborn mammals of many species to form glucuronides is associated with deficiencies in both glucuronosyltransferase and its cofactor, uridine diphosphate glucoronic acid (UDPGA). A combination of this deficiency, as well as slow excretion of the bilirubin conjugate formed, and the presence in the blood of pregnanediol, an inhibitor of glucuronidation, may lead to neonatal jaundice.

Glycine conjugations are also low in the newborn, due to a lack of available glycine, an amino acid that reaches normal levels at about 30 days of age in the rat and 8 weeks in the human. Glutathione conjugation may also be impaired, as in fetal and neonatal guinea pigs, due to a deficiency of available glutathione. In the serum and liver of perinatal rats, glutathione transferase is barely detectable, increasing rapidly until adult levels are reached at about 140 days (Figure 4.1). This pattern is not followed in all cases, since sulfate conjugation and acetylation appear to be fully functional and at adult levels in the guinea pig fetus. Thus, some compounds that are glucuronidated in the adult can be acetylated or conjugated as sulfates in the young.

The effect of senescence on the metabolism of xenobiotics has not been studied extensively. In rats, monooxygenase activity, which reaches a maximum at about 30 days of age, begins to decline some 250 days later, a decrease that may be associated with reduced levels of sex hormones. Glucuronidation also decreases in old animals, whereas monoamine oxidase activity increases.

These changes in the ability to metabolize xenobiotics are often reflected in changes in overall toxicity. The sleeping time for hexobarbital, which is detoxified by microsomal monooxygenase action, may be greatly extended in the newborn whereas the hepatotoxicity of paracetamol, which is activated by the same enzymes, is much lower in the newborn than in adults.

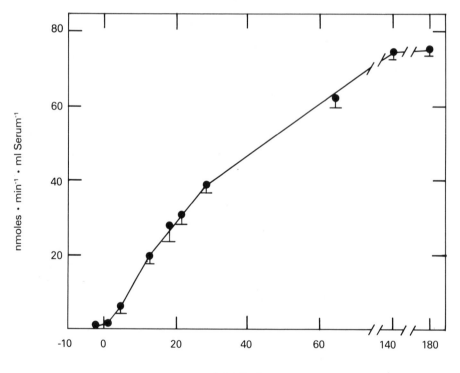

FIGURE 4.1.
Developmental pattern of serum glutathione *S*-transferase activity in female rats.
Source: Mukhtar and Bend. Life Sci. 1977; 21:1277. Used by permission.

4.3.2 Sex Differences

Metabolism of xenobiotics may vary with the sex of the organism. Sex differences become apparent at puberty and are usually maintained throughout adult life. Adult male rats metabolize many compounds at rates higher than females, eg, hexobarbital hydroxylation, aminopyrine N-demethylation, glucuronidation of o-aminophenol and glutathione conjugation of aryl substrates; with substrates such as aniline and zoxazolamine, however no sex differences are seen. In other species, including humans, the sex difference in xenobiotic metabolism is less pronounced.

The differences in microsomal monooxygenase activity between males and females have been shown to be under the control of sex hormones, at least in some species. Some enzyme activities are decreased by castration in the male, and administration of androgens to castrated males increases the activity of these sex-dependent enzyme activities without affecting the independent ones. Procaine hydrolysis is faster in male than female rats, and this compound is less toxic to the male.

Sex differences in enzyme activity may also vary from tissue to tissue. Hepatic microsomes from adult male guinea pigs are less active in the conjugation of p-nitrophenol than those from females, but no such sex difference is seen in the microsomes from lung, kidney, and small intestines.

Many differences in overall toxicity between males and females of various species are known (Table 4.1). Although it is not always known whether metabolism is the only or even the most important factor, such differences may be related to sex-related differences in metabolism. Hexobarbital is metabolized faster by male rats; thus, female rats have longer sleeping times. Parathion is activated to the cholinesterase inhibitor, paraoxon, more rapidly by female than male rats, and is thus more toxic to females.

Presumably many of the sex-related differences, as with developmental differences, are related to quantitative or qualitative differences in the isozymes of

TABLE 4.1
Sex-Related Differences in Toxicity

Species	Toxicant	Susceptibility
Rat	EPN	F > M
	Warfarin	F > M
	Strychnine	F > M
	Hexobarbital	F > M
	Parathion	F > M
	Aldrin	M > F
	Lead	M > F
	Epinephrine	M > F
	Ergot alkaloids	M > F
Cat	Dinitrophenol	F > M
Rabbit	Benzene	F > M
Mouse	Folic acid	F > M
	Nicotine	M > F
Dog	Digitoxin	M > F

those xenobiotic-metabolizing enzymes known to exist in multiple forms, but this aspect has not been extensively investigated.

4.3.3 Hormones

Hormones other than sex hormones are also known to affect the levels of xenobiotic metabolizing enzymes, but these effects are much less studied or understood.

4.3.3.1 Thyroid Hormone

Treatment of rats with thyroxin increases hepatic microsomal NADPH oxidation in both male and female rats, but the increase is greater in the female. Cytochrome P-450 content decreases in the male but not in the female. Hyperthyroidism causes a decrease in the sex-dependent monooxygenase reactions and appears to interfere with the ability of androgens to increase the activity of the enzymes responsible. Sex differences are not seen in the response of mice and rabbits to thyroxine. In the former, aminopyrine N-demethylase, aniline hydroxylase and hexobarbital hydroxylase are decreased, whereas p-nitrobenzoic reduction is unchanged. In the latter, hexobarbital hydroxylation is unchanged, whereas aniline hydroxylation and p-nitrobenzoic acid reduction increase.

Thyroid hormone can also affect enzymes other than microsomal monooxygenases. For example, liver monoamine oxidase activity is decreased whereas the activity of the same enzymes in the kidney is increased.

4.3.3.2 Adrenal Hormones

Removal of adrenal glands from male rats results in a decrease in the activity of hepatic microsomal enzymes, impairing the metabolism of aminopyrine and hexobarbital, but the same operation in females has no effect on their metabolism. Cortisone or prednisolone restores activity to normal levels.

4.3.3.3 Insulin

The effect of diabetes on xenobiotic metabolism is quite varied and, in this regard, alloxan-induced diabetes may not be a good model for the natural disease. The in vitro metabolism of hexobarbital and aminopyrine is decreased in alloxan-diabetic male rats, but is increased in similarly treated females. Aniline hydroxylase is increased in both males and females with alloxan diabetes. Studies of activity of the enzymes mentioned show no sex differences in the mouse; both sexes show an increase.

Some phase-two reactions, such as glucuronidation, are decreased in diabetic animals. This appears to be due to a lack of UDPGA caused by a decrease in UDPG dehydrogenase, rather than a decrease in transferase activity, and the effect can be reversed by insulin.

4.3.3.4 Other Hormones

Pituitary hormones regulate the function of many other endocrine glands and hypophysectomy in male rats results in a decrease in the activity of xenobiotic metabolizing enzymes. Administration of adrenocorticotropic hormone (ACTH) also results in a decrease of those oxidative enzyme activities that are sex dependent. In contrast, ACTH treatment of female rats causes in increase in aminopyrine *N*-demethylase but no change in other activities.

4.3.4 Pregnancy

Many xenobiotic metabolizing enzyme activities decrease during pregnancy. Catechol *O*-methyltransferase and monoamine oxidase decrease, as does glucuronide conjugation. The latter may be related to the increasing levels of progesterone and pregnanediol, both known to be inhibitors of glucuronosyltransferase in vitro. A similar effect on sulfate conjugation has been seen in pregnant rats and guinea pigs.

In some species, liver microsomal monooxygenase activity may also decrease during pregnancy, this decrease being accompanied by a concomitant decrease in cytochrome P-450 levels.

4.3.5 Disease

Quantitatively, the most important site for xenobiotic metabolism is the liver; thus, effects on the liver are likely to have a pronounced effect on the organism's overall capacity in this regard. At the same time, effects on other organs can have consequences no less serious for the organism. Patients with acute hepatitis frequently have an impaired ability to oxidize drugs, with a concomitant increase in plasma half-life. Impaired oxidative metabolism has also been shown in patients with chronic hepatitis or cirrhosis. The decrease in drug metabolism that occurs in obstructive jaundice may be a consequence of the accumulation of bile salts, which are known inhibitors of some of the enzymes involved.

Phase-two reactions may also be affected, decreases in acetylation, glucuronidation, and a variety of esterase activities having been seen in various liver diseases. Hepatic tumors, in general, have a lower ability to metabolize foreign compounds than does normal liver tissue, although in some cases the overall activity of tumor-bearing livers may be no lower than that of controls.

Kidney diseases may also affect the overall ability to handle xenobiotics, since this organ is one of the main routes for elimination of xenobiotics and their metabolites. The half-lives of tolbutamide, thiopental, hexobarbital, and chloramphenicol are all prolonged in patients with renal impairment.

4.3.6 Diural Rhythms

Diurnal rhythms, both in cytochrome P-450 levels and in the susceptibility to toxicants, have been described, especially in rodents. Although such changes appear to be related to the light cycle, they may, in fact, be activity dependent since feeding and other activities in rodents are themselves markedly diurnal.

4.4 COMPARATIVE AND GENETIC EFFECTS

Comparative toxicology is the study of the variation in toxicity of exogenous chemicals toward different organisms, either of different genetic strains or of different taxonomic groups. Thus, the comparative approach can be used in the study of any aspect of toxicology, such as absorption, metabolism, mode of action, and acute or chronic effects. Most comparative data exist in two areas, however—acute toxicity and the metabolism of toxic compounds. The value of the comparative approach can be summarized under four headings:

SELECTIVE TOXICITY.   If toxic compounds are to be used for controlling disease, pests, and parasites, it is important to develop selective biocides, toxic to the target organism but less toxic to other organisms, particularly humans.

EXPERIMENTAL MODELS.   Comparative studies of toxic phenomena are necessary to select the most appropriate model for extrapolation to humans and for testing and development of drugs and biocides. Taxonomic proximity does not necessarily indicate which will be the best experimental animal, since in some cases primates are less valuable for study than are other mammals.

ENVIRONMENTAL XENOBIOTIC CYCLES.   Much concern over toxic compounds springs from their occurrence in the environment. Different organisms in the complex ecological foodwebs metabolize compounds at different rates and to different products; the metabolic end-products are released back to the environment, either to be further metabolized by other organisms or to exert toxic effects of their own. Clearly, it is desirable to know the range of metabolic processes possible. Laboratory microecosystems have been developed, and with the aid of ^{14}C-labeled compounds, chemicals and their metabolites can be followed through the plants and terrestrial and aquatic animals involved. R.L. Metcalf of the University of Illinois pioneered this approach and has been one of its most successful practitioners.

COMPARATIVE BIOCHEMISTRY.   Some researchers believe that the proper role of comparative biochemistry is to put evolution on a molecular basis, and that detoxication enzymes, like other enzymes, are suitable subjects for study. Xenobiotic-metabolizing enzymes were probably essential in the early stages of animal evolution, since secondary plant products, even those of low toxicity, are frequently lipophilic and as a consequence would, in the absence of such enzymes, accumulate in lipid membranes and lipid depots.

4.4.1 Variations Among Taxonomic Groups

There are few differences in xenobiotic metabolism that are specific for large taxonomic groups. The formation of glucosides by insects and plants rather than the glucuronides of other animal groups is one of the most distinct. Although differences between species are common and of toxicological significance, they are usually quantitative rather than qualitative in nature and tend to occur within as well as between taxonomic groups. Although the ultimate explanation of such differences must be at the level of biochemical genetics, they are manifested at many other levels, the most important of which are summarized in the following sections.

4.4.1.1 In Vivo Toxicity

Toxicity is a term used to describe the adverse effects of chemicals on living organisms. Depending on the degree of toxicity, an animal may die or suffer injury to certain organs or have a specific functional derangement in a subcellular organelle. Sublethal effects of toxicants may be reversible.

Available data on the toxicity of selected pesticides to rats suggest that herbicide use, in general, provides the greatest human safety factor by selectively killing plants. Because the evolutionary position of the target species approaches that of humans, however, the human safety factor is narrowed considerably. Thus, as far as direct toxicity to humans and other mammals is concerned, biocide toxicity seems to be in the following progression:

herbicides = fungicides < molluscicides < acaricides < nematocides
< insecticides < rodenticides.

This relationship is obviously oversimplified, since marked differences in lethality are observed when different members of each group of biocides is tested against laboratory test animals and target species. One should also bear in mind that any chemical can be environmentally dangerous if misused since many possible targets are interrelated in complex ecological systems.

Interspecific differences are also known for some naturally occurring poisons. Nicotine, for instance, is used as an insecticide and kills many insect pests at low doses, yet tobacco leaves constitute a normal diet for several species. As indicated earlier, most strains of rabbit eat *Belladonna* leaves without ill effects, whereas other mammals are easily poisoned. Natural tolerance to HCN poisoning in millipedes and the high resistance to the powerful axonal blocking agent tetrodotoxin in puffer fish are examples of the tolerance of animals to the toxins they produce.

The specific organ toxicity of chemicals also exhibits wide species differences. Carbon tetrachloride, a highly potent hepatotoxicant, induces liver damage in many species, but chickens are almost unaffected by it. Dinitrophenol causes cataracts in humans, ducks, and chickens, but not in other experimental animals. The eggshell thinning associated with DDT poisoning in birds is observed in falcons and mallard ducks, whereas this reproductive toxicity is not observed in gallinaceous species. Delayed neurotoxicity caused by organophosphates such as leptophos and tri-*o*-cresyl phosphate can be easily demonstrated in chickens, but can be produced only with difficulty in most common laboratory mammals.

4.4.1.2 In Vivo Metabolism

Many ecological and physiological factors affect the rates of penetration, distribution, biotransformation, and excretion of chemicals, and thus govern their biological fate in the body. In general, the absorption of xenobiotics, their tissue distribution, and penetration across the blood-brain barrier and other barriers are dictated by their physicochemical nature and, therefore, tend to be similar in various animal species. The biological effect of a chemical depends on the concentration of its active form and its duration inside the body; this is governed in turn by the rates of its biotransformation and excretion and the magnitude and nature of its binding to tissue macromolecules. Thus, substantial differences in these variables should confer species specificity in the biological response to any metabolically active xenobiotic.

The biological half-life is governed by the rates of metabolism and excretion and thus reflects the most important variables explaining interspecies differences in toxic response. Striking differences between species can be seen in the biological half-lives of various drugs. Humans, in general, metabolize xenobiotics more slowly than do various experimental animals. For example, phenylbutazone is metabolized slowly in humans, with a half-life averaging three days. In the monkey, rat, guinea pig, rabbit, dog, and horse, however, this drug is metabolized readily, with half-lives ranging between three and six hours.

The interdependence of metabolic rate, half-life, and pharmacological action is well illustrated in the case of hexobarbital. The duration of sleeping time is directly related to the biological half-life and is inversely proportional to the in vitro degradation capacity of liver enzymes from the respective species. Thus, mice inactivate hexobarbital readily, as reflected in a brief biological half-life in vivo and short sleeping time, whereas the reverse is true in dogs.

Xenobiotics, once inside the body, undergo a series of biotransformations. Those reactions that introduce a new functional group into the molecule, either by oxidation, reduction, or hydrolysis, are designated phase-one reactions, whereas the conjugation reactions by which phase-one metabolites are combined with endogenous substrates in the body are referred to as phase-two reactions. Chemicals may undergo any one of these reactions or any combination of them, either simultaneously or consecutively. Because biotransformations are catalyzed by a large number of enzymes, it is to be expected that they will vary between species. Qualitative differences imply the occurrence of different enzymes, whereas quantitative differences imply variations in the rate of biotransformation along a common metabolic pathway, the variations resulting from differences in enzyme levels, in the extent of competing reactions, or in the efficiency of enzymes capable of reversing the reaction.

Even in the case of a xenobiotic undergoing oxidation primarily by a single reaction, there may be remarkable species differences in relative rates. Thus, in humans, rats, and guinea pigs, the major route of papaverine metabolism is O-demethylation to yield phenolic products, but very little of these products is formed in dogs.

Aromatic hydroxylation of aniline is another example. In this case, both *ortho* and *para* positions are susceptible to oxidative attack yielding the respective aminophenols. The biological fate of aniline has been studied in many species and striking selectivity in hydroxylation position has been noted (Table 4.2). These data show a trend, in that carnivores generally display a high aniline *ortho*-hydroxylase ability with a *para/ortho* ratio of ≤ 1, whereas rodents exhibit a striking preference for the *para* position, with a *para/ortho* ratio of from 2.5 to 15. Along with extensive p-aminophenol, substantial quantities of o-aminophenol are also produced from aniline administered to rabbits and hens. The major pathway is not always the same in any two animal species. 2-Acetylaminofluorene may be metabolized in mammals by two alternative routes, N-hydroxylation, yielding the carcinogenic N-hydroxy derivative, and aromatic hydroxylation, yielding the noncarcinogenic 7-hydroxy metabolite. The former is

TABLE 4.2
In Vivo Aromatic Hydroxylation of Aniline in Females of Various Animal Species

Class	Order	Species	Percent Dose Excreted as Aminophenol		Para/ortho Ratio
			Ortho	Para	
Mammalian	Carnivora	Dog	18.0	9.0	0.5
		Cat	32.0	14.0	0.4
		Ferret	26.0	28.0	1.0
	Rodentia	Rat	19.0	48.0	2.5
		Mouse	4.0	12.0	3.0
		Hamster	5.5	53.0	10.0
		Guinea pig	4.2	46.0	11.0
	Lagomorpha	Rabbit	8.8	50.0	6.0
Aves	Galliformes	Hen	10.5	44.0	4.0

Source: Reprinted by permission from Parke, D.V., Biochem. J. 77, p. 493, copyright © 1960 The Biochemical Society, London.

the metabolic route in the rat, rabbit, hamster, dog, and in humans in which the parent compound is known to be carcinogenic. In contrast, the monkey carries out aromatic hydroxylation and the guinea pig appears to deacetylate the *N*-hydroxy derivative; thus, both escape the carcinogenic effects.

The hydrolysis of esters by esterases and of amides by amidases constitutes one of the most common enzymatic reactions of xenobiotics in humans and other animal species. Because both the number of enzymes involved in hydrolytic attack and the number of substrates for them is large, it is not surprising to observe interspecific differences in the disposition of xenobiotics due to variations in these enzymes. The presence of a carboxylesterase in mammals that hydrolyzes malathion but is generally absent in insects explains the remarkable selectivity of this insecticide.

As with esters, wide differences exist between species in the rates of hydrolysis of various amides in vivo. Fluoracetamide is less toxic to mice than to the American cockroach. This is explained by the faster release of the toxic fluoroacetate in insects as compared with mice. The insecticide dimethoate is susceptible to the attack of both esterases and amidases, yielding nontoxic products. In the rat and mouse, both reactions occur, whereas sheep liver contains only the amidase and that of guinea pig only the esterase. The relative rates of these degradative enzymes in insects are very low as compared with those of mammals, however, and this correlates well with the high selectivity of dimethoate.

The various phase-two reactions are concerned with the conjugation of primary metabolites of xenobiotics produced by phase-one reactions. Factors that alter or govern the rates of phase-two reactions may play a role in interspecific differences in xenobiotic metabolism.

Xenobiotics, frequently in the form of conjugates, can be eliminated through urine, feces, lungs, sweat, saliva, milk, hair, nails, or placenta, although comparative data are generally available only for the first two routes. Interspecific variation in the pattern of biliary excretion may determine species differences in the relative extent to which compounds are eliminated in the urine or feces. Fecal excretion of a chemical or its metabolites tends to be higher in species that are good biliary excretors, such as the rat and dog, than in species that are poor biliary excretors, such as the rabbit, guinea pig, and monkey. For example, the fecal excretion of stilbestrol in the rat accounts for 75% of the dose, whereas in the rabbit about 70% can be found in the urine. Dogs, like humans, metabolize indomethacin to a glucuronide, but, unlike humans that excrete it in the urine, dogs excrete it primarily in the feces — apparently due to inefficient renal and hepatic blood clearance of the glucuronide. These differences may involve species variation in enterohepatic circulation, plasma levels, and biological half-life.

Interspecific differences in the magnitude of biliary excretion of a xenobiotic largely depend upon molecular weight, the presence of polar groups in the molecule, and the extent of conjugation. Conjugates with molecular weights of < 300 are poorly excreted in bile and tend to be excreted with urine, whereas the reverse is true for those with molecular weights > 300. The critical molecular weight appears to vary between species, and marked species differences are noted for biliary excretion of chemicals with molecular weights of about 300. Thus, the biliary excretion of succinylsulfathioazole is 20- to 30-fold greater in the rat and the dog than in the rabbit and the guinea pig, and > 100-fold greater than in the pig and the rhesus monkey. The cat and sheep are intermediate and excrete about 7% of the dose in the bile.

The evidence reported in a few studies suggests some relationship between the evolutionary position of a species and its conjugation mechanisms (Table 4.3). In humans and most mammals, the principal mechanisms involve conjugations with glucuronic acid, glycine, glutamine, and sulfate, mercapturic acid synthesis, acetylation, methylation, and thiocyanate synthesis. In some species of birds and reptiles, ornithine conjugation replaces that with glycine; in plants, bacteria, and insects, conjugation with glucose instead of glucuronic acid results in the formation of glucosides. In addition to these predominant reactions, certain other conjugative processes are found involving specific compounds in only a few species. These reactions include conjugation with phosphate, taurine, N-acetyl-glucosamine, ribose, glycyltaurine, serine, arginine, formic acid, and succinate. Certain species of spiders use glutamic acid and arginine for the conjugation of aromatic acids.

From the standpoint of evolution, similarity might be expected between humans and other primate species, as opposed to the nonprimates. This phylogenic relationship is obvious from the relative importance of glycine and glutamine in the conjugation of arylacetic acids. The conjugating agent in humans is exclusively glutamine, and the same is essentially true with Old World monkeys. New World monkeys, however, use both the glycine and glutamine pathways. Most nonprimates and lower primates selectively carry out glycine conjugation. A similar evolutionary trend is also observed in the N'-glucuronidation of sulfadimethoxine and in the aromatization of quinic acid; both reactions occur extensively in humans, and their importance decreases with increasing evolutionary divergence from humans. When the rela-

TABLE 4.3
Occurrence of Common and Unusual Conjugation Reactions

Conjugating Group	Common	Unusual
Carbohydrate	Glucuronic acid (animals) Glucose (insects and plants)	N-Acetylglucosamine (rabbit) Ribose (rats and mice)
Amino acids	Glycine Glutathione Methionine	Glutamine (insects and humans) Ornithine (birds) Arginine (ticks and spider) Glycyltaurine and glycylglycine (cat) Serine (rabbit)
Acetyl	Acetyl group from acetyl-CoA	
Formyl		Formylation (dog and rat)
Sulfate	Sulfate group from PAPS	
Phosphate		Phosphate monoester formation (dog and insects)

Source: Hodgson, E., Guthrie, F.E. Introduction to Biochemical Toxicology. New York: Elsevier, 1980.

tive importance of metabolic pathways is considered, one of the simplest cases of an enzyme-related species difference in the disposition of a substrate undergoing only one conjugative reaction is the acetylation of 4-aminohippuric acid. In the rat, guinea pig, and rabbit, the major biliary metabolite is 4-acetamido-hippuric acid; the cat excretes nearly equal amounts of free acid and its acetyl derivative; and the hen excretes mainly the unchanged compound. In the dog, 4-aminohippuric acid is also passed into the bile unchanged, since this species is unable to acetylate aromatic amino groups.

Defective operation of phase-two reactions usually causes a striking species difference in the disposition pattern of a xenobiotic. The origin of such species variations is usually either the absence or a low level of the enzyme(s) in question and/or its cofactors.

Glucuronide synthesis is one of the most common detoxication mechanisms in most mammalian species. The cat and closely related species have a defective glucuronide-forming system, however. Although cats form little or no glucuronide from *o*-aminophenol, phenol, *p*-nitrophenol, 2-amino-4-nitrophenol, 1- or 2-naphthol, and morphine, they readily form glucuronides from phenol-phthalein, bilirubin, thyroxine, and certain steroids. Recently, polymorphism of UDP glucuronyl-transferase has been demonstrated in rat and guinea pig liver preparations; thus, defective glucuronidation in the cat is probably related to the absence of the appropriate transferase rather than that of the active intermediate, UDPGA, which is known to occur in cat liver in normal concentrations. Insects are incapable of synthesizing glucuronide conjugates. This may be due to the lack of UDP glucuronyltransferase, UDPGA, or UDP glucose dehydrogenase, which converts UDP glucose into UDPGA.

Studies on the metabolic fate of phenol in several species have indicated that four urinary products are excreted (Figure 4.2). Although extensive phenol metabolism takes place in most species, the relative proportions of each metabolite produced varies from species to species. In contrast to the cat, which selectively forms sulfate conjugates, the pig excretes phenol exclusively as the glucuronide. This defect in sulfate conjugation in the pig is restricted to only a few substrates, however, and may be due to the lack of a specific phenyl sulfotransferase, since the formation of substantial amounts of the sulfate conjugate of 1-naphthol clearly indicates the occurrence of other forms of sulfotransferase.

Certain unusual conjugation mechanisms have been uncovered during comparative investigations, but this may be a reflection of inadequate data on other species. Future investigations may demonstrate a wider distribution.

A few species of birds and reptiles use ornithine for the conjugation of aromatic acids rather than glycine, as do mammals. For example, the turkey, goose, duck, and hen excrete ornithuric acid as the major metabolite of benzoic acid, whereas pigeons and doves excrete it exclusively as hippuric acid.

Taurine conjugation with bile acids, phenylacetic acid, and indolylacetic acid seems to be a minor process in most species, but in the pigeon and ferret it occurs extensively. Other infrequently reported conjugations include serine conjugation of xanthurenic acid in rats; excretion of quinaldic acid as quinaldylglycyltaurine and quinaldylglycylglycine in the urine of the cat, but not of the rat or rabbit; phosphate conjugation of 2-naphthylamine in the dog, but not in the rat or rabbit; and conversion of furfural to furylacrylic acid in the dog and rabbit, but not in the rat, hen, or human.

The dog and human but not the guinea pig, hamster, rabbit, or rat excrete the carcinogen 2-naphthyl hydroxylamine as a metabolite of 2-naphthylamine, which, as a result, has carcinogenic activity in the bladder of humans and dogs.

4.4.1.3 In Vitro Metabolism

Numerous variables simultaneously modulate the in vivo metabolism of xenobiotics; therefore, their relative importance cannot easily be studied. This problem is alleviated to some extent by in vitro studies of the underlying enzymatic mechanisms responsible for qualitative and quantitative species differences. Quantitative differences may be directly related to the absolute amount of active enzyme present and the affinity and specificity of the enzyme toward the substrate in question. Because many other factors alter enzymatic rates in vitro, caution must be exercised in interpreting data in terms of species variation. In particular, enzymes are often sensitive to the experimental conditions used in their preparation. Because this sensitivity varies from one enzyme to another, their relative effectiveness for a particular reaction can be somewhat miscalculated.

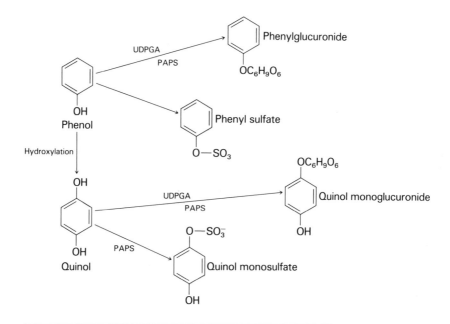

| | Percent of 24-Hr Excretion as | | | |
| Species | Glucuronide | | Sulfate | |
	Phenol	Quinol	Phenol	Quinol
Pig	100	0	0	0
Indian fruit bat	90	0	10	0
Rhesus monkey	35	0	65	0
Cat	0	0	87	13
Human	23	7	71	0
Squirrel monkey	70	19	10	0
Rat tail monkey	65	21	14	0
Guinea pig	78	5	17	0
Hamster	50	25	25	0
Rat	25	7	68	0
Ferret	41	0	32	28
Rabbit	46	0	45	9
Gerbil	15	0	69	15

FIGURE 4.2.
Species variation in the metabolic conversion of phenol in vivo.

Species variation in the oxidation of xenobiotics, in general, is quantitative (Table 4.4), whereas qualitative differences, such as the apparent total lack of parathion oxidation by lobster hepatopancreas microsomes, are seldom observed. Although the amount of cytochrome P-450 or the activity of NADPH-cytochrome P-450 reductase seems to be related to the oxidation of certain

TABLE 4.4
Species Variation in Microsomal Oxidation of Xenobiotics In Vitro

Substrate Oxidation	Rabbit	Rat	Mouse	Guinea Pig	Hamster	Chicken	Trout	Frog
Coumarin 7-hydroxylase (nmol/mg/h)	0.86	0.00	0.00	0.45	—	—	—	—
Biphenyl 4-hydroxylase (nmol/mg/min)	3.00	1.50	5.70	1.40	3.80	1.70	0.22	1.15
Biphenyl 2-hydroxylase (nmol/mg/min)	0.00	0.00	2.20	0.00	1.80	0.00	0.00	0.15
2-Methoxybiphenyl demethylase (nmol/mg liver/h)	5.20	1.80	3.40	2.20	2.30	2.00	0.60	0.40
4-Methoxybiphenyl demethylase (mnol/mg liver/h)	8.00	3.00	3.20	2.30	2.30	1.70	0.40	0.90
p-Nitroanisole O-demethylase (nmol/mg/15 min)	32.00	4.93	20.33	—	—	11.33	—	—
2-Ethoxybiphenyl deethylase (nmol/mg liver/h)	5.30	1.60	1.40	2.10	2.50	1.70	0.60	0.40
4-Ethoxybiphenyl deethylase (nmol/mg liver/h)	7.80	2.80	1.80	2.30	1.80	1.50	0.40	0.90
Ethylmorphine N-demethylase (nmol/mg/min)	4.00	11.60	13.20	5.40	—	—	—	—
Aldrin epoxidase (nmol/mg/min)	0.34	0.45	3.35	—	—	0.46	0.006	—
Parathion desulfurase (nmol/mg/min)	2.11	4.19	5.23	8.92	7.75	—	—	—

Source: Hodgson, E., Guthrie, F.E. Introduction to Biochemical Toxicology. New York: Elsevier, 1980.

substrates, this explanation is not always satisfactory since the absolute amount of cytochrome P-450 is not necessarily the rate-limiting characteristic.

Several lines of evidence indicate that there are multiple forms of microsomal cytochrome P-450 in each species, and that these forms differ from one species to another. This evidence includes both qualitative and quantitative species-related differences in the substrate difference spectra of microsomal cytochrome P-450. Difference spectra are presumed to be a direct reflection of enzyme–ligand complex formation. If the cytochromes P-450 of all animals were alike, similarity in spectral size and the ratio of type II/type I binding would be expected. A wide species variation is evident, however. Thus, in a closely related group of chlorinated hydrocarbons, DDT, dicofol, and DDD, DDT gives the smallest type I spectrum in all species tested; dicofol exhibits the largest type I difference spectrum with microsomes from sheep, rats, and Fchouseflies; and DDD exhibits the largest spectral response with microsomes from mice and rabbits. Several studies have failed to establish any relationship between spectral magnitude and substrate oxidation rate, however.

Reductive reactions, like oxidations, are carried out at different rates by enzyme preparations from different species. Microsomes from mammalian liver are ≤ 18 times higher in azoreductase activity and > 20 times higher in nitroreductase activity than those from fish liver. Although relatively inactive in nitroreductase, fish can reduce the nitro group of parathion, suggesting multiple forms of reductase enzymes.

Hydration of epoxides catalyzed by epoxide hydrolase is involved in both detoxication and intoxication reaction. With high concentrations of styrene oxide as a substrate, the relative activity of hepatic microsomal epoxide hydrolase in several animal species is rhesus monkey $>$ human $=$ guinea pig $>$ rabbit $>$ rat $>$ mouse. With some substrates, such as epoxidized lipids, the cytosolic hydrolase may be much more important than the microsomal enzyme.

Blood and various organs of humans and other animals contain esterases capable of acetylsalicylic acid hydrolysis. A comparative study has shown that the liver is the most active tissue in all animal species studied except for the guinea pig, in which the kidney is more than twice as active as the liver. Human liver is least active; the enzyme in guinea pig liver is the most active. The relatively low toxicity of some of the new synthetic pyrethroid insecticides appears to be related to the ability of mammals to hydrolyze their carboxyester linkages. Thus, mouse liver microsomes catalyzing (+)-*trans*-resmethrin hydrolysis are > 30-fold more active than insect microsomal preparations. The relative rates of hydrolysis of this substrate in enzyme preparations from various species are mouse $\gg$ milkweed bug $\gg$ cockroach $\gg$ cabbage looper $>$ housefly.

The toxicity of the organophosphorus insecticide dimethoate $[(CH_3O_2)_2P(S)SCH_2CONHCH_3]$ depends upon the rate at which it is hydrolyzed in vivo. This toxicant undergoes two main metabolic detoxication reactions, one catalyzed by an esterase and the other by an amidase. Although rat and mouse liver carry out both reactions, only the amidase occurs in sheep liver, and the esterase in guinea pig liver. The ability of liver preparations from different animal species to degrade dimethoate is as follows: rabbit $>$ sheep $>$ dog $>$ rat $>$ cattle $>$ hen $>$ guinea pig $>$ mouse $>$ pig, these rates being roughly inversely proportioned to the toxicity of dimethoate to the same species. Insects degrade this compound much more slowly than do mammals and hence are highly susceptible to dimethoate.

Hepatic microsomes of several animal species possess UDP glucuronyltransferase activity and, with *p*-nitrophenol as a substrate, a 12-fold difference in activity due to species variation is evident. Phospholipase-A activates the enzyme and results of activation experiments indicate that the amount of constraint on the activity of this enzyme is variable in different animal species.

Glutathione *S*-transferase in liver cytosol from different animal species also shows a wide variation in activity. Activity is very low in humans, whereas the mouse and guinea pig appear to be more efficient than other species. The ability of the guinea pig to form the initial glutathione conjugate contrasts with its inability to readily *N*-acetylate cysteine conjugates; consequently, mercapturic acid excretion is low in guinea pigs.

4.4.2 Selectivity

Selective toxic agents have been developed to protect crops, animals of economic importance, and humans from the vagaries of pests, parasites, and pathogens. Such selectivity is conferred primarily through distribution and comparative biochemistry.

Selectivity through differences in uptake permits the use of an agent toxic to both target and nontarget cells, provided that lethal concentrations accumulate only in target cells, leaving nontarget cells unharmed. An example is the accumulation of tetracycline by bacteria, but not by mammalian cells, the result being drastic inhibition of protein synthesis in the bacteria, leading to death.

Certain schistosome worms are parasitic in humans and their selective destruction by antimony is accounted for by the differential sensitivity of phosphofructokinase in the two species, the enzyme from schistosomes being more susceptible to inhibition by antimony than the mammalian enzyme.

Sometimes both target and nontarget species metabolize a xenobiotic by the same pathways but differences in rate determine selectivity. Malathion (Figure 1.2), a selective insecticide, is activated metabolically to the cholinesterase inhibitor, malaoxon. In addition to this activation reaction, several detoxicating reactions also occur. Carboxylesterase hydrolyzes malathion to form the monoacid, phosphatases hydrolyze the P—O—C linkages to yield nontoxic products, and glutathione *S*-alkyltransferase converts malathion to desmethylmalathion. Although all of these reactions occur both in insects and mammals and activation by oxidation desulfuration is rapid in both insects and mammals, hydrolysis is rapid in mammals but slow in insects. As a result, malaoxon accumulates in insects but not in mammals, resulting in selective toxicity.

A few examples are also available in which the lack of a specific enzyme in some cells in the human body has enabled the development of a therapeutic agent. For example, guanine deaminase is absent from the cells of certain cancers but is abundant in healthy tissue; as a result, 8-azaguanine can be used therapeutically.

Distinct differences in cells with regard to the presence or absence of target structures or metabolic processes also offer opportunities for selectivity. Herbicides such as phenylureas, simazine, etc., block the Hill reaction in chloroplasts and thereby kill plants without harm to animals. This is not always the case, since paraquat, which blocks photosynthetic reactions in plants, is a pulmonary toxicant in mammals, due apparently to analogous free-radical reactions (Section 6.3.4.3c) involving enzymes different from those involved in photosynthesis.

4.4.3 Genetic Differences

Just as the xenobiotic-metabolizing ability in different animal species seems to be related to evolutionary development and therefore to different genetic constitutions, different strains within a species may differ from one another in their ability to metabolize xenobiotics.

4.4.3.1 In Vivo Toxicity

The toxicity of organic compounds has been found to vary between different strains of laboratory animals. For example, mouse strain C_3H is resistant to histamine, the LD50 being 1,523 mg/kg in C_3H/Jax mice as compared with 230 in Swiss/ICR mice; ie, the animals of the former strain are 6.6 times less susceptible to the effects of histamine. Striking differences in the toxicity of thiourea, a compound used in the treatment of hyperthyroidism, are seen in different strains of the Norway rat. Harvard and wild Norway rats were 11 and 335 times more resistant, respectively, than rats of the Hopkins strain.

Genetic polymorphism is well known in the metabolism of drugs such as isoniazid. Such differences are related to the rate of acetylation of isoniazid and have a genetic basis. "Slow acetylators" are homozygous for a recessive gene; this is believed to lead to the lack of the hepatic enzyme acetyltransferase, which in normal homozygotes or heterozygotes (rapid acetylators) acetylates isoniazid as a step in the metabolism of this drug (Section 7.6.7 and Figure 7.12). This effect is also seen in humans, the gene for slow acetylation showing marked differences in distribution between different human populations. It is very low in Eskimos and Japanese, with 80–90% of these populations being rapid acetylators, whereas 40–60% of blacks and some European populations are rapid acetylators. Rapid acetylators often develop symptoms of hepatotoxicity and polyneuritis at the dosage necessary to maintain therapeutic blood levels of isoniazid.

The development of strains resistant to insecticides is an extremely widespread phenomenon that is known to have occurred in over 200 species of insects and mites and resistance of up to several hundred-fold has been noted. The different biochemical and genetic factors involved have been extensively studied and well characterized. Relatively few vertebrate species are known to have developed pesticide resistance. Susceptible and resistant strains of pine voles exhibit a 7.4-fold difference in endrin toxicity. Similarly, pine mice of a strain resistant to endrin were reported to be 12-fold more tolerant than a susceptible strain. Other examples include the occurrence of organochlorine insecticide-resistant and -susceptible strains of mosquito fish, and resistance to *Belladonna* in certain rabbit strains.

4.4.3.2 Metabolite Production

Strain variation in response to hexobarbital also depends on its degradation rate. For example, male mice of the AL/N strain are long sleepers, and this trait is correlated with slow inactivation of the drug. The reverse is true in CFW/N mice, which have a short sleeping time due to rapid hexobarbital oxidation. This close relationship is further evidenced by the fact that the level of brain hexobarbital at awakening is essentially the same in all strains. Similar strain differences have been reported for zoxazolamine paralysis in mice.

Studies on the induction of aryl hydrocarbon hydroxylase by 3-methylcholanthrene have revealed several responsive and nonresponsive mouse strains, and it is now well established that the induction of this enzyme is controlled by a single gene. In the accepted nomenclature, Ah^b represents the allele for responsiveness, whereas Ah^d denotes the allele for nonresponsiveness.

In rats, both age and sex seem to influence strain variation in xenobiotic metabolism. Male rats exhibit about twofold variation between strains in hexo-barbital metabolism, whereas female rats may display up to sixfold variation, depending on their age. As shown in Table 4.5, the ability to metabolize hexo-barbital is related to the metabolism of other substrates and the interstrain differences are maintained.

A well-known interstrain difference in phase-two reactions is that of glucu-ronidation in Gunn rats. This is a mutant strain of Wistar rats that is character-ized by a severe, genetically determined defect of bilirubin glucuronidation. Their ability to glucuronidate o-aminophenol, o-aminobenzoic acid, and a number of other substrates is also partially defective. This deficiency does not seem to be related to an inability to form UDPGA but rather to the lack of a specific UDP glucuronyltransferase. It has been demonstrated that Gunn rats can conjugate aniline by N-glucuronidation and can form the O-glucuronide of p-nitrophenol.

Rabbit strains may exhibit up to twentyfold variation, particularly in the case of hexobarbital, amphetamine, and aminopyrine metabolism. Relatively smaller differences between strains occur with chlorpromazine metabolism. Wild rabbits and California rabbits display the greatest differences from other rabbit strains in hepatic drug metabolism.

4.4.3.3 Enzyme Differences

The nature and amount of microsomal cytochrome P-450 have not been exten-sively studied in different strains of the same vertebrate. The only thorough investigations, those of the Ah locus, which controls aryl hydrocarbon hydrox-ylase induction, have shown that, in addition to quantitative differences in the amount of cytochrome P-450 after induction in the hepatic microsomes from different strains of mice, there is also a qualitative difference in the cytochrome induced.

The major difference in microsomal cytochrome P-450 between insecticide-

TABLE 4.5
Strain Variation in In Vitro Drug Metabolism in the Rat

Rat Strain	Hexobarbital Sleeping Time (min)	Substrate Metabolized (nmol/mg protein)			
		Hexobarbital	o-Nitroanisole	Aminopyrine	Acetanilide
Long-Evans	50	31.6	9.1	2.2	8.5
	26	41.5	11.1	3.6	10.0
Sprague-Dawley	55	30.0	6.6	1.1	8.8
	29	42.9	8.4	2.1	12.4
Buffalo	65	24.9	7.5	1.1	5.8
	32	36.4	8.9	2.0	7.4
Fischer	43	41.4	10.4	2.0	12.8
	19	47.9	12.2	2.9	16.6
Wistar	56	35.2	8.2	1.8	11.4
	30	44.6	10.2	3.0	15.4

Source: Mitoma et al. Proc. Soc. Exp. Biol. Med. 1967; 125:284. Used by permission.

resistant and insecticide-susceptible strains of the housefly are given in Table 4.6. A comparison of strains based on the size and peak location of the carbon monoxide, type I, type II, type III, *n*-octylamine, and ethyl isocyanide difference spectra reveal several points that provide strong evidence for both qualitative and quantitative differences between strains. Ligand interaction of > 100 other xenobiotics with cytochrome P-450 from resistant and susceptible housefly strains have been reported and lend strong support to the results given in Table 4.6.

Based on the data from crosses of houseflies of susceptible strains (with visible mutant markers) with those of resistant strains, it is apparent that at least four genes, three on chromosome II and one on chromosome V, are required to explain the spectral variants alone. Presumably, these genes are related to specific cytochrome P-450 isozymes, since such isozymes are known to occur in insects as they do in mammals.

4.5 CHEMICAL EFFECTS

With regard to both logistics and scientific philosophy, the study of the metabolism and toxicity of xenobiotics must be initiated by considering single compounds. Unfortunately, humans and other living organisms are not exposed in this way; rather, they are exposed to many xenobiotics simultaneously, involving different portals of entry, modes of action, and metabolic pathways. Some estimation of the number of chemicals in use in the United States are given in Table 4.7. Because it bears directly on the problem of toxicity-related interactions between different xenobiotics, the effect on chemicals on the metabolism of other exogenous compounds is one of the more important areas of biochemical toxicology.

Xenobiotics, in addition to serving as substrates for a number of enzymes, may also serve as inhibitors or inducers of these or other enzymes. Many examples are known of compounds that first inhibit and subsequently induce enzymes such as the microsomal monooxygenases. The situation is even further complicated by the fact that although some substances have an inherent toxicity and are detoxified in the body, others without inherent toxicity can be metabolically activated to potent toxicants. The following examples are illustrative of the situations that might occur involving two compounds.

TABLE 4.6
Spectral Characteristics of Microsomal Cytochrome P-450 in Insecticide-Resistant and Insecticide-Susceptible Strains of the Housefly, *Musca domestica*

Difference Spectrum	Susceptible	Resistant
CO spectrum (λ_{max} nm)	451–452	448–449
Relative P-450 level (CO spectrum)	100	150–200
Formation of type-I difference spectrum	Absent	Present
Type-II *n*-octylamine difference spectrum	Double trough	Single trough
Relative magnitude of type-III ethyl isocyanide 455-nm peak	100	60–70

TABLE 4.7
Some Estimates of the Number of Chemicals in Use in the United States

Number	Type	Source of Estimate
1,500	Active ingredients of pesticides	EPA
4,000	Active ingredients of drugs	FDA
2,000	Drug additives to improve stability, inhibit bacterial growth, etc.	FDA
2,500	Food additives with nutritional value	FDA
3,000	Food additives to promote product life	FDA
50,000	Additional chemicals in common use	EPA

Source: EPA, Environmental Protection Agency; FDA, Food and Drug Administration.

1. Compound A, without inherent toxicity, is metabolized to a potent toxicant. In the presence of an inhibitor of its metabolism, there would be a reduction in toxic effect.
2. Compound A, given after exposure to an inducer of the activating enzymes, would appear more toxic.
3. Compound B, a toxicant, is metabolically detoxified. In the presence of an inhibitor of the detoxifying enzymes, there would be an increase in the toxic effect.
4. Compound B, given after exposure to an inducer of the detoxifying enzymes, would appear less toxic.

In addition to the above cases, the toxicity of the inhibitor or inducer, as well as the time dependence of the effect, must also be considered since, as mentioned above, many xenobiotics that are initially enzyme inhibitors ultimately become inducers.

4.5.1 Inhibition

As previously indicated, inhibition of xenobiotic-metabolizing enzymes can cause either an increase or a decrease in toxicity. Several well-known inhibitors of such enzymes are shown in Figure 4.3 and are discussed in this section. Inhibitory effects can be demonstrated in a number of ways at different organizational levels.

4.5.1.1 Types of Inhibition: Experimental Demonstration

IN VIVO SYMPTOMS. The measurement of the effect of an inhibitor on the duration of action of a drug in vivo is the commonest method of demonstrating its action. These methods are open to criticism, however, since effects on duration of action can be mediated by systems other than those involved in the metabolism of the drug. Furthermore, they cannot be used for inhibitors that have pharmacological activity similar or opposite to the compound being used. The most used and most reliable of these tests involve the measurement of effects on the hexobarbital sleeping time and the zoxazolamine paralysis time.

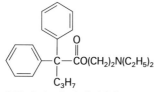

2(Diethylamino)ethyl-2,2-
diphenylpentanoate (SKF-525A)

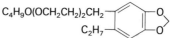

3,4-Methylenedioxy-6-propylbenzyl
n-butyl diethyleneglycol ether
(Piperonyl butoxide)

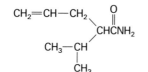

Allylisopropylacetamide

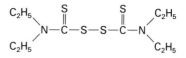

Tetraethylthiuram disulfide
(disulfiram, Antabuse)

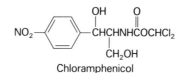

Chloramphenicol

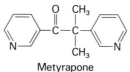

O-Ethyl-O-p-nitrophenyl
phenylphosphorothioate (EPN)

Metyrapone

FIGURE 4.3.
Some common inhibitors of xenobiotic-metabolizing enzymes.

Both of these drugs are fairly rapidly deactivated by the hepatic microsomal mixed-function oxidase system; thus, inhibitors of this system prolong their action.

For example, treatment of mice with chloramphenicol (Figure 4.3) 0.5 – 1.0 hours before pentobarbital treatment prolongs the duration of the pentobarbital sleeping time in a dose-related manner; it is effective at low doses (< 5 mg/kg) and has a greater than tenfold effect at high doses (100 – 200 mg/kg). The well-known inhibitor of drug metabolism SKF-525A causes an increase in both hexobarbital sleeping time and zoxazolamine paralysis time in rats and mice, as do the insecticide synergists piperonyl butoxide and tropital, the optimum pretreatment time being about 0.5 hours before the narcotic is given.

In the case of activation reactions, such as the activation of the insecticide azinphosmethyl to its potent anticholinesterase oxon derivative, a decrease in toxicity is apparent when rats are pretreated with SKF-525A, an inhibitor of the cytochrome P-450 monooxygenase system that catalyzes this reaction.

Cocarcinogenicity may also be an expression of inhibition of a detoxication reaction, as in the case of the cocarcinogenicity of piperonyl butoxide, a cytochrome P-450 monooxygenase activity inhibitor, and the carcinogens, freons 112 and 113.

DISTRIBUTION AND BLOOD LEVELS.   Treatment of an animal with an inhibitor of foreign compound metabolism may cause changes in the blood levels of an unmetabolized toxicant and/or its metabolites. This procedure may be used in the investigation of the inhibition of detoxication pathways; it has the advantage over in vitro methods of yielding results of direct physiological or toxicological interest since it is carried out in the intact animal. For example, if animals are first treated with either SKF-525A, glutethimide, or chlorcyclizine, followed in ≤ 1 hour by pentobarbital, it can be shown that the serum level of pentobarbital is considerably higher in treated animals than in controls within 1 hour of its injection. Moreover, the time sequence of the effects can be followed in individual animals, a factor of importance when inhibition is followed by induction—a not uncommon event.

EFFECTS ON METABOLISM IN VIVO.   A further refinement of the previous technique is to determine the effect of an inhibitor on the overall metabolism of a xenobiotic in vivo, usually by following the appearance of metabolites in the urine and/or feces. In some cases, the appearance of metabolites in the blood or tissue may also be followed. Again, the use of the intact animal has practical advantages over in vitro methods, although little is revealed about the mechanisms involved.

Studies of antipyrine metabolism may be used to illustrate the effect of inhibition on metabolism in vivo; in addition, these studies have demonstrated variation between species in the inhibition of the metabolism of xenobiotics. In the rat, a dose of piperonyl butoxide of at least 100 mg/kg was necessary to inhibit antipyrine metabolism, whereas in the mouse a single intraperitoneal (IP) or oral dose of 1 mg/kg produced a significant inhibition. An oral dose of 0.71 mg/kg had no discernible effect on the metabolism of antipyrine in humans.

Disulfiram (Antabuse) inhibits aldehyde dehydrogenase irreversibly, causing an increase in the level of acetaldehyde, formed from ethanol by the enzyme alcohol dehydrogenase. This results in nausea, vomiting, and other symptoms in the human—hence its use as a deterrent in alcoholism. Inhibition by disulfiram appears to be irreversible, the level returning to normal only as a result of protein synthesis.

EFFECTS ON IN VITRO METABOLISM FOLLOWING IN VIVO TREATMENT.   This method of demonstrating inhibition is of variable utility. The preparation of enzymes from animal tissues usually involves considerable dilution with the preparative medium during homogenization, centrifugation, and resuspension. As a result, inhibitors not tightly bound to the enzyme in question are lost, either in whole or in part, during the preparative processes. Therefore, negative results can have little utility since failure to inhibit and loss of the inhibitor give identical results. Positive results, on the other hand, not only indicate that the compound administered is an inhibitor but also provide a clear indication of excellent binding to the enzyme, most probably due to the formation of a covalent or slowly reversible inhibitory complex. The inhibition of esterases following treatment of the animal with phosphates, such as paraxon, is a good example, since the phosphorylated enzyme is stable and is still inhibited after the preparative procedures. Inhibition by carbamates, however, is greatly reduced by the same procedures, since the carbamylated enzyme is unstable and, in addition, the residual carbamate is highly diluted.

Microsomal monoozygenase inhibitors that form stable inhibitory complexes with cytochrome P-450, such as SKF-525A, piperonyl butoxide and other methylenedioxyphenyl compounds (see Figure 3.8), and amphetamine and its derivatives, can be readily investigated in this way since the microsomes isolated from pretreated animals have a reduced capacity to oxidize many xenobiotics.

Another form of chemical interaction, resulting from inhibition in vivo, that can then be demonstrated in vitro, involves those xenobiotics that function by causing destruction of the enzyme in question, so-called suicide substrates. Exposure of rats to vinyl chloride results in a loss of cytochrome P-450 and a corresponding reduction in the capacity of microsomes subsequently isolated to metabolize foreign compounds. Allyl isopropylacetamide and other allyl compounds have long been known to have a similar effect.

IN VITRO EFFECTS.   In vitro measurement of the effect of one xenobiotic on the metabolism of another is by far the commonest type of investigation of interactions involving inhibition. Although it is the most useful method for the study of inhibitory mechanisms, particularly when purified enzymes are used, it is of more limited utility in assessing the toxicological implications for the intact animal. The principal reason for this is that in vitro measurement does not assess the effects of factors that affect absorption, distribution, and prior metabolism, all of which occur before the inhibitory event under consideration.

Although the kinetics of inhibition of xenobiotic-metabolizing enzymes can be investigated in the same ways as any other enzyme mechanism, a number of problems arise that may decrease the value of this type of investigation. They include the following:

1. A particulate enzyme system, the cytochrome P-450-dependent monooxygenase system, has been investigated many times, with methods developed for single soluble enzymes. As a result, Lineweaver-Burke or other reciprocal plots are frequently curvilinear, and the same reaction may appear to have quite different characteristics from laboratory to laboratory, species to species, and organ to organ.
2. The nonspecific binding of substrate and/or inhibitor to membrane components is a further complicating factor affecting inhibition kinetics.
3. Substrates and inhibitors are frequently lipophilic, with low solubility in aqueous media.
4. Xenobiotic-metabolizing enzymes commonly exist in mutliple forms (eg, glutathione *S*-transferases and cytochromes P-450) that are all relatively nonspecific but differ from one another in the relative affinities of the different substrates.

The primary considerations in studies of inhibition mechanisms are reversibility and selectivity. The inhibition kinetics of reversible inhibition give considerable insight into the reaction mechanisms of enzymes and, for that reason, have been well studied. In general, reversible inhibition involves no covalent binding, occurs rapidly, and can be reversed by dialysis or, more rapidly, by dilution. Reversible inhibition is usually divided into competitive inhibition, uncompetitive inhibition, and noncompetitive inhibition, although these are not rigidly separated types, and many intermediate classes have been described.

Competitive inhibition is usually caused by two substrates competing for the same active site. Following classical enzyme kinetics, there should be a change in the apparent K_m but not in V_{max}. In microsomal monooxygenase reactions, type I ligands, which often appear to bind as substrates but do not bind to the heme iron, might be expected to be competitive inhibitors, and this frequently appears to be the case. Examples are the inhibition of the O-demethylation of p-nitroanisole by aminopyrene, aldrin epoxidation by dihydroaldrin, and N-demethylation of aminopyrene by nicotinamide. More recently, some of the polychlorinated biphenyls (PCBs), notably dichlorobiphenyl, but also, less effectively, tetrachlorobiphenyl and hexachlorobiphenyl, have been shown to have a high affinity as type I ligands for rabbit liver cytochrome P-450 and to be competitive inhibitors of the O-demethylation of p-nitroanisole.

Uncompetitive inhibition has seldom been reported in studies of xenobiotic metabolism. It occurs when an inhibitor interacts with an enzyme–substrate complex but cannot interact with free enzyme. Both K_m and V_{max} change by the same ratio, giving rise to a family of parallel lines in a Lineweaver-Burke plot.

Simple noncompetitive inhibitors can bind to both the enzyme and enzyme–substrate complex to form either an enzyme–inhibitor complex or an enzyme–inhibitor–substrate complex. The net result is a decrease in V_{max} but no change in K_m.

Metyrapone (Figure 4.3), a well-known inhibitor of monooxygenase reactions, can also, under some circumstances, stimulate metabolism in vitro. In either case, the effect is noncompetitive, in that the K_m does not change whereas V_{max} does, decreasing in the case of inhibition and increasing in the case of stimulation.

Irreversible inhibition, which is much more important toxicologically, can arise from various causes. In most cases, the formation of covalent or other stable bonds or the disruption of the enzyme structure is involved. In these cases, the effect cannot be readily reversed in vitro by either dialysis or dilution.

The formation of stable inhibitory complexes may involve the prior formation of a reactive intermediate that then interacts with the enzyme. An excellent example of this type of inhibition is the effect of the insecticide synergist piperonyl butoxide (Figure 4.3) on hepatic microsomal monooxygenase activity. This methylenedioxyphenyl compound can form a stable inhibitory complex that blocks CO binding to cytochrome P-450 and also prevents substrate oxidation. This complex causes the appearance of a characteristic difference spectrum that has two pH-dependent peaks in the Soret region and, apart from its stability, resembles that of ethyl isocyanide. This complex results from the formation of a reactive intermediate, which is shown by the fact that the type of inhibition changes from competitive to irreversible as metabolism, in the presence of NADPH and oxygen, proceeds. It appears probable that the metabolite in question is a carbene formed spontaneously by elimination of water following hydroxylation of the methylene carbon by the cytochrome (see Figure 3.8 for activation of methylenedioxyphenyl compounds). Piperonyl butoxide inhibits the in vitro metabolism of many substrates of the monooxygenase system, including aldrin, ethylmorphine, aniline, and aminopyrene, carbaryl, biphenyl, hexobarbital, *p*-nitroanisole, and many others. Although most of the studies carried out on piperonyl butoxide have involved rat or mouse liver microsomes, they have also been carried out on pig, rabbit, and carp liver microsomes, and in various preparations from houseflies, cockroaches, and other insects. Certain classes of monooxygenase inhibitors, in addition to methylenedioxyphenyl compounds, are now known to form "metabolic intermediate complexes," including amphetamine and its derivatives and SKF-525A and its derivatives.

The inhibition, by organophosphate compounds such as EPN, of the carboxylesterase that hydrolyzes malathion is a further example of xenobiotic interaction resulting from irreversible inhibition, since in this case the enzyme is phosphorylated by the inhibitor.

Another class of irreversible inhibitors of toxicological significance consists of those compounds that bring about the destruction of the xenobiotic-metabolizing enzymes, hence the designation "suicide substrate." The drug allylisopropylacetamide (Figure 4.3), as well as other allyl compounds, has long been known to cause the breakdown of cytochrome P-450 and the resultant release of heme. More recently, the hepatocarcinogen vinyl chloride has also been shown to have a similar effect, probably also mediated through the generation of a highly reactive intermediate. Much information has accumulated in the past decade on the mode of action of the hepatotoxicant carbon tetrachloride, which effects a number of irreversible changes in both liver proteins and lipids, such changes being generated by reactive intermediates formed during its metabolism.

The less specific disruptors of protein structure, such as urea, detergents, strong acids, etc., are probably of significance only in in vitro experiments.

4.5.1.2 Synergism and Potentiation

The terms synergism and potentiation have been variously used and defined but involve a toxicity that is greater when two compounds are given simultaneously or sequentially than would be expected from a consideration of the toxicities of the compounds given alone.

Some toxicologists have used the term synergism for cases that fit this definition but only when one compound is toxic alone while the other has little or no intrinsic toxicity. This is the case with the toxicity of insecticides to insects and mammals and the effects on this toxicity of methylenedioxyphenyl synergists such as piperonyl butoxide, sesamex, and tropital. The term potentiation is then reserved for those cases in which both compounds have appreciable intrinsic toxicity, such as in the case of malathion and EPN. Unfortunately, other toxicologists have used the terms in precisely the opposite manner, where even more of them use the terms interchangeably, without definition, leading to such statements as "potentiation of the toxicity of X by the synergist Y." Historically, pharmacologists used the term synergism to refer to simple additive toxicity and potentiation either as synonym or for examples of greater than additive toxicity or efficacy.

In an attempt to make uniform the use of these terms, it is suggested that insofar as toxic effects are concerned, they be used as defined above; ie, both involve toxicity greater than would be expected from the toxicities of the compounds administered separately, but in the case of synergism one compound has little or no intrinsic toxicity administered alone, whereas in the case of potentiation both compounds have appreciable toxicity when administered alone. It is further suggested that no special term is needed for simple additive toxicity of two or more compounds.

An example of synergism has already been mentioned. Piperonyl butoxide, sesamex, and related compounds increase the toxicity of insecticides to insects by inhibition of the insect monooxygenase system.

Other insecticide synergists that interact with the mixed-function oxidase system include aryloxyalkylamines such as SKF-525A, Lilly 18947, and their derivatives, compounds containing acetylenic bonds such as aryl-2-propynyl phosphate esters containing propynyl functions, phosphorothionates, benzothiadiazoles, and some imidazole derivatives.

The best known example of potentiation involving insecticides and an enzyme other than the monooxygenase system is the increase in the toxicity of malathion to mammals that is brought about by certain other organophosphates. Malathion has a low mammalian toxicity due primarily to its rapid hydrolysis by a carboxylesterase. EPN (Figure 4.3), another organophosphate insecticide, was shown to cause a dramatic increase in malathion toxicity to mammals at dose levels, that, given alone, caused essentially no inhibition of cholinesterase. In vitro studies further established that the oxygen analog of EPN, as well as many other organophosphate compounds, increases the toxicity of malathion by inhibiting the carboxylesterase responsible for its degradation.

4.5.1.3 Antagonism

In toxicology, antagonism may be defined as that situation in which the toxicity of two or more compounds administered together, or sequentially, is less than would be expected from a consideration of their toxicities when administered individually. Strictly speaking, this definition includes those cases in which the lowered toxicity results from induction of detoxifying enzymes; they are; however, considered separately in Section 4.5.2. Apart from the convenience of treating such antagonistic phenomena together with the other aspects of induction, they are frequently considered separately because of the significant time that must elapse between treatment with the inducer and subsequent treatment with the toxicant. The reduction of hexobarbital sleeping time and the reduction of zoxazolamine paralysis time by prior treatment with phenobarbital to induce drug-metabolizing enzymes are obvious examples of such induction effects at the acute level of drug action, whereas protection from the carcinogenic action of benzo(a)pyrene, aflatoxin B_1, and diethylnitrosamine by phenobarbital treatment are examples of inductive effects at the level of chronic toxicity. In the latter case, the cytochrome P-450 isozymes induced by phenobarbital metabolize the chemical to less toxic metabolites.

Antagonism not involving induction is a phenomenon often seen at a marginal level of detection and is consequently both difficult to explain and of marginal significance. In addition, several different types of antagonism of importance to toxicology that do not involve xenobiotic metabolism are known but are not appropriate for discussion in this chapter. They include competition for receptor sites, such as the competition between CO and O_2 in CO poisoning, or situations in which one toxicant combines nonenzymatically with another to reduce its toxic effects, such as in the chelation of metal ions. Physiological antagonism, in which two agonists act on the same physiological system but produce opposite effects, is also of importance.

4.5.2 Induction

About 25 years ago, during investigations on the *N*-demethylation of aminoazo dyes, it was observed that pretreatment of mammals with the substrate or, more remarkably, with other xenobiotics, caused an increase in the ability of the animal to metabolize these dyes. It was subsequently shown that this effect is due to an increase in the microsomal enzymes involved. A symposium in 1965 and a landmark review by Conney in 1967 established the importance of induction in xenobiotic interactions. Since then, it has become clear that this phenomenon is widespread and nonspecific. Several hundred compounds of diverse chemical structure have been shown to induce monooxygenase and other enzymes. These compounds include drugs, insecticides, polycyclic hydrocarbons, and many others; the only obvious common denominator is that they are all organic and lipophilic. It was already clear that enzymes of the monooxygenase pathway other than cytochrome P-450 were also increased in these situations. It was also apparent that, even though all inducers did not have the same effects, the effects tended to be nonspecific to the extent that any single inducer induced more than one enzymatic activity. It is now clear that other enzymes can also be induced, such as glutathione *S*-transferase, epoxide hydrolase, etc., and that induction can extend even to cellular organelles, such as smooth endoplasmic reticulum, peroxisomes, and mitochondria.

4.5.2.1 Specificity of Monooxygenase Induction

The many inducers of monooxygenase activity fall into two principal classes, one exemplified by phenobarbital and containing many types of chemicals, especially drugs and insecticides, and the other exemplified by 3-methylcholanthrene and benzo(a)pyrene and containing primarily polycyclic hydrocarbons. Many inducers require either fairly high dose levels or repeated dosing to be effective, frequently > 10 mg/kg and some as high as 100–200 mg/kg. Some insecticides, however, such as mirex, can induce at dose levels as low as 1 mg/kg, and the most potent inducer known, 2,3,7,8-tetrachlorodibenzo-*p*-dioxin (TCDD), is effective at 1 μg/kg in some species.

In the liver, phenobarbital-type inducers cause a marked proliferation of the smooth endoplasmic reticulum as well as an increase in the amount of cytochrome P-450. The cytochrome P-450 isozymes induced have approximately the same spectral characteristics as that of the liver of uninduced mammals. A wide range of oxidative activities are induced, including O-demethylation of p-nitroanisole, N-demethylation of benzphetamine, pentobarbital hydroxylation, and aldrin epoxidation.

Induction by polycyclic hydrocarbons, on the other hand, causes no increase in smooth endoplasmic reticulum although the cytochrome P-450 content is increased. The main isozyme induced is cytochrome P-448, (P_1-450), and it is characterized by a shift in the λ_{max} of the reduced cytochrome – CO complex from 450 nm to 448 nm. This cytochrome has a different pH equilibrium point for the reduced cytochrome P-450 – ethyl isocyanide complex than does the cytochrome P-450 induced by phenobarbital. A relatively narrow range of oxidative activities, primarily aryl hydrocarbon hydroxylase, is induced by polycyclic hydrocarbons, with the best known reaction being the hydroxylation of benzo(a)pyrene. The extremely potent inducer TCDD appears to fall in this class.

All inducers do not fall readily into one or the other of these two classes. Some oxidative processes can be induced by either type of inducer, such as the hydroxylation of aniline and the N-demethylation of chlorcyclizine. Some inducers, such as the mixture of PCBs designated Arochlor 1254, can induce a broad spectrum of cytochrome P-450 and P-448 isozymes. Many variations also exist in the relative stimulation of different oxidative activities within the same class of inducer, particularly of the phenobarbital type.

Pregnenolone-16α-carbonitrile (PCN) may represent a third type of inducer in that the substrate specificity of the microsomes from treated animals differs from that of the microsomes from either phenobarbital-treated or 3-methylcholanthrene – treated animals. Ethanol and isosafrole are known to induce specific forms of cytochrome P-450 not seen with other inducing agents.

It appears reasonable that since several types of cytochrome P-450 are associated with the hepatic endoplasmic reticulum, various inducers may induce one or more of them. Because each of these types has a relatively broad substrate specificity, differences may be caused by variations in the extent of induction of different cytochromes. Now that methods are available for gel electrophoresis of microsomes and for solubilization and characterization of different forms of cytochrome P-450, the complex array of inductive phenomena is being more logically explained in terms of specific isozymes.

Although the bulk of published investigations of the induction of monooxygenase enzymes have dealt with mammalian liver, induction has been observed in other mammalian tissues and in nonmammalian species, both vertebrate and invertebrate. Cytochromes characteristic of all of these types of inducers have now been purified from rabbit and rat liver and, in some cases, from other organisms. It is also clear that many of these induced cytochrome P-450s represent only a small percentage of the total cytochrome P-450 in the uninduced animal. For this reason, the "constitutive" isozymes, those already expressed in the uninduced animal, must be fully characterized, since they represent the available xenobiotic-metabolizing capacity of the normal animal.

Other anomalies of the induction phenomenon include the marked induction of aryl hydrocarbon hydroxylase activity in the placenta of human mothers who smoke cigarettes, an induction that is not accompanied by a discernible increase in the total amount of placental cytochrome P-450. Although feeding of chlordane to rats gives rise to an initial increase in aldrin epoxidase activity, there is a decline to control values despite continued induction of cytochrome P-450 and smooth endoplasmic reticulum, giving rise to a condition described by the investigators as "hypoactive, hypertrophic endoplasmic reticulum."

4.5.2.2 Mechanism and Genetics of Induction in Mammals

Although stress can affect the level of mammalian monooxygenase activities, the effect is secondary, since induction has been demonstrated following perfusion of the isolated liver with the inducer and also following treatment of isolated hepatocytes. It has not been duplicated in cell-free systems, however, presumably due to the time required for the process and the fact that several complex multienzyme processes are required simultaneously — notably the processes involved in gene expression and protein synthesis. It has been known for some time that the induction of monooxygenase activity is a true induction involving synthesis of new enzyme, and not the activation of enzyme already synthesized, since it is prevented by inhibitors of protein synthesis. For example, aryl hydrocarbon hydroxylase induction is inhibited by puromycin, ethionine, and cycloheximide. A simplified scheme for gene expression and protein synthesis is shown in Figure 4.4.

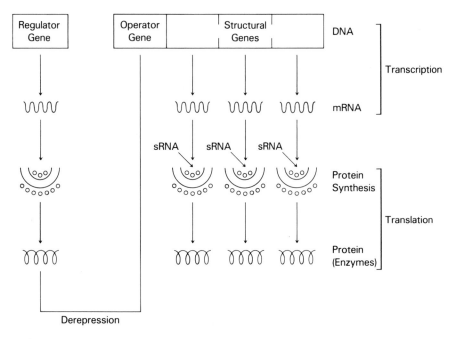

FIGURE 4.4.
Simplified scheme for gene expression in animals.

The use of suitable inhibitors of RNA and DNA metabolism has shown that inhibitors of RNA synthesis such as actinomycin D and mercapto(pyridethyl)-benzimidazole block aryl hydrocarbon hydroxylase induction, whereas hydroxyurea, at levels that completely block the incorporation of thymidine into DNA, has no effect. Thus, it appears that the inductive effect is at the level of transcription and that DNA synthesis is not required. Although induction by phenobarbital appears to take place by a similar mechanism to induction of aryl hydrocarbon hydroxylase by aromatic hydrocarbons, no receptor analogous to the Ah receptor has been identified.

These findings imply that compounds that induce xenobiotic-metabolizing enzymes play a role as derepressors of regulator or other genes in a manner analogous to steroid hormones — namely, combining with a cytosolic receptor followed by movement into the nucleus and then derepression of the appropriate gene. In the case of TCDD, the cytosolic receptor protein has been identified. The involvement of regulator and operator genes is more speculative; in view of the extremely variable results obtained with regard to the ratio of different enzymes induced by different inducers, it should be regarded with caution, particularly with inducers of the phenobarbital type.

The case is better argued with polycyclic hydrocarbon inducers, at least in the case of the mouse, since much genetic work has been done using "aromatic hydrocarbon-responsive" strains and "nonresponsive" strains. Thus, it has been demonstrated that facile inducibility of aryl hydrocarbon hydroxylase activity is due to a single dominant gene locus, Ah, even though it can be induced in so-called nonresponsive strains by the more potent inducers such as TCDD.

4.5.2.3 Effect of Induction

The effects of inducers are usually the opposite of those of inhibitors; thus, their effects can be demonstrated by much the same methods, that is, by their effects on pharmacological or toxicological properties in vivo or by the effects on enzymes in vitro following prior treatment of the animal with the inducer.

In vivo effects are frequently reported; the most common ones are the reduction of the hexobarbital sleeping time or zoxazolamine paralysis time. These effects have been reported for numerous inducers and can be quite dramatic. For example, in the rat, the paralysis time resulting from a high dose of zoxazolamine can be reduced from 11 hours to 17 minutes by treatment of the animal with benzo(a)pyrene 24 hours before the administration of zoxazolamine.

The induction of monooxygenase activity may also protect an animal from the effect of carcinogens by increasing the rate of detoxication. This has been demonstrated in the rat with a number of carcinogens including benzo(a)pyrene, N-2-fluorenylacetamide, and aflatoxin B_1. Effects on carcinogenesis may be expected to be complex since some carcinogens are both activated and detoxified by monooxygenase enzymes while, at the same time, epoxide hydrolase, which can also be involved in both activation and detoxication, may also be induced. For example, the toxicity of the carcinogen 2-naphthylamine, the hepatotoxic alkaloid monocrotaline, and the cytotoxin cyclophosphamide are all increased by phenobarbital induction — an effect mediated by the increased population of reactive intermediates.

Organochlorine insecticides are also well-known inducers. Treatment of rats with either DDT or chlordane, for example, will decrease hexobarbital sleeping time and offer protection from the toxic effect of warfarin.

Effects on xenobiotic metabolism in vivo are also widely known in both humans and animals. Cigarette smoke, as well as several of its constituent polycyclic hydrocarbons, is a potent inducer of aryl hydrocarbon hydroxylase in the rat placenta, liver, and other organs. Examination of the term placentas of smoking human mothers revealed a marked stimulation of aryl hydrocarbon hydroxylase and related activities — remarkable in an organ which, in the un-induced state, is almost inactive toward foreign chemicals. Similarly, cigarette smoking lowers the plasma levels of phenacetin by induction of the enzymes responsible for its oxidation to N-acetyl-p-aminophenol. Persons exposed to DDT and lindane metabolized antipyrine twice as fast as a group not exposed, whereas those exposed to DDT alone had a reduced half-life for phenylbuta-zone and increased excretion of 6-hydroxycortisol.

The effects of inducers on the metabolic activity of hepatic microsomes subsequently isolated from treated animals have often been reported. Whereas the polycyclic hydrocarbons primarily induce aryl hydrocarbon hyroxylase activity and a few related activities, inducers such as phenobarbital, DDT, etc., have been shown to induce many oxidative reactions, including benzpheta-mine N-demethylation, p-nitroanisole O-demethylation, N-demethylation of ethylmorphine, aldrin epoxidation, and many others.

Some enzyme activities, such as zoxazolamine hydroxylase, chlorpromazine N-demethylation, and aniline hydroxylation, are induced by both types of inducers.

4.5.2.4 Induction of Xenobiotic-Metabolizing Enzymes Other Than Monooxygenases

Although less well studied, xenobiotic-metabolizing enzymes other than the microsomal cytochrome P-450-dependent monooxygenase system are also known to be induced, frequently by the same inducers that induce the oxidases. These include glutathione S-transferases, epoxide hydrolase, and UDP glucu-ronyltransferase. The selective induction of one pathway over another can greatly affect the metabolism of a xenobiotic.

4.5.3 Biphasic Effects: Inhibition and Induction

Many inhibitors of mammalian monooxygenase activity can also act as in-ducers. Inhibition of microsomal monooxygenase activity is fairly rapid and involves a direct interaction with the cytochrome, whereas induction is a slower process. Therefore, following a single injection of a suitable compound, an initial decrease due to inhibition would be followed by an inductive phase. As the compound and its metabolites are eliminated, the levels would be expected to return to control values. Some of the best examples of such compounds are the methylenedioxyphenyl synergists, such as piperonyl butoxide. Because cytochrome P-450 combined with methylenedioxyphenyl compounds in the type III inhibitory complex cannot interact with CO, the cytochrome P-450 titer, as determined by the method of Omura and Sato (the CO-binding to reduced cytochrome), would appear to follow the same curve.

It is apparent from extensive reviews of the induction of monooxygenase activity by xenobiotics that many compounds other than methylenedioxyphenyl compounds have the same effect. It may be that any synergist that functions by inhibiting microsomal monooxygenase activity could also induce this activity on longer exposure, resulting in a biphasic curve as described previously for methylenedioxyphenyl compounds. This curve has been demonstrated for NIA 16824 (2-methylpropyl-2-propynyl phenylphosphonate) and WL 19255 (5,6-dichloro-1,2,3-benzothiadiazole), although the results were less marked with R05-8019 [2,(2,4,5-trichlorophenyl)-propynyl ether] and MGK 264 [N-(2-ethylhexyl)-5-norbornene-2,3-dicarboximide].

4.6 ENVIRONMENTAL EFFECTS

Because the in vitro effects of light, temperature, etc., on xenobiotic-metabolizing enzymes are not different from their effects on other enzymes or enzyme systems, we are not concerned with them now. This section deals with the effects of environmental factors on the intact animal as they relate to in vivo metabolism of foreign compounds.

4.6.1 Temperature

Although it might be expected that variations in ambient temperature would not affect the metabolism of xenobiotics in animals with homeothermic control, this is not the case. Temperature variations can be a form of stress and thereby produce changes mediated by hormonal interactions. Such effects of stress require an intact pituitary-adrenal axis and are eliminated by either hypothysectomy or adrenalectomy. There appear to be two basic types of temperature effect on toxicity: either with increase in toxicity at both high and low temperature or an increase in toxicity with an increase in temperature. For example, both warming and cooling increases the toxicity of caffeine to mice, whereas the toxicity of D-amphetamine is lower at reduced temperatures and shows a regular increase with increases in temperature.

In many studies, it is unclear whether the effects of temperature are mediated through metabolism of the toxicant or via some other physiological mechanisms. In other cases, however, temperature clearly affects metabolism. For example, in cold-stressed rats, there is an increase in the metabolism of 2-naphthylamine to 2-amino-1-naphthol.

4.6.2 Ionizing Radiation

In general, ionizing radiation reduces the rate of metabolism of xenobiotics both in vivo and in enzyme preparations subsequently isolated. This has occurred in hydroxylation of steroids, in the development of desulfuration activity toward azinphosmethyl in young rats, and in glucuronide formation in mice. Pseudocholinesterase activity is reduced by ionizing radiation in the ileum of both rats and mice.

4.6.3 Light

Because many enzymes, including some of those involved with xenobiotic metabolism, show a diurnal pattern that can be keyed to the light cycle, light cycles rather than light intensity would be expected to affect these enzymes. In the case of hydroxyindole-*O*-methyltransferase in the pineal gland, there is a diurnal rhythm with greatest activity at night; continuous darkness causes maintenance of the high level. Cytochrome P-450 and the microsomal monooxygenase system show a diurnal rhythm in both the rat and the mouse, with greatest activity occurring at the beginning of the dark phase.

4.6.4 Moisture

No moisture effect has been shown in vertebrates, but in insects it was noted that housefly larvae reared on diets containing 40% moisture had four times more activity for the epoxidation of heptachlor than did larvae reared in a similar medium saturated with water.

4.6.5 Altitude

Altitude can either increase or decrease toxicity. It has been suggested that these effects are related to the metabolism of toxicants rather than to physiological mechanisms involving the receptor system, but in most examples this has not been clearly demonstrated.

Examples of altitude effects include the observations that at altitudes of $\geq 5,000$ ft, the lethality of digitalis or strychnine to mice is decreased, whereas that of D-amphetamine is increased.

4.6.6 Other Stress Factors

Noise has been shown to affect the rate of metabolism of 2-napthylamine, causing a slight increase in the rat. This increase is additive with that caused by cold stress.

4.7 GENERAL SUMMARY AND CONCLUSIONS

It is apparent from the material presented in this chapter and the previous one that the metabolism of xenobiotics is complex, involving many enzymes, is susceptible to a large number of modifying factors, both physiological and exogenous, and that the toxicological implications of metabolism are important.

Despite the complexity, summary statements of considerable importance can be abstracted.

1. Phase-one metabolism generally introduces a functional group into a xenobiotic which enables conjugation to an endogenous metabolite to occur during phase-two metabolism.
2. The conjugates produced by phase-two metabolism are considerably more water-soluble than either the parent compound or the phase-one metabolite(s) and hence are more excretable.
3. During the course of metabolism, and particularly during phase-one reactions, reactive intermediates that are much more toxic than the parent compound may be produced. Thus, xenobiotic metabolism may be either a detoxication or an intoxication (activation) process.
4. Because the number of enzymes involved in phase-one and phase-two reactions is large and many different sites on organic molecules are susceptible to metabolic attack, the number of potential metabolites and intermediates that can be derived from a single substrate is frequently very large.
5. Because both qualitative and quantitative differences exist between species, strains, individual organs, and cell types, a particular toxicant may have different effects in different circumstances.
6. Because exogenous chemicals can be inducers and/or inhibitors of the xenobiotic-metabolizing enzymes of which they are substrates; such chemicals may interact to bring about toxic sequelae different from those that might be expected from any of them administered alone.
7. Because endogenous factors also affect the enzymes of xenobiotic metabolism, the toxic sequelae to be expected from a particular toxicant will vary with developmental stage, nutritional status, health or physiological status, stress, or environment.
8. It has become increasingly clear that most enzymes involved in xenobiotic metabolism occur as several isozymes and that these coexist within the same individual and, frequently, within the same subcellular organelle. An understanding of the biochemistry and molecular genetics of these isozymes may lead to an understanding of the variation between species, individuals, organs, sexes, developmental stages, etc.

4.8 SUGGESTED FURTHER READING

Albert, W. Selective Toxicity: The Physico-Chemical Basis of Therapy. 6th ed. London: Chapman and Hall, 1979.

Baker, S.B., Tripod, J., Jacob, J. (eds.). The problem of species difference and statistics in toxicology. In Proceedings of the European Society for the Study of Drug Toxicity, XI. Amsterdam: Excerpta Medica, 1970.

Caldwell, J., Jakoby, W.B. Biological Basis of Detoxication. New York: Academic Press, 1983.

Conney, A.H. Pharmacological implications of microsomal enzyme induction. Pharmacol. Rev. 1967; 19:317.

Conney, A.H., Pantuck, E.J., Hsiao, K.-C., Kuntzman, R., Alvares, A.P., Kappas, A. Regulation of drug metabolism in man by environmental chemicals and diet. Fed. Proc. 1977; 36:1647.

Elliott, R.W. Genetics of drug resistance. In Mihich, E. (ed.). Drug Resistance and Selectivity: Biochemical and Cellular Basis. New York: Academic Press, 1973, p. 41.

Engel, P.C. Enzyme Kinetics. New York: Wiley, 1977.

Franklin, M.K. Inhibition of mixed-function oxidations by substrates forming reduced cytochrome P-450 metabolic-intermediate complexes. Pharmacol. Ther. [A] 1977; 2:227.

Goldstein, A., Aronow, L., Kalman, S.M. Principles of Drug Action: The Basis of Pharmacology. 3d ed. New York: Wiley, 1985.

Hodgson, E. Comparative toxicology: Cytochrome P-450 and mixed-function oxidase activity in target and non-target organisms. Essays Toxicol. 1976; 7:73.

Hodgson, E., and Guthrie, F.E. (eds.). Introduction to Biochemical Toxicology. New York: Elsevier, 1980.

Hodgson, E., Philpot, R.M. Interaction of methylenedioxyphenyl (1,3-benzodioxole) compounds with enzymes and their effects on mammals. Drug Metab. Rev. 1974; 3:231.

Hucker, H.B. Species difference in drug metabolism. Annu. Rev. Pharmacol. 1970; 10:99.

Jollow, D.R., Kocsis, J.J., Snyder, R., Vainio, H. (eds.). Biological Reactive Intermediates: Formation, Toxicity and Inactivation. New York: Plenum Press, 1977.

Nebert, D.W., Felton, J.S. Importance of genetic factors influencing the metabolism of foreign compounds. Fed. Proc. 1976; 35:1133.

Parke, D.V. (ed.). Enzyme Induction. London: Plenum Press, 1975.

Sanvordeker, D.R., Lambert, H.J. Environmental modification of mammalian drug metabolism and biological response. Drug Metab. Rev. 1974; 3:201.

Schwartz, H.S., Mihich, E. Species and tissue differences in drug selectivity. In Mihich, E. (ed.). Drug Resistance and Selectivity: Biochemical and Cellular Basis. New York: Academic Press, 1973, pp. 413–452.

Snyder, R., Parke, D.V., Kocsis, J.J., Jollow, D.J., Gibson, C.G., Witmer, C.M. (eds.). Biological Reactive Intermediates II, Parts A and B. New York: Plenum Press, 1982.

Snyder, R., Jollow, D.J., Kocsis, J.J., Nelson, J.O. and Witmer, C.M. (eds). Biological Reactive Intermediates III: Animal Models and Human Disease. New York: Plenum Press, 1986.

Timbrell, J.A. Principles of Biochemical Toxicology. London: Taylor and Francis, 1982.

Testa, B. and Jenner, P. Inhibitions of cytochrome P-450s and their mechanisms of action. Drug Metab. Rev. 1981; 12:1.

Wilkinson, C.F. (ed.). Insecticide Biochemistry and Physiology. Chapter 15. New York: Plenum Press, 1976.

Williams, R.T. Interspecies variations in the metabolism of xenobiotics. Biochem. Soc. Trans. 1974; 2:359.

Williams, R.T., Millburn, P. Detoxication mechanisms — The biochemistry of foreign compounds. In Blaschko, H.K.F. (ed.). Physiological and Pharmacological Biochemistry, Biochemistry Series 1, vol. 12. Baltimore: University Park Press, 1975.

chapter five

ELIMINATION OF TOXICANTS

Frank E. Guthrie and Ernest Hodgson

5.1 INTRODUCTION

Simple forms of life eliminate toxicants ingested with food or otherwise passively absorbed due to a concentration gradient into the surrounding medium, which is usually water. As organisms evolved to fresh water, where water and CO_2 balance must be regulated, and to land, where, in addition, water must be conserved, elimination became a complex regulatory function. Thus, elimination of toxicants became a part of a broader specialized system of elimination that maintains a delicate balance of nutrients, minerals, and other substances necessary to life in terrestrial and other environments. Therefore, evolution of mechanisms for the elimination of endogenous and exogenous substances was a concomitant of the evolution of more complex forms of life, greater size, movement to fresh water and, ultimately, to land.

At first, it seems peculiar that a wide variety of synthetic organic chemicals that are very recent, relative to the evolutionary time scale, can be eliminated without special physiological systems. It has become apparent, however, that xenobiotics are not readily eliminated until they are in a form similar to that utilized for the elimination of endogenous substances. Thus, absorbed xenobiotics must first be metabolized by one or more reactions to progressively more polar forms, a process that eventually permits excretion, primarily by renal and hepatic routes. Other routes of excretion may serve to eliminate the parent compounds intact (for example, polychlorinated biphenyls (PCBs) in milk and ethanol in expired air).

Routes of elimination such as milk, lungs, alimentary excretion, sweat, hair, etc., are generally of minor importance as compared with urine and bile.

5.2 RENAL EXCRETION

The kidneys are primarily excretory organs. Elimination by this route not only accounts for most by-products of normal metabolism; the kidneys are also the primary organ for excretion of polar xenobiotics and the hydrophilic metabolites of any lipophilic xenobiotics that an animal has encountered. The nephron, the functional unit of the kidney, is depicted in Figure 5.1. Transport to the kidney may occur by solubilization in blood or by binding to blood proteins.

5.2.1 Glomerular Filtration

The initial step in urine formation is glomerular filtration. The plasma is passively filtered as it passes through numerous glomerular pores that are 70–100 Å in diameter. The system is under pressure generated by the heart. The rate of glomerular filtration is 180 Liters/day in an average human. No specificity is shown except for molecular size; any solute in the plasma small enough to pass the pores appears in the ultrafiltrate. Molecules too large to pass, or those bound to proteins, do not appear in the filtrate and must either be further altered or must be eliminated by other avenues. Any factor that affects the hydrostatic pressure of the glomerulus may affect the rate of filtration and perhaps result in elevated concentrations of excretory products in the plasma.

5.2.2 Tubular Reabsorption

The second major process occurring in the kidney is tubular reabsorption. The glomerular filtrate contains a large number of solutes necessary for normal

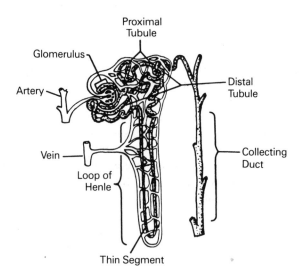

FIGURE 5.1.
Diagrammatic illustration of major components of a typical nephron in mammalian kidney. Source: Hodgson, E., Guthrie, F.E. Introduction to Biochemical Toxicology. New York: Elsevier, 1980.

body function—water, amino acids, glucose, salts, etc., solutes that must be recovered from the filtrate during the elimination process. Many resorption mechanisms take place in the cells of the proximal segment of the tubule; this portion of the tubule accounts for about 75% of reabsorption from the glomerular filtrate. For this reason, the proximal tubule is the site of toxic action of many reabsorbed toxicants. Both active and passive mechanisms permit varying degrees of selective action. Amino acids, and some cations, glucose, peptides, and organic acids are actively reabsorbed. Water, chloride, and other ions are passively reabsorbed due to osmotic and electrochemical gradients generated by active transport of sodium and potassium. Henle's loop functions to establish regulation of osmolarity of fluid in the collecting duct. The remainder of the water and ion reabsorption occurs in the distal tubule and collecting duct.

Reabsorption of xenobiotics is usually passive and regulated by the same principles that permit passage of similar endogenous molecules across membranes. Lipophilic compounds traverse cell walls more readily than do polar compounds. Thus, passive reabsorption of lipophilic toxicants is greater than reabsorption of more polar ones, and renal excretion of lipophilic xenobiotics is proportionally less.

5.2.3 Tubular Secretion

Another major mechanism whereby solutes may be excreted by the kidney is tubular secretion. This mechanism permits transport of solutes from the peritubular fluid to the lumen of the tubule, and the process may be either active or passive. One active mechanism permits secretion of a number of organic acids, including glucuronide and sulphate conjugates, whereas a second active process secretes strong organic bases. Passive secretion of some weak basic and acidic organic compounds occurs as a result of pH differences. The nonionized and therefore more lipophilic form is readily diffusible through the tubule walls. The pH in the tubular lumen, however, is such that the compounds become ionized and unable to diffuse back across the cell wall. This mechanism, diffusion trapping, is very sensitive to fluctuations of pH in the urine, and modification of the urine pH by, for example, the oral administration of bicarbonate can, in some cases, be used to help eliminate unwanted compounds.

5.2.4 Factors Affecting Renal Excretion

Toxicants are excreted by the same mechanisms that govern elimination of endogenous substances. Polar xenobiotics of a size permitting glomerular passage are removed from the plasma and concentrated in the tubules. Minimal tubular reabsorption of such polar compounds occurs, and they are readily secreted.

Xenobiotics bound to plasma proteins are unable to pass the glomerulus but are subject to tubular secretion as long as binding is readily reversible. As the free fraction of a toxicant in plasma is removed from the plasma and secreted by the tubular cells, more toxicant dissociates from the bound form to maintain the equilibrium of free and bound toxicant in the plasma. This equilibrium may be governed by pK_a and the solubility of the toxicant at the pH of plasma. The newly freed fraction is now available for tubular secretory processes. This process will eventually allow significant excretion of previously bound toxicants. Highly lipophilic toxicants would not be expected to be excreted by this mechanism since they easily diffuse back across the concentration gradient generated by tubular reabsorption.

5.3 HEPATIC EXCRETION

5.3.1 Bile Formation and Secretion

The second most significant route of elimination is biliary, or hepatic excretion. Although bile was first recognized as a route of excretion for xenobiotics > 100 years ago, only in recent years has it been recognized as a major mechanism of excretion, second only to urine. More than 200 foreign compounds have been detected in bile, and an appreciable fraction of many such chemicals appears in it.

A major problem in investigating hepatic excretion in humans is the difficulty of obtaining bile under physiological conditions. Surgery appreciably depresses bile flow, and studies are also greatly limited because relatively few drugs have warranted careful investigation. Within these constraints, evidence continues to mount for a significant role of the bile in the elimination of foreign compounds. Studies with laboratory animals are also confounded by the effects of anesthesia and surgery, and some investigators have implanted chronic cannulae in the bile duct to measure biliary excretion in unrestrained animals. This technique has the disadvantage of continued loss of bile salts and other biliary constituents, but recent experimental techniques, including a cannula that directs bile flow to the duodenum, promise to overcome these objections.

The liver is interposed between the intestinal tract and the general blood circulation and is ideally located to effect metabolism of endogenous and exogenous compounds. The products of metabolism may be released into the circulating blood or excreted in the bile. The bulk of the liver is comprised of hepatic cells arranged in plates two cells thick (Figure 5.2). These plates are arranged

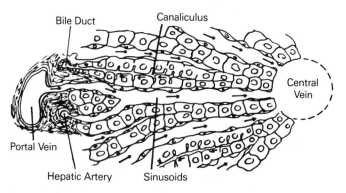

FIGURE 5.2.
Flow of blood from portal vein and hepatic artery into the sinusoids that empty into the central vein. Bile flows in the opposite direction through canaliculi to empty into bile ducts. Source: Hodgson, E., Guthrie, F.E. Introduction to Biochemical Toxicology. New York: Elsevier, 1980.

around the terminal branches of the hepatic veins and exposed to venous and arterial blood flowing through interconnecting spaces (hepatic sinusoids). The sinusoid walls are very permeable to relatively large molecules. Solutes may be transferred from the hepatic cells to the bile or blood by active or passive processes. There is little transfer of lipophilic compounds prior to metabolism to more water-soluble forms, however.

Bile secretion is relatively independent of hydrostatic pressure, and bile flow may be either bile salt-dependent, the most important mechanism, or bile salt-independent. Recently, a role for the Golgi apparatus has been suggested for optimal biliary secretion, but the depiction of intracellular events is sketchy.

The compounds actively secreted by bile are usually amphipathic molecules, having both polar and nonpolar moieties. Bile salts are classic examples of endogenous amphipathic molecules whereas conjugates of lipophilic xenobiotics are examples of amphipathic molecules of exogenous origin. As the pK_a of most conjugates is 3–4, they are 99% nonionized at physiological pH, thus facilitating active transport.

Brauer has classified compounds according to their bile/plasma concentration ratios. Class A compounds have a ratio of approximately 1 and are largely excreted by diffusion. They appear in blood or bile in approximately equal ratios. Class B compounds have a ratio greater than unity and tend to be concentrated in bile. These include conjugates of many xenobiotics, and active transport is involved. Class C compounds have a ratio < 1 and tend to be excluded from bile. These are usually macromolecules such as insulin, phospholipids, and protein.

Bile secreted by the liver cells into the bile canaliculi flows into the terminal branches of the bile duct and then to the hepatic duct and gall bladder. When an animal ingests a meal, hormonal action causes the gall bladder to release its contents into the duodenum. Some animals, such as rats, have no gall bladder, and release into the duodenum is continuous.

Compounds representing nearly every class of pharmacologic agent appear in bile to some extent. Most toxicants are found in the bile as metabolites. Biliary excretion has been studied in most common laboratory animals, fish, several domesticated and wild animals, and in humans; it varies considerably from one species to another.

Molecular weight is a major factor that determines the pathway of elimination. A threshold exists below which compounds are excreted primarily in the urine and above which they are excreted primarily in the bile. Such threshold figures are only approximations and vary widely between species. The approximate molecular-weight threshold is 325 in rats, 400 in guinea pigs, 475 in rabbits, and 500–700 in humans. This implies that a range of molecular weights may be excreted in both urine and bile to appreciable extents. Table 5.1 shows urinary versus biliary elimination for a series of compounds of increasing molecules weights. The molecular weight concept does not appear to be operative for all chemical classes, and some water-soluble compounds, such as certain highly water-soluble polymers, with molecular weights > 1,000, are readily eliminated in urine.

Induction of the monooxygenase system usually, but not always, causes increased biliary clearance, which is coupled with both increased liver size and increased bile flow. Inhibition of the monooxygenase system has been shown to

TABLE 5.1
Effect of Mol Wt on Route of Xenobiotic Excretion by the Rat

Xenobiotic	Molecular Weight	Percent of Total Excretion Detected in	
		Urine	Feces
Biphenyl	154	80	20
4-Monochlorobiphenyl	188	50	50
4,4'-Dichlorobiphenyl	223	34	66
2,4,5,2',5'-Pentachlorobiphenyl	326	11	89
2,3,6,2',3',6'-Hexachlorobiphenyl	361	1	99

Source: Matthews, H.B., in Hodgson, E., Guthrie, F.E. (eds.). Introduction to Biochemical Toxicology. New York: Elsevier, 1980.

decrease biliary elimination of such compounds as carbon tetrachloride. Sex and age are also known to be factors in altered biliary elimination.

5.3.2 Enterohepatic Circulation

An important aspect of biliary elimination concerns enterohepatic circulation. Following absorption and transfer to the liver, a nonpolar toxicant is usually conjugated. Depending on the molecular weight it is either eliminated in the urine or secreted in the bile. When conjugates enter the intestine, they may be hydrolyzed by microflora or other intestinal conditions. The compound is again in a less polar form and can be absorbed by the intestine and returned to the liver through the portal circulation. This process may be repeated a number of times, significantly increasing the biological half-life and possible adverse liver effects (Figure 5.3). Some of the compound may be excreted while in the intestinal lumen, and some of the reabsorbed compound may enter the general circulation. In many cases, however, most of the compound goes into enterohepatic circulation, and thus a much longer biological half-life is permitted. It may be possible to introduce compounds into the alimentary canal to bind to the newly hydrolyzed compound and thus hasten removal. Such therapy has been demonstrated for methyl mercury: a polythiol resin was introduced to remove the lipophilic toxicant.

5.4 PULMONARY EXCRETION

Although the renal and biliary systems are the most important routes of elimination, many volatile compounds are eliminated through the respiratory system. Some compounds temporarily taken into the respiratory system but not absorbed are eliminated, as discussed in the previous chapter on absorption.

The functional structure of the lungs consists of myriad, thin, highly vascularized alveoli. This highly specialized part of the lung with its great surface area and thin membranes has the primary function of exchanging O_2 from air to blood and CO_2 from blood to air (Figure 2.8). The exchange is primarily passive, and any toxicant in the blood with adequate volatility may pass from

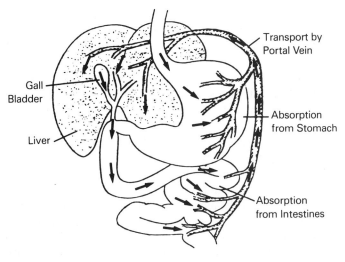

FIGURE 5.3.
Enterohepatic circulation.

blood to air for elimination. Ethanol is a well-recognized example, a fact that forms the basis for the forensic determination of inebriation.

The rate of elimination of volatile toxicants depends on solubility in blood, rate of respiration, and blood flow to the lungs. If a compound has considerable blood solubility, as does ether, hyperventilation will cause it to be eliminated more rapidly. If a compound has low blood solubility, as does ethylene, hyperventilation has little additional effect.

The best-known examples of respiratory elimination are among the anesthetic gases, but pesticide fumigants, many volatile organic solvents, and volatile metabolites of nonvolatile toxicants are eliminated to a significant extent by the lungs. In metabolic studies, carbon from compounds that are appropriately labeled with ^{14}C are often found in expired air, usually as $^{14}CO_2$. Disposition studies reveal that $\geq 50\%$ of some radiolabeled compounds is eliminated in expired air.

5.5 MINOR ROUTES OF ELIMINATION

The next most important routes of elimination may be categorized into two groups—minor routes of elimination of toxicants and obscure routes of elimination.

The minor routes are quite important in some specific instances, but are relatively inconsequential when one considers total elimination. The minor routes primarily concern sex-linked and alimentary elimination.

5.5.1 Sex-linked Routes

5.5.1.1 Milk

The route of excretion of some compounds becomes linked to reproductive functions of the female. When the mother has accumulated considerable quantities of highly lipid-soluble toxicants (such as DDT or PCBs in fatty depots), a ready route of elimination is in milk. An exchange of toxicants occurs between fatty depots and blood and those toxicants that readily cross the mammary cell membrane. A growing list of potentially adverse compounds have been shown to appear in milk: caffeine, alcohol, drugs, vitamins, hormones, and some pesticidal and industrial chemicals. Whereas the short half-lives of more polar compounds dictate a minor role for elimination in milk, for some compounds with long half-lives, milk may become an important mechanism of elimination. For example, in experimental studies with chlorinated insecticides, elimination in cow's milk of >25% of the administered dose may occur. In some South American countries, the DDT content of mother's milk is very close to the Acceptable Daily Intake (ADI) for DDT recommended by the World Health Organization. Although adverse effects to infants were not reported in this case, documented instances have resulted when nursing mothers were accidentally exposed to high concentrations of hexachlorobenzene or PCBs. In both cases, significant numbers of infants showed some level of intoxication.

5.5.1.2 Eggs

Another sex-linked route can be observed with the eggs of birds. Polar toxicants and metabolites may be eliminated primarily in the egg white. Adverse effects are usually quite transient or not noted in these cases. With lipophilic compounds, elimination may be noted in the egg yolk, and such compounds are metabolized with difficulty. The effect of such elimination on the survival of the young bird makes the use of these compounds as agricultural chemicals highly controversial.

5.5.1.3 Fetus

A final sex-linked route of elimination is in the fetus. The placental barrier may be important in preventing entry of a number of polar toxicants and their metabolites. The placental barrier is no longer considered an important barrier to entry of lipophilic compounds, however. Although the fetus contains relatively small amounts of toxicants in most cases, the tragic examples of teratologic effects of thalidamide, toxic effects of mercury, and carcinogenic effects of diethylstilbesterol are well documented.

5.5.2 Alimentary Elimination

A second grouping of minor route elimination concerns the alimentary canal. When toxicants equilibrate with body fluids and have the necessary lipophilicity to traverse membranes, they may move through the alimentary canal into the lumen. There is some evidence for active transport of penicillin through the salivary glands and of compounds of ammonia in the intestine, but usually the process is passive. Passive elimination in the alimentary canal usually results in the excretion of quantitatively unimportant amounts of toxicants; however, in some cases, this may be an important route of elimination. The contaminant chlordecone (kepone) appears to be primarily eliminated (although the rate is slow) in the intestine. The therapy for chlordecone poisoning is the administration of cholestyramine, which binds chlordecone and prevents its reabsorption (enterohepatic circulation); thus, in time, appreciable amounts of kepone may be eliminated.

5.5.3 Obscure Routes

Finally, elimination of toxicants may also involve some very obscure and poorly understood routes. Because diffusion of toxicants can occur across any of the cell membranes of the body, hair, feathers, oil glands, sweat glands, etc., all may be expected to be involved in the elimination of trace quantities of lipophilic compounds. Such elimination may also be possible when components of the body are continuously removed, for example in sloughing of skin when toxicants adhere to the tissue.

Cells that have a secretory function or much growth may be of some importance as routes of elimination. Such compounds as mercury, selenium, and arsenic are well-known examples of toxicants associated with hair. In recent studies with highly chlorinated biphenyls, which have extremely long half-lives, it has been suggested that hair growth may be an important route of elimination.

Extensive use of reviews by H.B. Matthews of the National Institute of Environmental Health Sciences is acknowledged with appreciation.

5.6 SUGGESTED FURTHER READING

Israili, Z.H. and Dayton, P.G. Enhancement of xenobiotic metabolism: Role of intestinal excretion. Drug Metab. Rev. 1984; 15:1123–1159.

Klaassen, C.D. Absorption, distribution and excretion of toxicants. In Doull, J., Klaassen, C.D. Amdur, M.O. (eds.). Toxicology: the Basic Science of Poisons. New York: Macmillan, 1980, 778 pp.

Lee, D.K., Falk, H.L., Murphy, S.D., Geiger, S.P. Handbook of Physiology, Section 9, Reactions to Environmental Agents. Baltimore: American Physiological Society, 1977.

Levine, W.G. Biliary excretion of drugs and other xenobiotics. In Jucher, E. (ed.). Progress in Drug Research, vol. 25. Berlin: Birkhauser Verlag, 1981.

Levine, W.G. Excretion mechanisms. In Caldwell, J., Jakoby, W.B. (eds.). Biological Basis of Detoxication. New York: Academic Press, 1983, 429 pp.

Matthews, H.B. Elimination of toxicants and their metabolites. In Hodgson, E., Guthrie, F.E. (eds.). Introduction to Biochemical Toxicology. New York: Elsevier, 1980, 436 pp.

Pritchard, J.B., James, M.O. Metabolism and urinary excretion. In Jakoby, W.B., Bend, J.R., Caldwell, J. (eds.). Metabolic Basis of Detoxication. New York: Academic Press, 1982, 375 pp.

chapter six

TOXIC ACTION

Patricia E. Levi

6.1 ROLE AND FORMATION OF REACTIVE METABOLITES

6.1.1 Metabolic Activation: Definition

During the processes between uptake from the environment and excretion from the body, many exogenous compounds undergo metabolism to highly reactive, electrophilic intermediates. These products may interact with cellular constituents in numerous ways, such as binding covalently to macromolecules and/or stimulating lipid peroxidation. This biotransformation of relatively inert chemicals to highly reactive intermediary metabolites is commonly referred to as "metabolic activation" or "bioactivation" and is known to be the initial event in several kinds of chemical-induced toxicities. Some toxicants are direct-acting, however, and require no activation, eg, CN^-, whereas others may be activated nonenzymatically.

6.1.2 Activation Enzymes

Most of these activations are catalyzed by the cytochrome P-450–dependent monooxygenase system, which is most highly concentrated in the liver, but which has also been detected in other tissues, including skin, kidney, intestine, lung, placenta, and nasal mucosa. Because cytochrome P-450 exists as multiple isozymes with different substrate specificities, the presence or absence of a particular cytochrome P-450 isozyme may contribute to tissue-specific toxicity. Many drugs and other foreign compounds are known to induce one or more of the cytochrome P-450 isozymes, resulting in an increase, decrease, or alteration of metabolism of certain chemicals. Specific examples of these types of interactions are given later in this section. In addition to activations catalyzed by cytochrome P-450, phase-two conjugations, cooxidation during prostaglan-

133

din biosynthesis, oxidation by the FAD-containing monooxygenase, and metabolism by intestinal microflora may also lead to the formation of reactive, toxic products. Most known activation reactions occur via the cytochrome P-450 pathways, however.

With some chemicals, only one enzymatic reaction is involved; with other compounds, several reactions, occasionally involving multiple pathways, are necessary for the production of the "ultimate" reactive metabolite.

6.1.3 Chemical Classes of Reactive Metabolites

Active metabolites include such diverse groups as epoxides, quinones, free radicals, reactive oxygen species, and unstable conjugates. Figure 6.1 gives some examples of activation reactions, the reactive metabolites that are formed, and the enzymes that catalyze their bioactivation.

6.1.4 Fate of Reactive Metabolites

6.1.4.1 Binding to Cellular Macromolecules

Most reactive toxic metabolites are electrophiles that can bind covalently to nucleophilic sites on cellular macromolecules such as proteins, polypeptides, RNA, and DNA. This covalent binding is considered to be the initiating event for many toxic processes such as mutagenesis, carcinogenesis, and cellular necrosis, and will be discussed in greater detail in subsequent sections.

6.1.4.2 Lipid Peroxidation

Radicals such as $CCl_3^{\bullet}$, produced during the oxidation of carbon tetrachloride, may induce lipid peroxidation and subsequent destruction of cellular components. This mechanism is discussed more fully in Section 6.3.4.1b. Biochemically, more is known about the metabolic reactions producing reactive intermediates than about how these metabolites interact with cellular components or how these interactions may cause subsequent cell alterations.

6.1.4.3 Trapping and Removal: Role of Glutathione

Once reactive metabolites are formed, mechanisms within the cell may bring about their rapid removal and inactivation. Toxicity then depends primarily on the balance between the rate of metabolite formation and the rate of removal. With some compounds, reduced glutathione plays an important protective role by trapping electrophilic metabolites and preventing their binding to hepatic proteins and enzymes. Although conjugation reactions occasionally result in bioactivation of a compound (see discussion of 2-acetyl-aminofluorene in Section 6.1.5.2), the acetyl, glutathione-, glucuronyl-, or sulfotransferases usually result in the formation of a nontoxic, water-soluble metabolite that is then easily excreted. The availability of the conjugating chemical may be an important factor in determining the fate of the reactive intermediate however (see discussion of acetaminophen toxicity in Section 6.1.5.3).

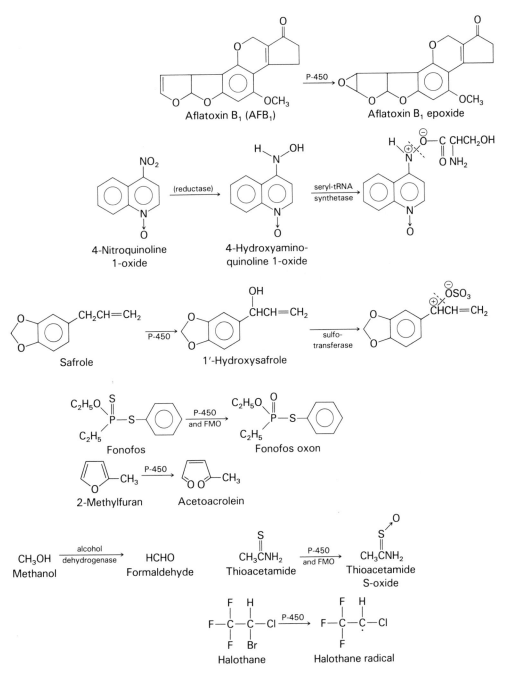

FIGURE 6.1.
Reactive metabolites of some foreign compounds. P-450, cytochrome P-450 monooxygenase system; FMO, FAD-containing monooxygenase.

6.1.5 Specific Examples of Activation Reactions

6.1.5.1 Aflatoxin B₁

Aflatoxin B$_1$ (AFB$_1$) is one of the mycotins produced by *Aspergillus flavus* and *A. parasiticus* and is a well-known hepatotoxicant and hepatocarcinogen. It is generally accepted that the activated form of AFB$_1$ that binds covalently to DNA is the 2,3-epoxide (Figure 6.1). AFB$_1$-induced hepatotoxicity and carcinogenicity varies among species of livestock and laboratory animals. The selective toxicity of AFB$_1$ appears to be dependent on quantitative differences in formation of the epoxide. Table 6.1 shows the relative rates of AFB$_1$ metabolism by liver microsomes from different species. Because the epoxides of foreign compounds are frequently further metabolized by epoxide hydrolases or are nonenzymatically converted to the corresponding dihydrodiols, formation of the dihydrodiol may be considered as evidence for prior formation of the epoxide. Epoxide formation is catalyzed by the cytochrome P-450–dependent monooxygenase system. The amount of AFB$_1$-dihydrodiol produced in microsomes in which specific cytochrome P-450 isozymes have been induced by phenobarbital (PB) is fivefold higher than that in control microsomes.

6.1.5.2 Acetylaminofluorene

In the case of the hepatocarcinogen 2-acetylaminofluorene (2-AAF), two activation steps are necessary to form the reactive metabolites (Figure 6.2). The initial reaction, *N*-hydroxylation, is a cytochrome P-450–dependent phase-one reaction, whereas the second reaction, formation of the unstable sulfate ester, a phase-two conjugation, results in the formation of a reactive intermediate. An alternate phase-two reaction, glucuronide conjugation, on the other hand, is a detoxification step, with this product being readily excreted. 2-AAF is known to be carcinogenic in some animal species and noncarcinogenic in others, and its carcinogenic potential can be correlated with the ability to form *N*-hydroxy-2-AAF or the sulfate ester of the *N*-hydroxy-2-AAF. Sulfotransferase activity, as well as hepatocarcinogenicity, is considerably higher in male rats than in female rats. In addition to *N*-hydroxylation, 2-AAF can undergo various ring hydroxylations that are, however, detoxification pathways. Because both *N*-hydroxylation and ring hydroxylation are catalyzed by cytochrome

TABLE 6.1
Formation of Aflatoxin B$_1$ Dihydrodiol by Liver Microsomes

Source of Microsomes	Dihydrodiol Formation[a]
C57 mouse	1.3
Rat	0.7
PB-induced rat	3.3
Guinea pig	2.0
Chicken (6 weeks)	4.8

[a] Microgram dihydrodiol formed per milligram microsomal protein/30 minutes.
Source: Neal, G.E., et al. Toxicol. Appl. Pharmacol. 1981; 58:431–437. Used by permission.

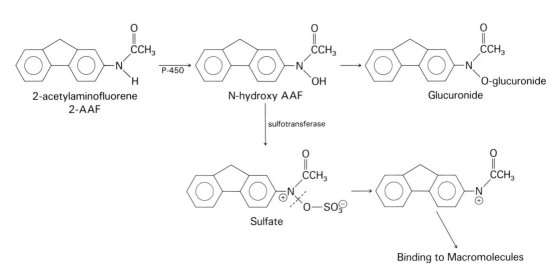

FIGURE 6.2.
Bioactivation of 2-acetylaminofluorene.

P-450, the difference in the levels of the various cytochrome P-450 isozymes will affect the balance between activation and detoxification and thus the carcinogenicity of the compound.

6.1.5.3 Acetaminophen

A good example of the importance of the concentration in the cell of the conjugating chemical is found with acetaminophen. At normal therapeutic doses, acetaminophen is safe, but can be extremely hepatotoxic at high doses. The major portion of acetaminophen is conjugated with either sulfate or glucuronic acid to form water-soluble, readily excreted metabolites. Significant amounts of a reactive intermediate, believed to be a quinoneimine, are formed by the cytochrome P-450–dependent monooxygenase system, however (Figure 6.3). When therapeutic doses of acetaminophen are ingested, the reactive intermediate is efficiently deactivated by conjugation with glutathione. When large doses are taken, however, the concentration of glutathione in the liver is depleted, resulting in an increased interaction of the reactive metabolite with cellular proteins, giving rise to acute hepatic necrosis, which can be fatal.

6.1.5.4 Cycasin

While studying a neurotoxic syndrome that occurs on South Pacific islands among residents who use flour from the cycad nut, Laquer discovered that flour from this nut, when fed to rats, led to cancers of the liver, kidney, and digestive tract. The active compound was found to be cycasin, the β-glucoside of methylazoxymethanol (Figure 6.4). If this compound was injected intraperitoneally (IP) rather than given orally, however, or if it was fed to germ-free rats, no tumors formed. It was later shown that the intestinal microflora possess the necessary enzyme, β-glucosidase, to form the active compound, methylazoxy-

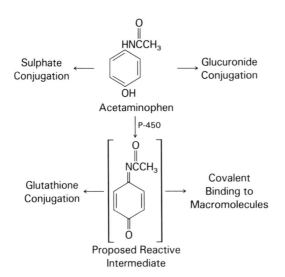

FIGURE 6.3.
Formation of a reactive metabolite from acetaminophen that may bind to tissue macro-molecules, resulting in necrosis.

methanol. Indeed, methylazoxymethanol will lead to tumors in both normal and germ-free animals regardless of the route of administration.

6.1.6 Factors Affecting Toxicity of Reactive Metabolites

In summary, a number of factors influence the balance between the rate of formation of reactive metabolites and the rate of removal:

1. The level of activating enzymes. Specific isozymes of cytochrome P-450 may be very important in determining metabolic activation of a foreign compound. As mentioned previously, many xenobiotics induce specific forms of cytochrome P-450. Thus, PB pretreatment of animals induces a cytochrome P-450 that converts bromobenzene to the highly toxic 3,4-epoxide (Figure 6.23), whereas pretreatment with 3-methylcholanthrene induces an isozyme of cytochrome P-450 that catalyzes primarily the formation of the nontoxic 2,3-epoxide (Section 6.3.4.1c).
2. Levels of conjugating enzymes. Levels of conjugating enzymes, such as glutathione transferases, are also known to be influenced by drugs and

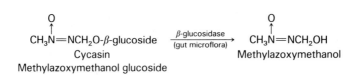

FIGURE 6.4.
Bioactivation of cycasin by intestinal microflora to the carcinogen, methylazoxymeth-anol.

other environmental factors; this will in turn affect the detoxication process.

3. Level of cofactors or conjugating chemicals. Treatment of animals with N-acetylcysteine, a precursor of glutathione, protects animals against acetaminophen-induced hepatic necrosis, possibly by reducing covalent binding to tissue macromolecules. On the other hand, depletion of glutathione potentiates covalent binding and hepatotoxicity.

6.2 ACUTE TOXICITY

6.2.1 Introduction

Acute effects are those that occur soon after a brief exposure to a chemical agent. Acute exposure can be either a single exposure or multiple exposures occurring within a short time (generally ≤ 24 hours). The acute effect is an effect that is observed within the first few days after exposure and, in most cases, within the first 2 weeks. Chronic effects, on the other hand, are those that appear only after repetitive exposure to a substance: many compounds require months of continuous exposure. Acute exposure to agents that are rapidly absorbed is likely to produce immediate toxic effects, but acute exposure can also produce delayed toxicity.

6.2.2 Nervous System Toxicants

6.2.2.1 Cholinesterase Inhibitors: Insecticides, Nerve Gases

Cholinesterase inhibitors used commercially as insecticides and nematocides include both the organophosphates and N-methyl carbamates (Figures 7.6 and 7.7). Organophosphate and carbamate compounds impair the function of the nervous system, their acute toxic effects being a result of binding to and inhibition of the enzyme, acetylcholinesterase (AChE), which is found at synapses within the central and autonomic nervous systems and at the nerve endings in striated muscles. Normally, acetylcholine, a neurotransmitter, is released from the presynapse and then binds to a protein receptor at the postsynapse, leading to opening of ionic channels and a depolarization of the postsynaptic membrane. When acetylcholine is released by the receptor, it is hydrolyzed by AChE to choline and acetate (Figure 6.5a), and its stimulatory activity is terminated. If AChE is inhibited, hydrolysis is prevented, and acetylcholine accumulates, resulting in excessive nerve excitation.

Exposure to organophosphates produces a broad spectrum of clinical effects indicative of overstimulation of the cholinergic system. These effects fall into three categories: Inhibition of AChE at the neuromuscular junctions leads to muscular twitching from excessive contraction of muscles, extreme weakness, and often paralysis (nicotinic effects). The main muscles of concern in acute poisoning are respiratory muscles, because paralysis of the diaphragm and chest muscles can result in respiratory failure. Inhibition in the autonomic nervous system (muscarinic receptors) results in abdominal pain, diarrhea, involuntary urination, increased secretions in the respiratory system filling the bronchioles with fluids, spasms of the smooth muscles in the respiratory tract causing

140

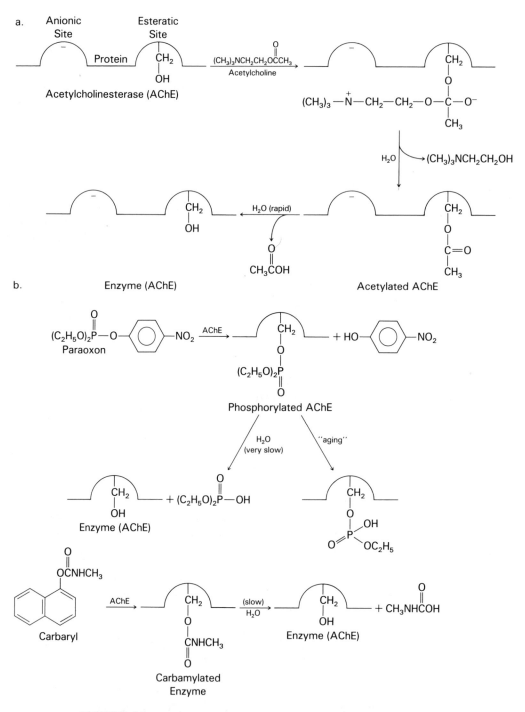

FIGURE 6.5.
a. Hydrolysis of acetylcholine by acetylcholinesterase (AChE). The esteratic site shows the —CH₂OH of the serine molecule at the active site. b. Reactions of paraoxon and carbaryl with acetylcholinesterase. Hydrolysis of carbamylated AChE occurs more readily than hydrolysis of phosphorylated enzyme.

constriction of the airways, and a marked construction of the pupils (miosis). Effects on the central nervous system cause tremors, confusion, slurred speech, lack of coordination, and convulsions in very high exposure.

Inhibition of cholinesterase results from blockage of the active site normally occupied by acetylcholine. The organophosphates, if they are used as the P=S compound, such as parathion (Figure 3.7) or malathion, first require metabolic activation to the P=O analog, termed the oxon, to possess anticholinesterase activity. Most organophosphates are activated by the cytochrome P-450–dependent monooxygenase system; however, fonofos (Figure 6.1) is activated by both the cytochrome P-450–dependent monooxygenase and the FAD-containing monooxygenase. The oxon then becomes bound at the active site and undergoes cleavage to release the corresponding alcohol or thiol, leaving behind the phosphorylated enzyme (Figure 6.5b). The inactivation of the enzyme will persist until hydrolysis of the phosphorylated enzymes occurs. The time required for reactivation of free enzyme varies with different organophosphorates from a few hours to several days. In addition, with some compounds such as paraoxon, a dealkylation reaction occurs, stabilizing the phosphorylated enzyme ("aging"), and the enzyme is irreversibly inhibited. In such cases, synthesis of new AChE is necessary for enzyme activity to be restored.

The treatment for organophosphate poisoning is a combination of atropine to counter the cholinergic stimulation and 2-pyridine aldoxime methiodide (2-PAM), which will accelerate the hydrolysis of the phosphorylated enzyme by removing and binding the phosphate moiety from the enzyme. The effectiveness of 2-PAM is dependent on its being administered early as the "aged" phosphorylated enzyme is not reversible by the oximes (see Sections 11.4.2.5 and 11.4.2.6 on Treatment of Toxicity).

Carbamate pesticides are similar to organophosphate pesticides in that they act by binding to the active site of AChE, forming a carbamylated enzyme (Figure 6.5b). The carbamylated enzyme, however, is rapidly hydrolyzed and reactivated. The signs and symptoms of carbamate poisoning are typical of cholinesterase inhibition: lightheadedness, nausea and vomiting, increased sweating, blurred vision, increased salivation, weakness, chest pains, miosis and, in severe cases, convulsions. Atropine is the recommended antidote for poisoning by carbamates; however, 2-PAM is not given since the reversal of the carbamylation of the enzyme is so rapid.

6.2.2.2 Other Nervous System Toxicants

Many exogenous chemicals can affect the presynaptic and postsynaptic binding sites of the neuromuscular junction, and some highly poisonous compounds owe their toxic action to their ability to alter nerve impulse transmission at this junction.

6.2.2.2a Tubocurarine

Tubocurarine from the plant *Chondrodendron tomentosuni* is a deadly poison that owes its toxic action to its ability to block irreversibly the cholinoreceptor (the receptor site that binds acetylcholine as the neurotransmitter) of certain motor neurons. Curare and similar drugs that act as competitive antagonists of acetylcholine at the postjunctional membrane of muscle fibers, reducing or blocking acetylcholine's transmitter action, are used as "muscle relaxants."

6.2.2.2b Botulinum Toxins

Botulinum toxins are heat-labile neurotoxins produced by the microorganism *Clostridium botulinum*. Botulinum toxin binds irreversibly to the axon terminal, thus preventing release of acetylcholine. Botulism, one of the most dreaded of the bacterial foodborne diseases because it is so frequently fatal, results primarily from eating improperly preserved canned food in which the bacterium grew and produced the toxin.

6.2.2.2c Tetrodotoxin

Tetrodotoxin has been responsible for deaths in humans as a result of consumption of improperly prepared puffer fish (Tetraodontidae). In Japan, puffer fish, known as fugu, are considered a great delicacy and are widely sold in restaurants. The toxins are found in the roe, liver, and skin of puffer fish, and workers must be specially trained in the preparation of this fish. It is thought that tetrodotoxin selectively blocks sodium channels along the nerve axon, preventing the inward sodium current of the action potential while leaving unaffected the outward potassium current. Approximately 60% of all cases of poisoning due to puffer fish result in death.

6.2.2.2d Batrachotoxin

Batrachotoxin has been used as an arrow poison and is found in the skin of the South American frog *Phyllobates aurotaenia*. The action of batrachotoxin is opposite to the effects of tetradotoxin on the sodium channels in that batrachotoxin increases the permeability of the resting membranes to sodium ions.

6.2.3 Inhibitors of Oxidative Phosphorylation

6.2.3.1 Electron Transport Inhibitors

6.2.3.1a Cyanide

Cyanide is one of the most rapidly acting of all poisons. It is readily absorbed through all routes, including skin and mucous membranes, and by inhalation. Ingestion of very small amounts of cyanide causes death within minutes or hours, depending on the route of exposure. Inhalation of hydrogen cyanide gas leads to death in a few minutes. The chemist, Karl Wilhelm Scheele, discoverer of hydrocyanic acid (prussic acid), was killed by its vapors. Cyanide is a common component in some rat and pest poisons, silver and metal polishes, ore refining processes, photographic solutions, and fumigating products. Cyanide is also present in the seeds of apples, peaches, plums, apricots, cherries, and almonds in the form of amygdalin, a cyanogenic glycoside.

Amygdalin, also an ingredient of Laetrile, an alleged anticancer drug, is composed of glucose, benzaldehyde, and cyanide moieties. Cyanide can be released from the glucoside by the action of β-glucosidase (emulsin), present in the pulp from crushed seeds and in mammalian intestinal microflora. For this reason, amygdalin may be much more toxic orally than intravenously (IV).

Laetrile has been responsible for cases of human cyanide poisoning, as have apricot kernels, the latter being widely available in health food stores.

Another potential source of cyanide poisoning is the drug sodium nitroprusside, which is used in the treatment of hypertension. Overdoses of this drug have led to cyanide toxicity.

Cyanide exerts its toxic effect by interrupting electron transport in the mitochondrial cytochrome chain at the cytochromes $a-a_3$ step (Figure 6.6). These cytochromes, which are isolated as a single, large protein molecule containing both cytochromes a and a_3, are referred to as cytochrome a_3 or cytochrome oxidase. Cyanide complexes with the heme of cytochrome a_3, thus preventing the heme's binding with oxygen. As a result of cyanide inhibition, electron transfer from cytochrome a_3 to molecular oxygen is blocked and cell death occurs. Death from cyanide poisoning is due to respiratory arrest.

The symptoms, which occur in quick succession, are salivation, giddiness, headache, palpitation, difficulty in breathing, and unconsciousness. Typically, cyanide has a bitter, burning taste; in addition, there is a faint odor of almonds. It has been estimated, however, that 20–40% of the population are genetically unable to detect the cyanide odor and thus are insensitive to this property.

The accepted treatment for cyanide poisonings is a three-step procedure. First, amyl nitrite is given to the patient by inhalation followed by IV administration of sodium nitrite. These chemicals oxidize the heme iron of hemoglobin from the ferrous (Fe^{2+}) to the ferric (Fe^{3+}) state; the resulting greenish-brown to black pigment is known as methemoglobin. The ferric iron of the methemoglobin combines with CN^- from the plasma, causing dissociation of cyanide already bound to cytochrome oxidase. After administration of nitrite, sodium thiosulfate is injected. Thiosulfate provides a substrate for the enzyme rhodanese (thiosulfate sulfur transferase) that catalyzes the conversion of cyanide to thiocyanate, which is nontoxic and readily excreted (Figure 6.6). For additional discussion of cyanide toxicity and treatment, see Section 11.4.2.2.

6.2.3.1b Other Inhibitors

Azide, like cyanide, inhibits cytochrome oxidase and produces similar biochemical lesions. Hydrogen sulfide is also an inhibitor of cytochrome oxidase in vitro and is thought to have the same mode of action as hydrogen cyanide.

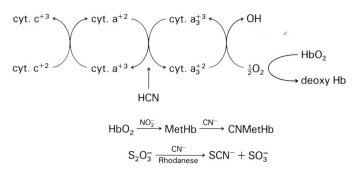

FIGURE 6.6.
Cyanide poisoning and treatment.

Carbon monoxide, on the other hand, combines directly with hemoglobin, forming a stable carboxy–hemoglobin complex, thus preventing the association of O_2 with hemoglobin.

6.2.3.2 Uncouplers of Oxidative Phosphorylation

Uncoupling agents allow electron transport to continue but prevent the phosphorylation of ADP to ATP. In vitro uncouplers can be shown to stimulate the rate of oxygen uptake by mitochondria, even in the absence of ADP or inorganic phosphate ions, and induce ATPase activity, which is normally low in mitochondria. The first uncoupling agent described was the herbicide 2,4-dinitrophenol. Most uncoupling compounds are lipophilic, weak acids, usually containing an aromatic ring. Many different uncoupling agents are known, including halogenated and nitrophenols, dicoumarin, carbonylcyanide phenylhydrazone, salicylanilides, atebrin (an antimalarial drug), and arsenate (Figure 6.7). Uncoupling agents are thought to function by breaking down or discharging a high energy state or intermediate generated by electron transport. They can "short-circuit" the proton current by transporting protons directly through the mitochondrial membrane, which normally is impermeable.

This "uncoupling" increases oxygen consumption and heat production. In humans, the result is hyperthermia, and the symptoms include fast respiratory and heart rates, flushed skin, sweating, nausea, and coma. The illness runs a rapid course, with either death due to fatal hyperthermia or recovery generally occurring within 24–48 hours.

6.2.4 Lethal Synthesis: Fluoroacetate

Compounds that interfere in intermediary metabolism may lead to depletion of energy-rich intermediates and thus result in the failure of energy supply.

An example of this is monofluoroacetic acid (fluoroacetate), a compound found naturally in certain plants from South Africa, where it has been known to cause livestock poisoning. It is also used as a rodenticide (Compound 1080, sodium fluoroacetate and Compound 1081, fluoroacetamide). Because of their extreme toxicity to most animals, these chemicals are not available for household or general use. The mechanism of toxicity was established by Sir Rudolph Peters who coined the term "lethal synthesis" to describe this type of biochemical lesion. Fluoroacetate produces its toxic action by inhibiting the citric acid cycle (Figure 6.8). The fluorine-substituted acetate becomes incorporated, by the mechanism for endogenous acetate, into fluoroacetyl coenzyme A, which

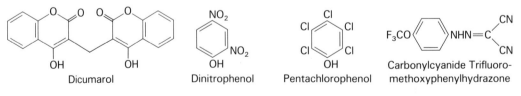

Dicumarol   Dinitrophenol   Pentachlorophenol   Carbonylcyanide Trifluoro-
                                                          methoxyphenylhydrazone

FIGURE 6.7.
Examples of some compounds that uncouple oxidative phosphorylation.

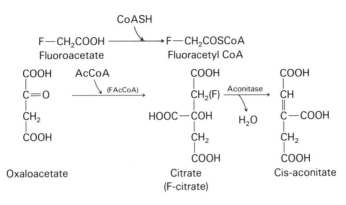

FIGURE 6.8.
Inhibition of citric acid cycle by fluoroacetate. The enzyme aconitase is inhibited by the intermediate fluorocitrate.

combines with oxaloacetate to form fluorocitrate. The next enzyme in the cycle, aconitase, is inhibited by fluorocitrate, resulting in a large accumulation of citrate and disruption of the mitochondrial energy supply. The heart and nervous system are the most critical tissues involved in poisoning caused by a general inhibition of oxidative energy metabolism. The symptoms of fluoroacetate poisoning include nausea, convulsions, and defects in cardiac rhythm, leading to death from ventricular fibrillation or respiratory failure.

6.3 CHRONIC TOXICITY

6.3.1 Carcinogenesis

6.3.1.1 Historical Perspective

The fact that certain agents in the environment may lead to various forms of cancer has been known for >200 years. The evidence that environmental chemicals had the potential to cause cancer usually came first from observations of a high cancer incidence among certain occupational groups, but it was not until much later that direct experimental evidence confirmed these suggestions (Table 6.2). One of the first of these recorded observations was that of Sir Percivall Pott in 1775. The London doctor observed that many of his patients with cancer of the scrotum were chimney sweeps, and he related this cancer to their exposure to soot and coal tar. His observation was not confirmed until 1916, however, when it was shown that skin cancer could be produced on rabbit's ears by application of coal tar. In the 1920s, coal tar was fractionated, and the active components were shown to be polycyclic aromatic hydrocarbons such as dibenzo(a,h)anthracene and benzo(a)pyrene.

In the 1860s, Germany became the center for the manufacture of synthetic dyes that were based on aromatic amines or their products. About 30 years later came the first warning that exposure to the dyes or their intermediates was hazardous. In 1895, Ludwig Rehn, a surgeon in Frankfurt, reported a cluster of bladder carcinomas in workmen from nearby dye factories. Epidemiologic evidence suggested that 2-naphthylamine was the probable carcinogen, but this

TABLE 6.2
History of the Discovery of Environmental Agents Causing Human Cancer

Suspected Carcinogen	Organ	Discoverer	Year
Soot	Scrotum	Pott	1775
Pipe smoking	Lips	Sommering	1795
Coal tar	Skin	Volkman	1875
Dye intermediates	Bladder	Rehn	1895
X-rays	Skin	Van Trieben	1902
Tobacco juices	Oral cavity	Abbe	1915
Radioactive watch dial dyes	Bone	Martland	1929
Sunlight	Skin	Molesworth	1937
Tobacco (cigarette) smoking	Lung	Muller	1939
Asbestos	Pleura	Wagner	1960
Cadmium	Prostate	Kipling; Waterhouse	1967

was not directly confirmed until 1938 when Hueper and coworkers demonstrated bladder tumors in dogs fed 2-naphthylamine. Figure 6.9 gives the structure of some synthetic chemical carcinogens, and Figure 6.10 shows the structure of some naturally occurring carcinogens.

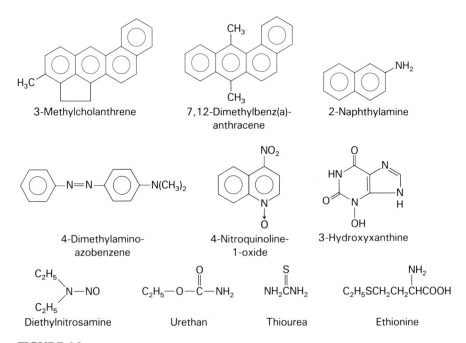

FIGURE 6.9.
Structures of some synthetic chemical carcinogens.

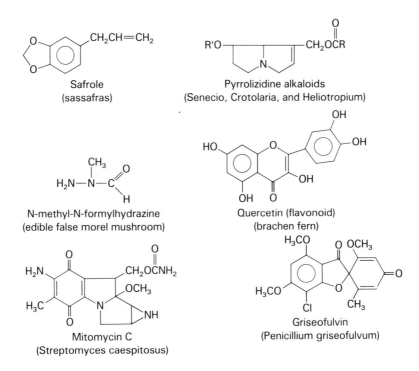

FIGURE 6.10.
Structures of some naturally occurring chemical carcinogens.

6.3.1.2 Carcinogenic Process

The induction of cancer by chemicals is a complex multistep process involving interactions between environmental and endogeneous factors. Carcinogenesis often proceeds through several discernible sequential stages leading to a malignant neoplasm (Figure 6.11). At least three stages are commonly recognized: initiation, promotion, and progression.

6.3.1.2a Initiation

The initiation stage is considered to be a rapid, essentially irreversible alteration in the cell that "primes" the cell for subsequent neoplastic development. The initiator chemical is either an electrophile or is metabolically activated to an electrophile. This reactive chemical then binds to DNA to form a permanent and heritable, but not yet expressed, change in the cell genome. Most initiators are mutagens and thus are classified as genotoxic carcinogens (Section 6.3.1.3).

6.3.1.2b Promotion

Promoting agents are chemicals that are not in themselves carcinogens, but which, when given after a low dose of an initiating agent, increase cancer incidence. Promoters may either increase the number of tumors or decrease the latency period. Promoters are not usually electrophiles and thus do not bind to DNA (see epigenetic carcinogens, Section 6.3.1.4).

This step-wise nature of carcinogenesis was first shown in mouse skin, and

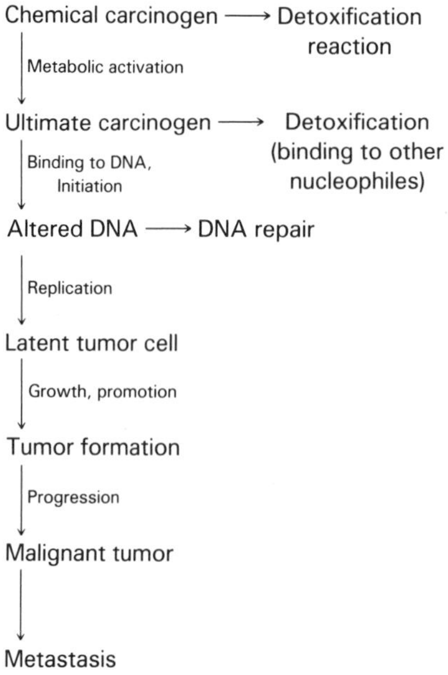

Chemical carcinogen ⟶ Detoxification
         reaction
 ⎥ Metabolic activation
 ↓

Ultimate carcinogen ⟶   Detoxification
        (binding to other
 ⎥ Binding to DNA, nucleophiles)
 ⎥   Initiation
 ↓

Altered DNA ⟶ DNA repair

 ⎥ Replication
 ↓

Latent tumor cell

 ⎥ Growth, promotion
 ↓

Tumor formation

 ⎥ Progression
 ↓

Malignant tumor

 ⎥
 ↓

Metastasis

FIGURE 6.11.
Sequence of events in chemical carcinogenesis.

this model has now been well characterized. In a typical experiment, an initiating chemical such as 7,12-dimethylbenz(a)-anthracene is applied to mouse skin at a low dose so that very few tumors are produced in the animal's lifetime. After an interval of 1 week to 1 year, the treated skin is exposed to multiple applications of a promoter such as the phorbol esters found in croton oil. Tumors begin to appear within 5–6 weeks of application of the promotor, and all mice yield tumors by 10–12 weeks after application.

6.3.1.2c   Essential Features of Initiation and Promotion

1. The initiator must be given first; no tumors or very few tumors result if the promoter is given first.
2. The initiator, if given once at a subcarcinogenic dose, does not produce tumors during the life of the animal; however, repeated doses of the initiator may elicit tumors even in the absence of the promoter.
3. The action of the initiator is irreversible; tumors result in nearly the same yield if the interval between initiation and promotion is extended from 1 week to 1 year.
4. The initiator is an electrophile, or is metabolically activated to an electrophile, which binds covalently to DNA to bring about a mutagenic change.
5. The essential function of the tumor promoter is to complete the carcinogenic process started by the initiator.
6. Promoters have not been found to be electrophilic, and there is no evidence of covalent binding to macromolecules.

7. The action of the promoter is reversible at an early stage and usually requires repeated exposure; thus, there is probably a threshold level of exposure.

6.3.1.2d Examples of Promoters

In addition to promotion of skin carcinogenesis by the phorbol esters, there are known or suspected promoters for tumors in other organs. Bile acids are known to be promoters of colon carcinogenesis in experimental animals. In humans, there is a strong association between high intake of dietary fat and cancer of the colon; since ingestion of fat increases the amount of bile acids in the colon, the increased colon cancer may be due to the promotion effect of the bile acids.

In rat bladder, saccharin and cyclamate are promoters for tumors after an initiating dose of methylnitrosourea; tryptophan is a promoter for urinary bladder tumors in dogs treated with an initiating dose of 4-aminobiphenyl or 2-naphthylamine.

Hormones are also known modifiers of chemical carcinogenesis. An oral or IV injection of dimethylbenzanthracene (DMBA) produces mammary tumors in susceptible female mice. Prolactin will increase tumor development, whereas animals in which the ovaries have been removed yield very few tumors.

6.3.1.2e Cocarcinogenesis

A cocarcinogen is an agent that is applied either just before or together with a carcinogen and results in significantly higher tumor yields than with the carcinogen alone. Sometimes promoters can also act as cocarcinogens. Cocarcinogenesis can result from such factors as hormones, viruses, immunological factors, nutritional factors, physical trauma, and skin abrasion. Several possible mechanisms by which cocarcinogens may affect the initiating process are summarized in Table 6.3.

Several cocarcinogens have been investigated in connection with tumors of the respiratory tract. Silicon dioxide dust in combination with benzo(a)pyrene is cocarcinogenic for carcinoma of the larynx, trachea, and lungs in experimental animals. Among uranium miners, uranium dust exposure has a synergistic effect on the formation of lung tumors among cigarette smokers. A similar effect occurs in connection with lung carcinoma among asbestos workers. An extensive study showed that, as compared with controls who neither smoked nor worked with asbestos, asbestos workers had a death rate from lung cancer

TABLE 6.3
Possible Mechanisms of Cocarcinogenesis

Increased cellular uptake of carcinogen
Increased proportion of carcinogen activated
Depletion of competing nucleophiles
Inhibition of DNA repair mechanisms
Enhanced conversion of DNA lesions to permanent alterations

Source: Williams, G. Modulation of chemical carcinogenesis by xenobiotics. Fund. Appl. Tox. 1984; 4:325–344. Used by permission.

that was five times higher. For smokers who were not asbestos workers, the rate was 11 times higher, but for asbestos workers who also smoked, it was 53 times higher.[1]

Hormones may also play an important role as modulators of carcinogenesis. For example, male rats are generally more susceptible to tumor induction by 2-AAF than are female rats. This is due in part to higher sulfotransferase activity in male rats, (Section 6.1.5.2). Activity can be depressed in castrated males by the administration of $17\text{-}\beta\text{-estradiol}$.

Tobacco smoke contains only relatively small amounts of genotoxic carcinogens such as polycyclic hydrocarbons and nitrosamines. Tobacco smoke also includes cocarcinogens and promoters in the form of catechol and other phenolic compounds, however. The cocarcinogenic and promotional factors in tobacco smoke are thought to play an important role in the overall induction of cancer in cigarette smokers.

The concepts of initiation, promotion, and cocarcinogenesis are extremely important because many chemicals that are structurally unrelated to known carcinogens and appear not to be carcinogenic may turn out to be promoters or cocarcinogens. In the future, hazard assessment may require testing for promotion activity of many substances that are currently believed to be harmless and that are not related to known classes of chemical carcinogens.

6.3.1.3   Genotoxic and Epigenetic Carcinogens

In the study of chemical carcinogenesis, two important ideas have evolved. First, many carcinogenic chemicals irreversibly alter cellular DNA, resulting in a heritable change; such chemicals are known as mutagens. Second, cancer formation is a multistep process, with the simplest model being that of initiation and promotion. In this multistep process, at least one step must involve a change in the DNA; the additional steps affect the growth and development of tumor cells. Thus, a carcinogen may be defined as any agent that induces neoplasms not usually observed, the earlier appearance of neoplasms, or a greater number of tumors. A proposed mechanistic classification of carcinogens by Williams (Table 6.4) categorizes carcinogenic agents into two main types, genotoxic and epigenetic.

Genotoxic chemicals are those that are capable of damaging or modifying DNA, whereas epigenetic carcinogens exert their oncogenic effect by means other than genotoxic action. This includes such indirect mechanisms as immunosuppression, hormonal imbalances, cytotoxicity, cocarcinogenic action, and promoting effects. The differences in chemical actions and mechanisms between the two types of carcinogens suggest that chemical reactivity and short-term tests for genetic effects could be used to distinguish genotoxic from epigenetic chemicals.

6.3.1.4   Activation of Carcinogens and Binding to Macromolecules

An important advance in understanding chemical carcinogenesis came from the investigations of Drs. Elizabeth and James Miller who demonstrated that

---

[1] Selikoff, I.J., et al. J. Am. Med. Assoc. 1968; 204:106.

TABLE 6.4
Classification of Carcinogens

Genotoxic carcinogens	Examples
Primary carcinogens (direct-acting)	Alkylating agents
Procarcinogens (require activation)	Benzo(a)pyrene
	Vinyl chloride
	Dimethylnitrosamine (DMN)
Inorganic	Nickel
	Chromium
Epigenetic carcinogens	
Solid state	Plastics, asbestos
Hormone	Estrogen, androgen
Immunosuppressor	Purine analog
Cocarcinogen	Phorbol ester
	Catechol
Promoter	Phorbol ester
	Bile acid
	Organochlorine compounds
	Saccharin, drugs

Source: Williams, G. Ann. N.Y. Acad. Sci. 1983a; 407:328–333. Used by permission.

many carcinogens are not intrinsically carcinogenic but require metabolic activation in order to express their carcinogenic potential. The Millers introduced the terms precarcinogen, proximate carcinogen, and ultimate carcinogen to describe the initial inactive compound, its more active products, and the product that is actually responsible for carcinogenesis. Not all carcinogens, however, require metabolic activation, and those compounds that do not are referred to as direct acting or primary carcinogens (Figure 6.12). Generally, these chemicals are extremely reactive or are converted nonenzymatically to reactive electrophilies. Frequently, direct-acting carcinogens cause tumors at the site of exposure. Such compounds are usually too reactive to pose an environmental problem.

Most chemical carcinogens do require metabolic activation in vivo to exert their carcinogenic action (see Section 6.1.1, Metabolic Activation). The reactive metabolites, or ultimate carcinogens, are strong electrophiles, such as carbonium and nitrenium ions. These chemicals can form covalent adducts nonenzymatically with a wide variety of nucleophilic sites in cellular macromolecules such as peptides, proteins, RNA, and DNA. Binding to proteins, because of their relative abundance in cells, is usually the major macromolecular interaction of carcinogens. Electrophilic carcinogens also bind to nucleic acids, and this covalent binding to DNA is considered the critical reaction of genotoxic carcinogens in the initiation of tumor formation.

Such electrophiles attack nucleophilic oxygen as well as nitrogen atoms of the DNA bases. The most reactive groups in adenine, guanine, cytosine, and thymine (the four bases of DNA) are the N-7 of guanine, and N-3 and N-7 of adenine. In addition to these sites, chemical carcinogens also interact to a lesser extent at several other positions in the purine and pyrimidine bases of DNA. (See Section 6.3.2, Mutagenesis).

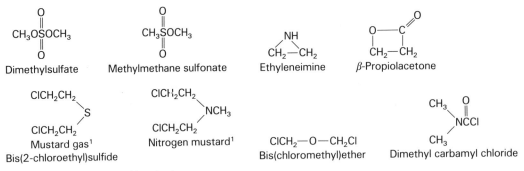

FIGURE 6.12.
Structures of some primary carcinogens.

The mechanism by which this interaction with DNA brings about carcinogenesis is unknown but may involve activation of cellular oncogenes. Because the transformation of a normal cell into a neoplastic one involves a permanent, heritable change that is passed on to daughter cells, it is not surprising that cancer has historically been suspected of arising as a result of mutation.

6.3.1.5 DNA Repair

Experimental and clinical evidence indicates that the development of cancer following exposure to chemical carcinogens is a relatively rare event. In part, this can be explained by the cell's ability to recognize and repair damaged DNA (excision repair). The DNA region containing the adduct is removed, and a new area of DNA is synthesized, using the opposite intact strand as a template. The new segment is then spliced into the DNA molecule in place of the defective one. To be effective in restoring the cell to normal, DNA repair must occur prior to cell division. If repair is not complete before DNA replication, the presence of the adducts can give rise to mispairing of bases and probably other genetic effects such as rearrangements and translocations of segments of DNA. Thus, an agent that alters the repair process or the rate of cell division can itself affect the frequency of neoplastic transformation.

Clinical studies have shown that persons with an impaired ability to repair damaged DNA frequently develop cancers at an early age. In one syndrome, xeroderma pigmentosum, the person is unable to excise thymine dimers induced by ultraviolet (UV) light from the sun. These people are extremely sensitive to sunlight, and their incidence of skin cancer is nearly 100% by early adulthood.

Agents that promote cell proliferation can enhance carcinogenesis, presumably because the time available for repair of DNA damage is shortened. Increased cell proliferation may account in part for the cocarcinogenicity of some compounds such as ferric oxide and asbestos in lung cancer and mycotoxins in chronic hepatitis and liver carcinogenesis.

6.3.1.6 Radiation Carcinogenesis

The effects of ionizing radiations on cells are initiated by the absorption of energy sufficient to expel electrons from molecules, resulting in the formation of positively charged ions. The expelled electrons react with nearby molecules, forming negatively charged ions. Because water is the principle component of the cell, it absorbs most of the ionizing radiation, forming free radicals that then can react with each other, with other water molecules, or with macromolecules within the cell. These "active" oxygen molecules such as superoxide, hydroperoxy radical, hydroxyl radical, and hydrogen peroxide, cause general oxidative damage to cellular macromolecules, including DNA. Ionizing radiation has been known to be mutagenic and carcinogenic for many years.

6.3.1.7 Oncogenes and a Common Pathway

Oncogenes are genes that, when activated in cells, can transform the cells from normal to cancerous. Sometimes oncogenes are carried into normal cells by infecting viruses, particularly RNA viruses, or retroviruses. In some cases, however, the oncogene is already present in the normal human cell, and it needs only a mutation or other activating event to change it from a harmless, and possibly essential gene, called a proto-oncogene, into a cancer-producing gene. More than 30 oncogenes have now been identified in humans; however, not all the oncogenes bring about cell transformation in the same way. At least three distinct classes of oncogenes have been recognized, and a fourth class includes oncogenes that do not seem to fit into any of the first three classes.

Infection of cells by oncogenic viruses results in the physical integration of virus-specific genetic information into the DNA of host cells. In the case of DNA tumor viruses, the viral genome is integrated directly into the host DNA, whereas that of the RNA viruses is first transcribed into DNA by the enzyme RNA-dependent polymerase, and the corresponding viral DNA is then integrated. With both DNA and RNA viruses, transformation of the host cell appears to depend on certain viral genes, called transformation genes, and the production of specific gene products.

DNA sequences identical to those of many viral oncogenes have been identified as constituents of the normal cellular DNA from a wide variety of species including birds, fish, mammals, and humans. The apparently wide distribution and conservation of viral oncogene sequences in normal cellular DNA has led to the suggestion that perhaps retrovirus oncogenes have extracted cellular genes and, after acquiring them, have activated the sequence to give rise to cancer-forming genes.

Inactive oncogenes (proto-oncogenes) are postulated to be normal genetic constituents of many if not all cells. Their high degree of conservation suggests that they may have important functions during embryogenesis and perhaps during certain periods of adult life. For example, one cellular oncogene that is expressed during regeneration of normal rat liver cells is turned off when regeneration ceases.

The various means by which inactive cellular oncogenes are turned on during oncogenesis and how these genes effect cell transformation is still not understood. Some preliminary insights are emerging, however. For example, the c-*src* gene is functional in normal cells and produces minute amounts of *src*-protein, a protein identical to that produced by viral *src* gene of the Rous sarcoma virus. Apparently, this protein is necessary for cellular transformation. Because cells infected with the retrovirus produce tenfold or more *src* protein than do noninfected cells, it is thought that neoplastic transformation may be mediated by production of excessive amounts of *src* protein. This increase in protein production in malignant cells may be related to a dysfunction of a repressor–operator complex in the gene which controls the level of *src* protein synthesis.

With other oncogene products, it appears that the formation of an abnormal protein may be a critical factor in tumor formation. In the case of bladder epithelial cells, a relatively minor change in the bases of the DNA of a normal cellular proto-oncogene is sufficient to change the gene to an oncogene. In this case, the mutation does not increase the level of the protein produced by the gene, but instead changes the structure of the protein.

Such minute base changes are precisely what occurs when chemicals or ionizing radiation induce mutations in DNA. The potential for neoplastic behavior appears to exist in all cells and needs to be activated either directly by a mutation of the cellular oncogene itself, or of a nearby regulatory gene that normally keeps the oncogene at a low level of activity or even completely shut down. In other cases, the mutation may lead to the synthesis of an abnormal gene protein.

6.3.2 Mutagenesis

6.3.2.1 Introduction

Mutations are hereditary changes produced in the genetic information stored in the DNA in all cells. Various physical and chemical agents known to produce such alterations include ionizing radiation, sulphur and nitrogen mustards, epoxides, ethyleneimine, and methylsulfonate.

Such alterations in DNA are not necessarily harmful, since mutations are the building blocks for evolutionary change and enable the species to adapt to a changing environment. The danger is that mutations are undirected, and the effects on the individual organism are usually negative. The harmful effects of mutations include fertility disorders, embryonic and perinatal death, malformations, hereditary diseases, and cancers. A goal of toxicologists working in this area is to minimize human exposure to exogenous mutagens in order to avoid adding to the existing "genetic load."

In general, the alterations in the genetic material can be divided into two categories: (1) point mutations, which involve a change in a single base such as base-pair exchange or addition or deletion of a base; and (2) chromosomal aberrations such as gaps, breaks, translocations, and changes in the number of chromosomes.

6.3.2.2 Point Mutations: Base-Pair Transformation

The smallest unit of mutation is the transformation of a single base-pair and is called a point mutation. If the replacement involves the same type of base — for example, purine to purine, or pyrimidine to pyrimidine — the mutation is called a base-pair transition. If the change is a purine to pyrimidine replacement, it is termed a base-pair transversion. These point mutations can occur in at least three ways: by chemical modification, by incorporation of abnormal base analogs into DNA, and by alkylating agents.

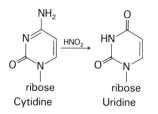

FIGURE 6.13.
Deamination of cytidine to uridine by the action of nitrous acid.

6.3.2.2a Chemical Transformation

An example of chemical transformation of bases is that caused by nitrous acid, HNO_2, which results in the transformation of cytosine to uracil or adenine to hypoxanthine (Figure 6.13). Nitrous acid is known to be mutagenic in phage, bacteria, and fungi. In humans, however, the greater risk is the potential carcinogenicity of nitroso compounds formed by the reaction of nitrites with organic compounds in the acid conditions prevailing in the stomach.

6.3.2.2b Incorporation of Abnormal Base Analogs

Most of the chemicals active in this respect were developed as drugs for cancer therapy and owe their effectiveness to their ability to produce lethal mutations in rapidly dividing cancer cells. Some examples of base analogs are 5-bromouracil, 5-fluorodeoxyuridine, 2-aminopurine, and 6-mercaptopurine. The effect of incorporation of abnormal bases and the resulting base transformations is illustrated with 5-bromouracil (Figure 6.14).

6.3.2.2c Alkylating Agents

Alkylating agents are chemicals that can add alkyl groups to DNA. These chemicals yield positively charged carbonium ions (eg, CH_3^+) that combine with the electron-rich bases in the DNA. This is an example of an electrophilic–nucleophilic interaction. Some examples of alkylating agents are shown in Figure 6.15 and the reaction of dimethylnitrosamine to form a DNA adduct is illustrated in Figure 6.16. Alkylation of DNA results both in mispairing of bases and in chromosome breaks.

Adenine can be alkylated at three ring nitrogens: N-1, N-3, or N-7; guanine

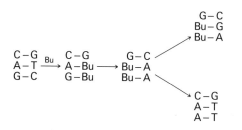

FIGURE 6.14.
Replication of a nucleic acid in the presence of the base analog bromouracil (Bu). This analog will pair with both adenine and guanine. In this case, the result is a transition of G–C to A–T.

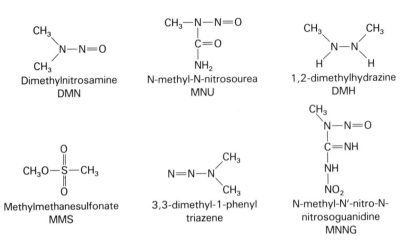

FIGURE 6.15.
Structures of some simple alkylation carcinogens.

can undergo alkylation at either N-3, N-7, or O-6 (Figure 6.17). Cytosine can be alkylated at N-3 and O-2, and thymine can be alkylated at N-3, O-2, and O-4. In addition to alkylation of the purine and pyrimidine bases, the phosphates in the DNA may also undergo alkylation. Although the most frequent site of alkylation is the N-7 of guanine, alkylation at the O-6 position of guanine has most frequently been associated with the mispairing of bases and induction of cancer.

6.3.2.3 Frameshift Mutations

Addition or deletion of a base in the DNA molecule puts the triplet code out of sequence and results in what is known as a frameshift mutation (Figure 6.18). If the addition of another base follows in close proximity to a deletion, the production of functional or partially functional proteins may occur. Some chemicals, such as acridine, are known to induce frameshifts. In addition, errors occurring during chromatid crossover may also lead to frameshift mutations.

6.3.2.4 DNA Repair

Enzymes that are able to correct or repair many of the mutations that have occurred to the original DNA molecule exist within the cells (Section 6.3.1.5).

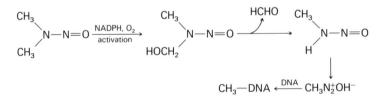

FIGURE 6.16.
Generation of a methylating agent from dimethylnitrosoamine (DMN). The first step requires metabolic activation to form a highly reactive intermediate that combines nonenzymatically with DNA.

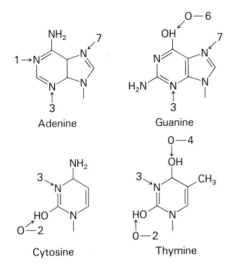

FIGURE 6.17.
Sites of alkylation of DNA under physiological conditions.

Consequently, fewer mutations are retained in the replicated DNA molecules than occur originally. If the mutation is not recognized and repaired, the incorrect information may be transcribed into RNA, and the mutation is expressed as an altered protein. The change may be critical or insignificant depending on the position of the amino acid or the amount and function of the protein affected. It is also possible that the mutations may lead to an improvement in the gene product.

The protein that repairs O^6-methylguanine is a methyltransferase that removes the methyl group and restores the DNA structure in a single step. Other enzymes that repair DNA are glycosylases which split the bond between the N-9 position of the purine and the deoxyribose forming an apurinic site in the DNA. These sites and those generated by spontaneous hydrolysis of methylated bases are then restored by the action of an endonuclease that breaks the DNA chain, excising 3–4 nucleotides, including the damaged site. Subsequently, the gap is filled by nucleotide polymerization by DNA polymerase, followed by closing of the strand by DNA ligase.

AC$\boxed{A}$	AAG	AGU	CCA	UCA
threonine	lysine	serine	provaline	serine

		↓	
ACA	AGA	GUC	CAU
threonine	lysine	serine	histidine

FIGURE 6.18.
Formation of frameshift mutations by addition or deletion of a base in DNA. Deletion of the base adenine (A) shifts the reading of the triplet code so that different amino acids are coded for. In a long-chain protein produced from such a template, substantial errors may occur.

6.3.2.5 Chromosome Aberrations

The term clastogenesis is used to refer to the process resulting in additions, deletions, or rearrangements of parts of the chromosomes that are detectable by light microscopy. Gaps, which are achromatic lesions in a chromosome, may vary in length and are thought to be due to loss of DNA. Breaks are broken ends of chromatids that are dislocated but still contained within the metaphase. Several genetic diseases such as Bloom's syndrome and Falconi's anemia are correlated with chromosomal breaks, but it is uncertain whether the breaks are a cause or a symptom of the disease. Many chemicals, as well as ionizing radiation, can cause breakage of chromosomes. Alkylating agents, especially bifunctional chemicals, may cause breaks by cross-linking with DNA.

Chromosomal mutations refer to changes in chromosomes that arise from incorrect reincorporation of broken parts. The main types of change are deletions, translocations, duplications, and inversions. Deletions and translocations are relatively easy to detect by microscopy and assume more importance in practical mutagenicity testing.

Numerical aberrations are a consequence of unequal division of chromosomes and result in a cell with either more or fewer chromosomes than normal. Such cells may or may not be viable. Several genetic diseases are a result of the unequal division (nondisjunction) of chromosomes. Down's syndrome (mongolism) is associated with a trisomy of chromosome 21, and the condition is characterized by small flattened skull, short, flat-bridged nose, short phalanges, and moderate to severe mental retardation. Two disorders related to nondisjunction of the sex chromosomes are Klinefelter's syndrome (XXY), characterized by small testes with fibrosis and hyalinization of the seminiferous tubules and impairment of function, and Turner's syndrome (XO), characterized by short stature, undifferentiated gonads, and variable abnormalities, include low posterior hairline and cardiac defects.

Several chemicals are known to induce polyploidy. The best known examples are the metaphase poisons, such as colchicine, a specific spindle poison, which binds to the spindle protein tubulin and inhibits its polymerization. Thus, colchicine stops mitosis at metaphase, leaving the cell with the doubled quantity of chromosomal material, resulting in a polyploid cell. Other compounds that can cause similar effects are the vinca alkaloids, vincristine and vinblastine, and podophyllotoxin, which binds to the same site as colchicine. Polyploidy is well known in plants and is used extensively in plant breeding; however, polyploidy in animals is not as viable and is generally a lethal mutation.

6.3.2.6 Relationship of Mutagenesis to Carcinogenesis

A large body of work on chemical carcinogenesis has now demonstrated that the carcinogenic potency of a compound is correlated with its mutagenic ability, suggesting that DNA is the ultimate target of carcinogenic initiation (Sections 6.3.1.2a, 6.3.1.3 and 6.3.1.4). In recent years, many chemicals known to be carcinogenic have been found to be mutagenic as well; likewise, many known mutagens have been found to be carcinogenic. Because of the high correlation of mutagenicity of chemicals to carcinogenic potential, the testing of chemicals as mutagens has now become an important screening tool in assessing potential carcinogenic risk of compounds (see Section 8.6).

6.3.3 Teratogenesis

6.3.3.1 Introduction

The word teratogenesis literally means the production of a monstrous or mis-shapen organism and comes from the Greek teras, teratos meaning monster or marvel. At different times in the past and in various cultures, the appearance of unusual or deformed infants was attributed to causes such as hybridization between humans and gods or humans and demons. Among the ancient Greeks and Romans, there was a tendency to consider monstrous infants divine, and some mythological figures appear to have been derived from terata. At other times, such as in Europe during the fifteenth and sixteenth centuries, malformations were believed to be the result of association with demons, witches, or other evil creatures, and both the infant and mother were put to death.

Modern experimental teratology gained impetus in the 1940s with the work of Warknay and his colleagues, who demonstrated that environmental factors such as maternal dietary deficiencies and irradiation could affect the intrauterine growth and development of mammals. Earlier studies with fish, amphibians, and chick embryos had shown them to be very susceptible to adverse conditions, but it was not generally believed that mammals were as vulnerable. Rather, it was widely believed that the mother and ultimately the placenta provided an effective barrier to environmental factors, and that most aspects of normal as well as abnormal development were genetically determined.

In the 1920s accounts were published of pregnant women who had been exposed to ionizing radiation and who later gave birth to children with central nervous system and skeletal defects. In 1941, Gregg reported the association of maternal rubella (German measles) infection with death, blindness, and deafness among their offspring. Neither of these reports nor the experiments of Warknay, however, aroused much concern that other extrinsic agents might pose a risk to the developing human fetus.

Then, in the late 1950s and early 1960s, the concept of the placental barrier was shattered when thousands of severely malformed infants were born to women who had been taking the presumably harmless sedative thalidomide during their pregnancy. This incident vividly called attention to the fact that human and other mammalian embryos can be highly vulnerable to certain environmental agents, even though these have either negligible or no maternal effects.

6.3.3.2 General Principles of Teratology

As the study of teratology has expanded, some important generalizations have emerged, been accepted, and modified. At least six generalizations have been defined by Wilson and Fraser (1977) as principles of teratology.

6.3.3.2a Genetic Factors/Influences

Susceptibility to teratogens depends on the genotype of the organism, including species as well as strain differences. This variation in response may be due in part to differences in maternal metabolism, distribution, or transplacental passage of the compound that results in differential exposure to the ultimate teratogenic agent. For example, rabbits and mice are very susceptible to cleft palate induction by cortisone, whereas rats are not. Thalidomide is another teratogen that is very species specific; humans, certain higher primates (macaque monkeys, baboons, and marmosets) and certain white rabbit strains are extremely sensitive to the effects of thalidomide, whereas most other mammals are quite resistant, with only some strains of rats and mice reacting to large doses that must be administered at a very specific time.

6.3.3.2b   Critical Periods

The complex process of embryogenesis involves cell proliferation, differentiation, migration, and finally organogenesis, all of which must occur in a precisely timed sequence. The first 2 weeks in human embryonic development is a time of rapid cell proliferation. After fertilization, the cells divide rapidly, forming the blastocyst, with very little morphologic differentiation occurring at this time, except that some cells are on the surface and some are internal. Very few specific teratogenic effects are known to occur at this time, the major effect being death of the embryo due to substantial damage to undifferentiated cells.

The time of greatest susceptibility to teratogens, as far as the induction of gross anatomic defects, occurs during the period of germ-layer formation and organogenesis (Figure 6.19). The time span of organ development varies among species (Table 6.5); in all species, however, organogenesis is the period between germ-layer differentiation and completion of major organ formation. The type of teratogenic response is determined by the developmental stage of the fetus at the time of exposure, ie, there are "critical periods" for different malformations of organ systems. Because the early events in organ formation are the most sensitive, during testing the teratogen is administered during or just prior to the development of that organ.

Histogenesis and functional development generally begin before organogenesis is completed and continue into the subsequent growth phases. Adverse influences at this time do not usually result in gross malformations but can result in functional abnormalities. This type of physiological or biochemical defect may be manifested only by growth retardation or, more seriously, the defect may result in fetal death due to interference with some critical biological function.

6.3.3.2c   Initiating Mechanisms

The literature on experimental teratogenesis shows that many different types of compounds frequently cause similar abnormalities if they are administered during the same critical period. This observation has lead to the proposal that teratogenic agents are able to initiate abnormal developments by a number of mechanisms (Section 6.3.3.3 and Figure 6.20). The teratogenic agent initiates one or more of these mechanisms, resulting in abnormal embryogenesis. This in turn leads to pathways that seem to be characterized by too few cells or cell products for normal morphogenesis or functional development. This cell death or tissue necrosis is one of the most frequent signs of chemical or physical damage to the developing embryo. Although cell death above normal physio-

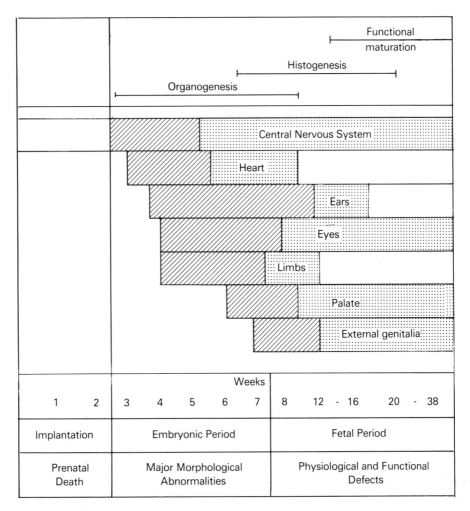

FIGURE 6.19.
Sequence of events in human development showing sensitive periods for developmental defects. Dark areas, most sensitive times; lighter areas, less sensitive times.

TABLE 6.5
Comparison of Gestation in Several Species

| Species | Number of Days After Conception | | |
	Implantation	Embryonic Period[a]	Fetal Period
Human	6–7	20–56	56–280
Rabbit	7–8	8–16	17–32
Rat	6–8	9–17	18–22
Mouse	4–6	7–16	17–20

[a] Period of organogenesis and greatest teratogenic risk.

Initial change ⟶ Pathogenesis ⟶ Common pathways ⟶ Final defect

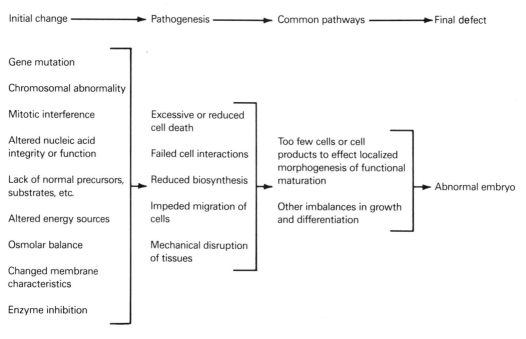

FIGURE 6.20.
Successive stages in the formation of a development defect, beginning with the initial changes in the developing cells or tissues (the mechanism) and continuing to the final defect. *Source:* Adapted from Wilson, J.G., and Fraser, F.C., eds., Current status of teratology, in Handbook of Teratology. New York: Plenum Press, 1977.

logical levels does not inevitably lead to malformation, if a critical mass of cells is destroyed, there may be too few cells or cell products to effect localized morphogenesis or functional developments.

6.3.3.2d Consequences of Abnormal Development

There are four manifestations of abnormal development: death, malformation, growth retardation, and functional disorder. Prior to differentiation, the embryo is not usually damaged by most agents; however, a sufficiently high dosage frequently results in death of the embryo. Xenobiotics that are embryotoxic are not usually called teratogens, but if administered at a lower dose or at a different time period, they may be teratogenic. The time of organogenesis is the most sensitive time for induction of specific malformations, whereas structural defects at the tissue level or functional deficits are most likely to occur when damage occurs during the fetal period. Structural defects are usually considered the main criterion in estimating teratological risks since they are more obvious; however, functional disorders may be as incapacitating and result in as great a mortality rate among offspring as morphologic abnormalities.

6.3.3.2e Access to Embryo and Fetus

Only a few agents, such as radiation or ultrasound, pass directly through the maternal tissue. For chemical compounds and their metabolites, the route of access is by way of the maternal body through fluids surrounding the embryo or by way of the blood after formation of the placenta. Prior to the thalidomide disaster, it was commonly believed that the placental barrier protected the fetus from drugs given to the mother. It is now known, however, that many pharmacologic substances and other chemicals can readily pass from the maternal blood to the fetal blood. Generally, most unbound compounds with a molecular weight of < 600 and a low ionic charge will readily pass through the placenta by simple diffusion. The chemical half-life of a compound determines whether it can travel from its site of metabolism, usually the maternal liver, to the embryonic tissue; very reactive intermediates will be unstable and react at the site of formation. Other compounds, however, may pass through the maternal blood and be activated by fetoplacental tissue.

6.3.3.2f Dose–Response Relationship

Most teratogens appear to have a threshold or "no-effect" level below which no malformations are observable. Abnormal development frequently seems to depend on the destruction of a critical number of cells above that level which the embryo can restore quickly; destruction of less than this critical mass by a low or moderate dose of teratogen produces no persistent effect, whereas destruction of an excessive number results in fetal death.

6.3.3.3 Teratogenic Mechanisms

Because the initiating events of abnormal development usually occur at the subcellular or molecular level, the damage is not readily detected until cell death, morphologic damage, or functional disability is observed. As summarized in Figure 6.20, probably eight to ten mechanisms are responsible for the initial molecular damage.

6.3.3.3a Mutation

It has been estimated that some 20–30% of human developmental errors are due to mutations in the germ cells; such changes are hereditary. If the mutations occur in somatic cells, the alteration will be transmitted to all descendants of that cell, but it will not become an inherited change. Somatic mutations in the early embryo may affect enough cells to produce a structural or functional defect, however. Mutagens include such agents as ionizing radiation, chemicals such as nitrous acid, alkylating agents, most carcinogens, and agents that interfere with normal DNA repair mechanisms (see Section 6.3.2, Mutagenesis).

6.3.3.3b Chromosomal Abnormalities

Chromosomal abnormalities, such as excess of chromosomes, deficiencies, and rearrangements result from nondisjunction or breaks in the chromosomes. These abnormalities probably account for $< 3\%$ of human developmental errors, probably because an excess or deficiency of chromosomal material is usually lethal, the exception being an excess or deficiency of sex chromosomes. Advanced maternal age is known to be a factor in nondisjunction of germ cells, as is aging of germ cells in the genital tract prior to fertilization. Other causes of chromosomal abnormalities include viral infection, irradiation, and chemical agents.

6.3.3.3c Mitotic Interference

Certain "cytotoxic" chemicals, such as hydroxyurea, or irradiation are known to slow or arrest DNA synthesis, thereby inhibiting mitosis. Other chemicals, such as colchicine and vincristine, interfere with spindle formation and prevent the chromosomes from separating at anaphase. The resulting tetraploid cells usually lead to fetotoxicity. Still other agents such as irradiation or radiomimetic chemicals lead to "stickiness" or "bridges" between chromatids, which prevents proper separation of chromosomes.

6.3.3.3d Interference with Nucleic Acid Function

Many antibiotics and antineoplastic drugs are teratogenic by interfering with nucleic acid replication, transcription, or RNA translation. They include cytotoxic chemicals such as cytosine arabinoside, which inhibits DNA polymerase, and 6-mercaptopurine, which blocks incorporation of adenine and guanine into DNA. Agents that block protein synthesis are generally embryolethal above the no-effect dose; ie, at lower doses some growth retardation occurs, but at higher doses significant blockage of protein synthesis leads to death of the embryo rather than malformation.

6.3.3.3e Nutritional Deficiencies

The lack of precursors or substrates is a well-established mechanism of teratogenesis. Specific dietary deficiencies, especially of vitamins and minerals, are known to be growth inhibiting, teratogenic, and embryolethal. Embryos frequently show teratogenic symptoms before the mother shows signs of deficiencies, contrary to the widespread belief that the embryo will receive nutrients at the mother's expense. A disease in lambs known as "swayback," investigated in western Australia, was found to be primarily due to copper deficiency in pregnant sheep. The disease is characterized by paralysis of the hind limbs, lack of coordination and, in some cases, blindness. The disease can be prevented by giving copper supplements to pregnant ewes.

Endemic cretinism, characterized by mental and physical retardation, potbelly, large tongue, and facial characteristics similar to those of Down's syndrome, occurs in areas where the iodine content of the soil is extremely low. The incidence of cretinism is almost eliminated by addition of iodine to the diet in the form of iodized salt.

Deficiencies can also occur in the presence of analogs or antagonists to vitamins, amino acids, or nucleic acids, which may result in the utilization of the abnormal metabolites in biosynthesis. Other causes of deficiencies may include failure of materials to be absorbed from the maternal digestive system, as with excess zinc or sulfate preventing adequate copper absorption, or the failure of placental transport of essential metabolites as in the teratogenic action of azo dyes in rodents and rabbits, which are dependent for early placental transport of nutrients on the inverted yolk sac placenta.

6.3.3.3f Deficient or Altered Energy Supply

The growth of the embryo requires high levels of energy, and factors that interfere with the energy supply are associated with teratogenesis. These are known to include inadequate glucose supply (dietary deficiency, induced hypoglycemia), interference with glycolysis (iodoacetate, 6-aminonicotinamide), inhibition of the citric acid cycle (riboflavin deficiency, 6-aminonicotinamide), and blockage of the terminal electron transport system (hypoxia, cyanide, dinitrophenol). See Section 6.2 for discussion of these mechanisms.

6.3.3.3g Changes in Osmolarity

Abnormal fluid accumulations are known to cause tissue distortions sufficient to lead to malformations. For example, hypoxia in chick embryos leads to edema, hematomas, and blisters, which subsequently give rise to abnormal embryogenesis in eye, brain, and limbs. Agents such as trypan blue, hypertonic solutions, and adrenal hormones are also known to give rise to this "edema syndrome" and resulting malformations.

6.3.3.3h Ultrastructural Changes in Cell Membrane

Altered membrane permeability can lead to osmolar imbalance and result in changes such as those previously described. It has been suggested that agents such as the solvent dimethylsulfoxide (DMSO) and excess vitamin A act in this way.

6.3.3.3i Enzyme Inhibition

Chemicals that inhibit enzymes, especially those involved in intermediary metabolism, are able to alter fetal growth and development. Other agents are known to be mutagenic and teratogenic agents by inhibiting DNA repair enzymes or by inhibiting polymerases necessary for formation of the mitotic spindle. Some enzyme inhibitors thought to be involved in teratogenesis are: 5-fluorouracil, an inhibitor of thymidylate synthetase; hydroxyurea, an inhibitor of ribonucleoside diphosphate reductase; and cytosine arabinoside, an inhibitor of DNA polymerase.

6.3.3.4 Human Teratogenesis: Some Specific Examples

In terms of human developmental abnormality, about 3–7% of human babies are born with malformations serious enough to require treatment. Etiologically, these can be divided into several categories: genetic causes (mutant gene), chromosomal abnormalities, environmental agents, multifactorial causes, and unknown. These causes are summarized in Table 6.6.

6.3.3.4a Folic Acid Antagonists

Folic acid antagonists (aminopterin), which had been shown to be embryolethal in laboratory animals, were developed as abortifacients to be used for therapeutic abortions. In the trial tests, not all of the fetuses were aborted, and most of those that survived (about 30%) were malformed, being born with hydrocephalus, absent or ossified skull bones, palate defects, and anomalies of the extremities.

6.3.3.4b Androgenic Hormones

Progesterone and synthetic progesterones, which were used to treat breast cancers, to prevent spontaneous abortions, and to control bleeding during

TABLE 6.6
Causes of Human Developmental Defects

Cause		Percent of Defects
Known genetic transmission		20
Chromosomal aberration		3–5
Environmental		
Ionizing radiations		<1
Therapeutic	Nuclear	
Infections		2–3
Rubella virus	Varicella virus(?)	
Cytomegalovirus	Toxoplasma	
Herpes virus hominis	Syphilis	
Maternal metabolic imbalance		1–2
Endemic cretinism	Phenylketonuria	
Diabetes	Virilizing tumors	
Drug and environmental chemicals		4–5
Androgenic hormone	Alcohol	
Folic antagonists	Anticonvulsants	
Thalidomide	Oral hypoglycemics(?)	
Oral anticoagulants	Organic mercury	
Combinations and interactions		
Unknown		65–70

Estimates based on surveys and case reports in the medical literature.
Source: Wilson, J.G. Embryotoxicity of drugs in man. In Handbook of Teratology. Vol. 1. 1977. Plenum Press, New York. Used by permission.

pregnancy led to the birth of a number of masculinized female fetuses. This masculinization was due to the androgenic activity of many of the synthetic progestins.

6.3.3.4c Thalidomide
Thalidomide, one of the most potent human teratogens known, was introduced as a sedative-tranquilizer in West Germany, England, and some other European countries in the early 1960s. The drug was effective in producing a teratogenic effect even if taken on only a single day any time from the third to the seventh week of pregnancy. The most pronounced defect was phocomelia—shortening or complete absence of limbs. Altogether, > 10,000 cases were seen before the drug was withdrawn. The drug was never approved for use in the United States. Thalidomide is very species specific: humans show teratogenic effect at doses as low as 0.5–1.0 mg/kg, whereas there is no or very little effect in most mouse or rat strains at doses as high as 4,000 mg/kg. The only animals showing similar responses to humans are certain strains of rabbits and some species of monkeys, baboons, and marmosets.

6.3.3.4d Alcohol
Suspicion that alcohol possessed teratogenic potential stretches back many centuries. During the eighteenth century, England was the scene of what was

called the "gin epidemic" as a result of very cheap readily available gin. In 1736, a report was submitted to Parliament:

> The contagion has spread even to the female sex. Unhappy mothers habituate themselves to these distilled liquors, whose children are born weak and sickly, and often look shrivel'd and old as though they had numbered many years.

Only recently, however, has the direct involvement of alcohol in abnormal fetal development been firmly established. Fetal alcohol syndrome (FAS) refers to a pattern of defects in children born to alcoholic women. For a diagnosis of FAS to be made, there are three criteria: (1) prenatal or postnatal growth retardation; (2) characteristic facial anomalies (microcephaly, small eye opening, thinned upper lip); and (3) central nervous system dysfunction (mental retardation, developmental delays).

If only one or two of these criteria are met, a diagnosis of possible FAS, or fetal alcohol effects (FAE) may be made if the mother is suspected of drinking during pregnancy. Prenatal alcohol exposure is suspected of causing a broad spectrum of effects ranging from barely perceptible effects to FAS and spontaneous abortion. One important unanswered question is why some alcoholic women give birth to children with FAS whereas other women who drink the same amount do not.

The overall incidence of FAS among the general population is relatively low; estimates range between 0.4 and 3.1 per 1,000; however, if patients showing FAE are included, the incidence is much higher.

Although there is little doubt that alcohol is a teratogen, the mechanism by which its effects are produced is not known. One of the most likely ways appears to be induced hypoxia to the embryo or fetus, although other mechanisms such as direct toxicity of alcohol or acetaldehyde may also be contributing factors.

6.3.3.4e Methyl Mercury

Methyl mercury is one of the few environmental contaminants that has been established as embryotoxic in humans. Between 1954 and 1960, at Minamata Bay and elsewhere in Japan, many infants were born with severe neurological symptoms resembling cerebral palsy. Fetal Minamata disease was traced to the consumption of mercury-contaminated fish by the mothers.

6.3.3.4f Infectious Diseases

Gregg, in 1941, first recognized the association between maternal rubella infection (German measles) and infant cataracts. Additional malformations caused by the virus are now known to include eye abnormalities, deafness, cardiac defects, and mental retardation. An epidemic of rubella in 1971 resulted in the birth of > 20,000 defective children. Other viruses, such as cytomegalovirus (CMV) and herpes simplex, are also known to cause central nervous system defects.

Syphilis during pregnancy is also known to lead to malformations, including hydrocephalus, seizure, and mental retardation due to direct invasion and destruction of fetal tissue by the spirochete, causing syphilis palladiura.

6.3.3.4g Transplacental Carcinogenesis

Transplacental carcinogenesis is the induction of cancer in the offspring resulting from the exposure of the pregnant female to the teratogenic agent. The best known example is the appearance of vaginal cancer in females born to mothers given the drug diethylstibestrol (DES) during pregnancy to prevent spontaneous abortion. The carcinogenicity of DES was first recognized because of the occurrence of an unusual type of vaginal adenocarcinoma in young women between 15 and 22 years of age instead of the expected postmenopausal age. The stilbestrols were in widespread use between 1950 and 1970; by 1976, > 400 cases of DES-related carcinoma of the vagina and cervix had been recorded.

One of the critical questions in terms of human teratogenic risks is whether pregnancy can be recognized soon enough to avoid exposure to potentially damaging agents. Because organogenesis begins about day 20, many women may be unaware that they are pregnant, especially teenaged women with irregular menstrual cycles.

6.3.4 Organ Toxicity

6.3.4.1 Hepatotoxicity

6.3.4.1a Susceptibility of Liver

The liver, the largest organ in the body, is often the target organ for chemically induced injuries, and several important factors are known to contribute to the liver's susceptibility. First, most xenobiotics enter the body through the GI tract and, after absorption, are transported by the hepatic portal vein to the liver; thus, the liver is the first organ perfused by chemicals absorbed in the gut. A second factor is a high concentration in the liver of xenobiotic-metabolizing enzymes, primarily, the cytochrome P-450–dependent monooxygenase system. Although most biotransformations are detoxication reactions, many oxidative reactions produce reactive metabolites (Section 6.1) that can induce lesions within the liver. Often areas of damage are in the centrilobular region, and this localization has been attributed to the higher concentration of cytochrome P-450 in that area of the liver.

6.3.4.1b Types of Liver Injury

FATTY LIVER.   Some agents that produce liver injury cause an abnormal accumulation of fats, mainly triglycerides, in the parenchymal cells (Table 6.7). Although many toxicants cause lipid accumulation in the liver, the mechanisms may differ. Excess lipid can result from oversupply of free fatty acids from adipose tissues, or more commonly, from impaired release of triglycerides from the liver into the plasma. Triglycerides are secreted from the liver as lipoproteins (VLDL, very-low-density lipoprotein), and a number of factors may affect this reaction:

1. Interference with synthesis of the protein moiety;
2. Impaired conjugation of triglyceride with lipoprotein;
3. Interference with transfer of VLDL across cell membranes, eg, K^+ loss from hepatocytes;
4. Decreased synthesis of phospholipids;
5. Impaired oxidation of lipids by mitochondria.

TABLE 6.7
Some Examples of Hepatotoxic Agents and Associated Liver Injury

Necrosis and Fatty Liver
Carbon tetrachloride	Acetaminophen
Chloroform	Dimethylnitrosamine
Trichloroethylene	Tannic acid[a]
Tetrachloroethylene	Mitomycin[b]
Bromobenzene[a]	Puromycin
Thioacetamide[a]	Phosphorous
Pyrrolizidine alkaloids	Beryllium[a]
Aflatoxin	Allyl alcohol[a]
Ethionine[b]	Galactosamine
Cycloheximide[b]	Azaserine
Tetracycline[b]	

Cholestasis (drug-induced)
Chlorpromazine	Mestranol
Promazine	Estradiol
Thioridazine	Carbarsone
Mepazine	Chlorthiazide
Amitriptyline	Methimazole
Imipramine	Sulfanilamide
Diazepam	Phenindione
Methandrolone	

Hepatitis (drug-induced)
Iproniazid	Phenyl butazone
Isoniazid	Cholchicine
Imipramine	Halothane
6-Mercaptopurine	Zoxazolamine
Methoxyfluorane	Indomethacin
Papaverine	Methyldopa

Carcinogenesis (in experimental animals)
Aflatoxin B_1	Dialkyl nitrosamines
Pyrrolizidine alkaloids	Polychlorinated biphenyls
Cycasin	Vinyl chloride
Safrole	Acetylaminofluorene
Dimethylbenzanthracene	Urethane

[a] Primary effect is necrosis.
[b] Primary effect is fatty liver.

The importance of fatty liver in liver injury is not clearly understood, and fatty liver in itself does not necessarily mean liver dysfunction.

CELL NECROSIS.   Cell necrosis or cell death is usually an acute injury and may be focal (central, midzonal, or peripheral) or massive. Because of the regenerating capability of the liver, necrotic lesions are not necessarily critical. Cell death occurs, along with rupture of the plasma membrane, and is preceded by a number of morphologic changes such as cytoplasmic edema, dilation of endoplasmic reticulum, disaggregation of polysomes, accumulation of triglycerides, swelling of mitochondria with disruption of cristae, and dissolution of organelles and nucleus. Biochemical events that may lead to these changes include binding of reactive metabolites to proteins and unsaturated lipids (inducing lipid peroxidation and subsequent membrane destruction), disturbance of cellular Ca^{2+} homeostasis, interference with metabolic pathways, shifts in Na^+ and K^+ balance, and inhibition of protein synthesis.

CHOLESTASIS.   This is the stoppage or suppression of the flow of bile and may have either intrahepatic or extrahepatic causes. Inflammation or blockage of the bile ducts results in retention of bile salts as well as bilirubin accumulation causing jaundice. Cholestasis is usually drug induced (Table 6.7) and is difficult to produce in experimental animals.

CIRRHOSIS.   This progressive disease is characterized pathologically by the presence of collagen throughout most of the liver. Cirrhosis is often associated with liver dysfunction, frequently resulting in jaundice. In humans, chronic use of ethanol is the single most important cause of cirrhosis, although there is some dispute as to whether the effect is due to ethanol alone or is also related to the nutritional deficiencies that usually accompany alcoholism.

HEPATITIS.   Hepatitis or inflammation of the liver, is usually viral in origin; however, certain chemicals, usually drugs, can induce a hepatitis that closely resembles that produced by viral infections (Table 6.7). This type of liver injury is not usually demonstrable in laboratory animals and is often manifest only in susceptible individuals.

CARCINOGENESIS.   The most common type of primary liver tumor is hepato-cellular carcinoma; other types include cholangiocarcinoma, angiosarcoma, glandular carcinoma, and undifferentiated liver cell carcinoma. Although a wide variety of chemicals are known to induce liver cancer in laboratory animals (Table 6.7) only a few, such as vinyl chloride which causes angiosarcoma, are known to be human carcinogens.

6.3.4.1c   Mechanisms

Chemically induced cell injury can be thought of as involving a series of events occurring in the affected animal and often in the target organ itself:

1. The chemical agent being activated to form the initiating (toxic) agent followed by;
2. Either detoxication of the toxic agent, or early molecular changes in the cell followed by;
3. Either recovery or irreversible changes and finally;
4. The altered cell, culminating in cell death.

Cell injury can be initiated by a number of mechanisms, such as inhibition of enzymes, depletion of cofactors or metabolites, interaction with receptors, and alteration of cell membranes. In recent years, attention has focused on the role of biotransformation of chemicals to highly reactive metabolites that initiate cellular toxicity.

Many compounds, including clinically useful drugs, can cause cellular damage through metabolic activation of the chemical to highly reactive compounds, such as free radicals, carbenes, and nitrenes (see Section 6.1, Role and formation of reactive metabolites). These reactive metabolites may bind covalently to cellular macromolecules such as nucleic acids, proteins, cofactors, lipids, and polysaccharides, thereby changing their biological properties. The liver is particularly vulnerable to toxicity produced by reactive metabolites since it is the major site of xenobiotic metabolism.

Most activation reactions are catalyzed by the cytochrome P-450 monooxygenase system, and pretreatment with agents that induce these enzymes, such as phenobarbital and 3-methylcholanthrene, usually increases toxicity. Conversely, pretreatment with inhibitors of cytochrome P-450, such as SKF-525A and piperonyl butoxide, frequently decreases toxicity. Mechanisms such as conjugation of the reactive chemical with glutathione exist within the cell for the rapid removal and inactivation of many potentially toxic compounds. Thus, cellular toxicity depends primarily on the balance between the rate of formation of reactive metabolites and the rate of their removal. Most of these mechanisms are illustrated in the following discussion of specific hepatotoxicants. Frequently, the area of tissue damage is most severe in the regions containing the highest concentration of activating enzymes. For example, the centrilobular region of the liver contains the highest concentration of cytochrome P-450, and is often the site of focal necrosis following toxic chemical injury.

6.3.4.1d Carbon Tetrachloride

Carbon tetrachloride is the classic example of a hepatotoxicant activated by the cytochrome P-450–dependent monooxygenase system to a free radical. This chemical has probably been studied more extensively, both biochemically and pathologically, than any other hepatotoxicant. From these studies have come many insights into the mechanisms of hepatotoxicity. Carbon tetrachloride is converted to the trichloromethyl radical ($CCl_3^{\cdot}$) and the trichloromethylperoxy radical (CCl_3O_2) (Figure 6.21). Such radicals are highly reactive and generally have a small radius of action; the necrosis induced by CCl_4 is most severe in the centrilobular liver cells that contain the highest concentration of cytochrome P-450.

Typically, free radicals may initiate chin reactions such as lipid peroxidation and also participate in other potentially damaging events such as covalent binding to lipids, proteins, or nucleotides (Figure 6.22). It is now thought that CCl_3, which forms relatively stable adducts, is responsible for covalent binding

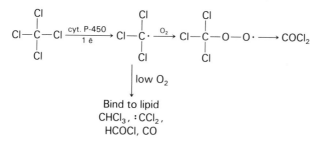

FIGURE 6.21
Some possible metabolites of CCl_4 produced by the cytochrome P-450–dependent monooxygenase system.

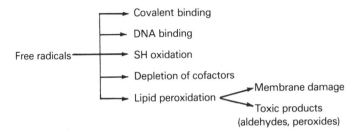

FIGURE 6.22.
Summary of some of the damaging effects of free radicals.

to macromolecules, and the more reactive CCl_3O_2, which is formed when CCl_3 reacts with oxygen, is the prime initiator of lipid peroxidation. Lipid peroxidation in turn leads to a cascade of events, starting with the oxidation of unsaturated fatty acids to form lipid hydroperoxides, which then break down to yield a variety of end-products, mainly aldehydes which can produce toxicity in distal tissues. Thus, cellular damage results both from the breakdown of membranes such as those of the endoplasmic reticulum, mitochondria, and lysosomes, and indirectly by the production of reactive aldehydes that can produce toxicity in distal tissues. It is now thought that many types of tissue injury, including inflammation, may involve lipid peroxidation.

6.3.4.1e Bromobenzene

Bromobenzene is a toxic industrial solvent that is known to produce centrilobular hepatic necrosis through the formation of reactive epoxides as the toxic intermediates. Figure 6.23 summarizes the major pathways of bromobenzene metabolism. Both bromobenzene 2,3-epoxide and bromobenzene 3,4-epoxide are produced on oxidation by cytochrome P-450 monooxygenases; the 2,3-epoxide that readily forms 2-bromophenol is nontoxic. Several pathways exist that can detoxify the reactive 3,4-epoxide: rearrangement to the 4-bromophenol, hydration to the 3,4-dihydrodiol catalyzed by epoxide hydrolase, or conjugation with glutathione. When more 3,4-epoxide is produced than can readily be detoxified, cell injury increases. Pretreatment of animals with inhibitors of cytochrome P-450 is known to decrease tissue necrosis by slowing down the rate of formation of the reactive metabolite, whereas pretreatment with the cytochrome P-450 inducer, phenobarbital, increases hepatotoxicity. Pretreatment with another cytochrome P-450 inducer, 3-methylcholanthrene, decreases bromobenzene hepatotoxicity, however, by inducing a form of cytochrome P-450 which produces primarily the nontoxic 2,3-epoxide rather than the more toxic 3,4-epoxide.

6.3.4.1f Acetaminophen

Acetaminophen is a widely used analgesic that normally is safe when taken in therapeutic doses, but an overdose may cause acute centrilobular hepatic necrosis, which can be fatal. Although acetaminophen is eliminated primarily by formation of glucuronide and sulfate conjugates, a small proportion is metabolized by cytochrome P-450 to a reactive, electrophilic intermediate (Section

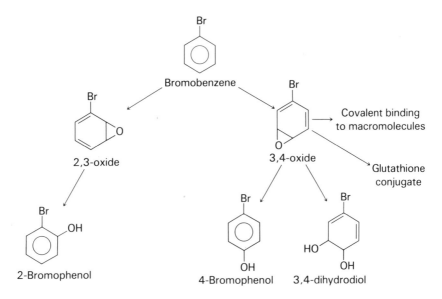

FIGURE 6.23.
Metabolism of bromobenzene. Oxidation may yield the nontoxic 2,3-oxide, which rapidly forms the phenol, or the toxic 3,4-oxide. As levels of glutathione (GSH) are depleted by the 3,4-oxide, covalent binding is increased. Other detoxication pathways are formation of 4-bromophenol and hydration to 3,4-dihydrodiol.

6.1.5.3 and Figure 6.3). This reactive intermediate is usually inactivated by conjugation with reduced glutathione and excreted. Higher doses of acetaminophen will progressively deplete hepatic glutathione levels, however, resulting in extensive covalent binding of the reactive metabolite to liver macromolecules with subsequent hepatic necrosis. The early administration of sulphydryl compounds such as cysteamine, methionine, and N-acetylcysteine is very effective in preventing the liver damage, renal failure, and death that would ctherwise follow an acetaminophen overdose. These agents are thought to act primarily by stimulating glutathione synthesis.

In laboratory animals, the formation of the acetaminophen-reactive metabolite, the extent of covalent binding, and the severity of hepatotoxicity can be influenced by altering the activity of the cytochrome P-450 monooxygenases. Induction of cytochrome P-450 with phenobarbital, 3-methylcholanthrene, or ethanol increases toxicity, whereas inhibition of cytochrome P-450 with piperonyl butoxide, cobalt chloride, or metyrapone decreases toxicity. Consistent with these effects in animals, it appears that the severity of liver damage after acetaminophen overdose is greater in chronic alcoholics and patients taking enzyme-inducing drugs. Thus, factors that selectively induce or inhibit metabolism of acetaminophen may enhance or reduce hepatotoxic effects in humans.

Studies of liver toxicity by bromobenzene, acetaminophen, and other compounds have led to some important observations concerning liver necrosis: (1) hepatotoxicity may be correlated with the formation of a minor, but highly reactive intermediate; (2) a threshold tissue concentration of the reactive metabolite must be attained before liver injury occurs; (3) endogenous substances, such as glutathione, play an essential role in protecting the cell from injury by removing chemically reactive intermediates (thus preventing the metabolite from reaching a critical concentration) and by protecting the sulfhydral groups of proteins by keeping them in the reduced state; (4) other pathways, such as glutathione transferase and epoxide hydrolases play an important role in protecting the cell; (5) agents that selectively induce or inhibit the oxidative enzymes may alter the hepatotoxicity of exogenous chemicals. These same principles are applicable to the toxicity caused by reactive metabolites in other organs, such as kidney and lung.

6.3.4.2 Nephrotoxicity

6.3.4.2a Susceptibility of the Kidney

The kidney appears to be particularly sensitive to a variety of nephrotoxicants. Several factors may be involved in this sensitivity (Table 6.8), but perhaps the most important is the high renal blood flow. Although the two kidneys comprise <1% of the total body mass, they receive approximately 25% of the cardiac output. Because of this high blood flow to the kidneys, any drug or chemical in the systemic circulation will be delivered to the kidney in significant amounts.

A second factor affecting the kidney's sensitivity to chemicals is its ability to concentrate substances. First, as salt and water are reabsorbed from the glomerular filtrate, the substances remaining in the tubular fluid become more concentrated. Thus, a nontoxic concentration in the plasma may reach toxic concentrations in the tubular fluid. Second, the transport characteristics of the kidney also contribute to concentration of substances within the cells. If the chemical is actively secreted from the blood into the tubular urine, it will be accumulated initially within the cells of the proximal tubules or, if the substance is readsorbed from the urine, it will pass through the epithelial cells in a relatively high concentration.

Another factor to consider in nephrotoxicity is the biotransformation of the parent compound to a toxic metabolite. Although the kidney does not possess the high levels of xenobiotic metabolizing enzymes (such as the cytochrome P-450–dependent monooxygenase system) that are found in the liver, many of the same enzymatic reactions have been shown to occur in the kidney. The levels of cytochrome P-450 are highest in the cells of the pars recta of the proximal tubule, an area that is particularly susceptible to toxic damage. Considering the unstable nature of many reactive metabolites, it seems most likely that covalent binding to tissue macromolecules is in close proximity to the site of activation. Thus, chemicals that exert their toxicity by a reactive interme-

TABLE 6.8
Factors Influencing Susceptibility of the Kidney to Xenobiotics

High renal blood flow
Concentration of tubular fluid and chemicals in fluid
Renal transportation of chemicals into tubular cells
Biotransformation of parent compound to toxic metabolite

diate are probably activated directly in the kidney rather than being activated in the liver and then transported to the kidney. As with hepatotoxicity, an important determinant in kidney toxicity is the balance between the rate of generation of reactive metabolites and the rate of their removal. The levels of glutathione in renal tissue also play an important role in the detoxification process.

6.3.4.2b Metals
Many of the heavy metals are potent nephrotoxicants, with metal ion-induced kidney damage being specific for individual metals rather than a general cytotoxic effect.

URANIUM. About 50% of plasma uranium is bound, as the uranyl ion, to bicarbonate, which is filtered by the glomerulus. As a result of acidification in the proximal tubule, the bicarbonate complex dissociates followed by reabsorption of the HCO_3^- ion; the released UO_2^{++} then becomes attached to the membrane of the proximal tubule cells. Loss of cell function follows, evidenced by increased concentration of glucose, amino acids, and proteins in the urine.

CADMIUM. Cadmium is excreted in the urine mainly as its metallothionein complex (CdMT). Metallothionein is a low molecular weight protein containing a large number of sulfhydryl groups that bind certain metals. The CdMT complex is reabsorbed and, once inside the cell, the cadmium is released, presumably by decomposition of the complex within the lysosomes. Cadmium has a long biological half-life, 20–30 years in the kidney; thus, low levels of chronic exposure will eventually result in accumulation to toxic levels. In Japan, a disease called Itai-itai Byo occurs primarily among women who eat rice grown in soils very high in cadmium. The disease is characterized by anemia, damage to proximal tubules, and severe bone and mineral loss.

LEAD. Lead, as Pb^{2+}, is taken up readily by proximal tubule cells where it damages mitochondria and inhibits mitochondrial function, thus altering the normal absorptive functions of the cell. Complexes of lead with acidic proteins appear as inclusion bodies in the nuclei of the tubular epithelium cells. These bodies, which are formed before signs of lead toxicity occur, appear to serve as a detoxication mechanism.

MERCURY. Mercury exerts its principle toxic effect on the membrane of the proximal tubule cell. In low concentrations, Hg^{2+} binds to the sulfhydryl groups of membrane enzymes and thus acts as a diuretic by inhibiting sodium reabsorption. Organomercurial diuretics were introduced in the 1920s, and were used into the 1960s. In spite of their widespread acceptance as effective therapeutic agents, it was known that there were problems of severe kidney toxicity. In the absence of other drugs that were as effective, however, the organomercurials proved to be valuable, even life-saving, therapeutic agents.

6.3.4.2c Antibiotics
Certain antibiotics, most notably the aminoglycosides, are known to be nephrotoxic in humans, especially in high doses or after prolonged therapy. This group of compounds include the drugs streptomycin, neomycin, kanany-

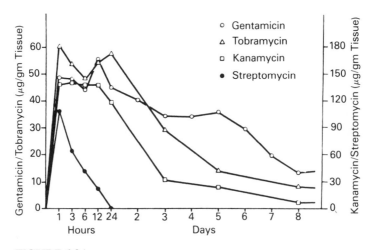

FIGURE 6.24.
Concentration of some aminoglycosides in the kidney over a period of several days after a single dose of the drug. In contrast to the persistence in the kidney, none of the antibiotics could be detected in the liver after 1 hour; by 3 hours, none was detected in the serum. Source: Luft, F.C., Kleit, S.A., J. Infect. Dis. 1974; 130:656. Used by permission.

cin, and gentamicin. As with most toxicants, a critical factor in initiating renal damage appears to be the tissue concentration of the antibiotic. Figure 6.24 shows the persistence in the kidney for some of the aminoglycosides following a single injection of antibiotic. With gentamicin, 5–6 days elapse before the tissue concentration is reduced by half. In contrast, streptomycin is completely cleared within 24 hours. In comparison with the kidney, gentamicin cannot be detected in the lungs, liver, or plasma after 3 hours, suggesting that the drug is tightly bound to renal tissue and that accumulation occurs when multiple doses are given over a period of days. As would be expected, toxicity parallels the rate of clearance of the antibiotics, with streptomycin being the least toxic, and gentamicin the most toxic. Recent evidence suggests that gentamicin is taken up by the cells of the proximal tubule, where it accumulates in the lysosomes. When a threshold (toxic) concentration is reached, the lysosomes rupture, releasing hydrolytic enzymes that damage the cells, thus causing tissue necrosis.

With certain other drugs, the damage may be related to the biochemical mechanism of action. For example, the polymycins, such as amphotericin B, are surface-active agents that bind to membrane phospholipids, disrupt the integrity of the membrane, and thereby cause leaky cells.

6.3.4.2d Reactive Metabolites

Still other nephrotoxins are activated in the kidney by the cytochrome P-450 monooxygenase system to produce strong electrophiles or free radicals that can cause cell necrosis by binding to cell macromolecules or initiating lipid peroxidation. Many of these toxicants are the same as those that are activated in the liver and cause hepatotoxicity: acetaminophen, bromobenzene, chloroform, and carbon tetrachloride.

6.3.4.3 Pulmonary Toxicity

6.3.4.3a Susceptibility of the Lungs

The principal function of the lungs is gas exchange, providing O_2 to the tissues and removing CO_2. Because the lung has such a large surface area and because such a large volume of air is passed over its surface (10,000–20,000 L/day for the average adult), the lung is the major interface between an organism and the environment. Pulmonary diseases caused by agents in the environment have been known for centuries and have been associated with occupations such as stone quarrying, coal mining, and textiles. The problem is more complex and widespread today because new agents are constantly being added to our environments, including gasoline additives and exhaust particles, pesticides, plastics, solvents, deodorant and cosmetic sprays, and construction materials. In addition, the entire blood volume passes through the lung one to five times a minute, exposing the lung to circulating toxins and drugs. Thus, the possibility of damage from inhaled or circulating agents is clearly enormous.

6.3.4.3b Toxic Responses of the Lungs

Although many different agents may damage the lung, the patterns of cellular injury and repair are relatively constant. Perhaps one of the most obvious and familiar is irritation caused by volatile compounds such as ammonia or chlorine gas. Such irritation, especially if severe or persistent, may lead to constriction of airways and edema of lung tissue. Intense damage to cells lining the airways often results in increased permeability of membranes, edema, and even necrosis; such damage is known to follow exposure to agents such as ozone, nitrogen oxides, and phosgene.

Fibrosis, or formation of collagenous tissue, was perhaps one of the earliest recognized forms of occupational diseases. Silicosis resulting from inhalation of silica (SiO_2) is thought to involve first the uptake of the particles by macrophages and lysosomal incorporation, followed by rupture of the lysosomal membrane and release of lysosomal enzymes into the cytoplasm of the macrophages. Thus, the macrophage is digested by its own enzymes. After lysis, the free silica is released to be ingested by fresh macrophages, and the cycle continues. It is also thought that the damaged macrophages release a chemical that is instrumental in initiating collagen formation in the lung tissue. Asbestosis was recognized as long ago as 1907; however, the magnitude of the risk has become apparent only recently, primarily due to the increased incidence of lung cancer among asbestosis sufferers, especially those who are also cigarette smokers.

Numerous agents, including microorganisms, spores, dust, and chemicals, are known to elicit allergic responses. Several diverse examples are farmer's lung resulting from spores of a mold that grows on damp hay and releases its spores when the temperature is 40–60 °F; mushroom picker's lung; maple bark stripper's disease, from spores of a fungus growing on maple trees; and cheese washer's lung from penicillin spores.

Perhaps the most severe response of the lung to injury is cancer; today, the primary causative agent is inhaled cigarette smoke.

6.3.4.3c Metabolic Activation of Toxicants

The activation of pulmonary toxicants can be classified into three main categories or mechanisms depending either on the site of formation of the activated compound or on the nature of the reactive intermediate.

1. The parent compound may be activated in the liver, with the reactive metabolite then transported by the circulation to the lung. Such metabolites, although very reactive, have sufficient stability that a part of that formed in the liver can persist long enough to enter the lung. As would be expected, these activated compounds lead to covalent binding and damage to both liver and lung tissues. Perhaps the best known example of lung toxicity by this mechanism is damage to pulmonary endothelial cells caused by certain pyrrolizidine alkaloids from various plant species, such as monocrotaline.

2. A foreign chemical entering the lung, either from inhaled air or the circulatory system, may be metabolized to the ultimate toxic compound directly within the lung itself. Although the total concentration of activating enzymes of the cytochrome P-450 monooxygenase system is less in the lung than in the liver, the concentration varies considerably in the different cell types in the lung, with the highest concentration being found in the nonciliated bronchiolar epithelial (Clara) cells of the terminal bronchioles. In addition, the complement of cytochrome P-450 isozymes in the lung is quite different from that in the liver; in the rabbit, for example, two of the cytochrome P-450 isozymes that make up >70% of pulmonary cytochrome P-450, are minor components of the hepatic cytochrome P-450 monooxygenase system.

   The best known example of a toxic compound activated in the lung is 4-ipomeanol (Figure 6.25). This naturally occurring furan derivative was isolated and shown to be the major toxic substance in moldy sweet potatoes that had been responsible for severe lung injury and death in cattle. Pulmonary injury by 4-ipomeanol is caused, not by the parent compound, but by a highly reactive, alkylating metabolite — probably an epoxide — produced by cytochrome P-450 isozymes. The two major lung cytochrome P-450 isozymes readily metabolize 4-ipomeanol. Consequently, activation

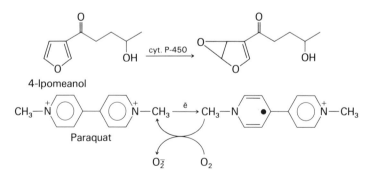

FIGURE 6.25.
Bioactivation of two pulmonary toxicants: 4-ipomeanol and paraquat.

by the lung is much greater than that in the liver, which contains significantly lower levels of these two isozymes. In addition, these isozymes are highly concentrated in the Clara cells, which are most affected by 4-ipomeanol toxicity. Other toxic lung furans, such as the atmospheric contaminants, 2-methylfuran and 3-methylfuran (Figure 6.1), may exert their toxicity through the formation of reactive metabolites, probably reactive aldehydes.

The presence of the cytochrome P-450 system in Clara cells is of considerable toxicological significance since many cytotoxic and carcinogenic chemicals require activation by this enzyme system. In this case, the Clara cells may be a major site for the formation of the ultimate toxicant or carcinogen as well as a primary target for the effects of activated chemicals.

3. Another means of metabolic activation is the cyclic reduction/oxidation of the parent compound resulting in high rates of consumption of NADPH and production of superoxide anion. Either the depletion of NADPH and/or the formation of reactive oxygen radicals could lead to cellular injury. Pulmonary injury by this mechanism is best illustrated by the herbicide paraquat (Figure 6.25).

Systemic administration of paraquat initiates a progression of degenerative and potentially lethal lesions in the lung. The redox cycling of paraquat produces two damaging events within the cell. One is the generation of active oxygen species (superoxide anion, hydrogen peroxide, and hydroxy radical), which are highly reactive toward tissue macromolecules; a second is the depletion of cellular reducing equivalents (NADPH, reduced glutathione) that are essential for normal function. Several other lung toxicants such as oxygen, bleomycin (a cancer therapeutic agent) and nitroflurantoin (an antibiotic used for urinary tract infections) may have similar mechanisms.

6.3.5 Behavioral Effects

6.3.5.1 Introduction and Definition

Behavioral toxicology is the science dealing with the effects of nonphysiological chemicals on the behavior of intact organisms. The term "behavior" has been defined in many ways: by Skinner in 1938 as "what an organism is doing—or more accurately, what it is observed to be doing." Today, behavioral toxicologists have extended that definition to say that behavior represents nervous system output, or the functioning of the CNS, and thus behavioral tests offer a sensitive way to monitor damage to this organ system. Figure 6.26 is a simplified schematic representation of the nervous system showing several points at which a chemical may act to disrupt the input/output relations. Altered behavior could thus be an indicator for either a direct or an indirect toxic effect on the nervous system. A chemical may act to disrupt these input/output relationships either directly by affecting some level of neuronal organization or indirectly by interacting with another organ system which, in turn, affects nervous system function. Chemicals that damage the nervous system directly are called neurotoxicants. Neurobehavioral techniques are not limited to the effects of neuro-

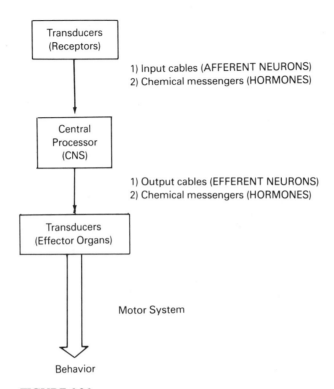

FIGURE 6.26.
Schematic representation of the nervous system showing the various locations which are subject to disruption by toxic agents. Source: Reiter. Environ. Health Perspect. 1978; 26:5.

toxicants, however, but may provide an indication of toxicity to other organs, which then manifests itself as a behavioral effect. Thus, the

> Behavior of an organism is the endpoint of the functional integration of the nervous system, encompassing sensory, motor, and cognitive aspects. The functional capacity of the central nervous system cannot be determined by histological or even physiological studies independent of behavioral analysis (Mello, 1975).

6.3.5.2 Behavioral Teratology

The central nervous system (CNS) appears to be especially vulnerable to adverse factors during its development; these alterations in neurodevelopment may then be manifested as changes in behavior. There is some indication that these functional alterations can be produced at lower exposure levels than those that lead to gross morphologic defects. The developmental period of the central nervous system is long, and vulnerability to toxic insult continues into the postnatal period. Thus, the nervous system is at least as susceptible to teratogenic influence as other developing systems. Unlike structural birth defects, however, subtle behavioral abnormalities are not readily evident at birth and may be revealed only by special tests during postnatal life. Particularly at low levels, teratogens may cause behavioral changes in the absence of gross functional or structural defects. Some type of ultrastructural or biochemical abnormality most underlie the abnormal behavior, however.

In looking for behavioral effects following prenatal exposure, factors affecting both teratology and behavioral toxicology testing must be considered. In many behavioral teratologic tests, the dose level used is low enough not to cause gross structural malformations, and the organism is exposed during all stages of development.

Other factors to be considered in behavioral teratology are "latent" effects, ie, defects in a developmental process that may not become expressed until later in life as a behavioral disorder or mental deficiency. Determination of such long-term or delayed effects requires the use of a "longitudinal" research designed to follow individuals from birth through maturity and to look for certain developmental processes, such as those that might occur at sexual maturity.

The major concern with drugs administered prenatally has been the risk of structural malformation. Teratogenic agents can produce a range of effects, however, including intrauterine death, growth retardation, and behavioral effects. Several agents that are teratogenic to the developing central nervous system in animals have been shown to produce learning and motor impairment when administered during embryogenesis at doses too low to produce structural malformations. Of the agents known to be teratogenic in humans, alcohol produces the most serious postnatal behavioral consequences. These include delayed development, hyperactivity, fine motor dysfunction, and mental retardation (see Section 6.3.3.4.d, FAS discussion). The environmental contaminant, methyl mercury, causes cerebral palsy-like symptoms in infants whose mothers ate mercury-contaminated fish while pregnant (Section 6.3.3.4e).

6.3.5.3 Behavioral Testing

Behavioral testing procedures must not only be sensitive indicators of toxicity, but also simple, rapid, and inexpensive. For these reasons, locomotor activity measurements have been used extensively. In addition, many of the locomotor activities occur naturally in the test animal, and different types of activities occur at various developmental times. Examples of such activities include righting, swimming, grooming, walking backward, rope and rod climbing. More sophisticated techniques are also used to assess deficits in "learning" that involve acquisition, retention, and recall of skills.

In some cases, function, as monitored by behavior, may be the easiest phenomenon to measure in the intact organism, especially humans.

6.3.5.4 Summary

Increasing evidence indicates that nervous tissue, especially in developing organisms, is very sensitive to many foreign chemicals; the toxic effects from such substances may result in behavioral changes that can be measured to give useful information on the toxicity of the chemical. Such behavioral assessment is an important component in evaluating the toxic action of a chemical for the following reasons: (1) subtle behavioral changes may serve as early indicators of later, more severe, consequences; (2) behavioral deficits themselves may be extremely disadvantageous to an organism; (3) these behavioral changes are indicative of some physical, chemical, or biological alterations that may not be readily apparent by classical testing methods; (4) behavioral changes, especially following in utero exposure, may occur at very low concentrations of the chemical. This type of exposure is more likely to reflect the exposure humans normally encounter and may be an important criterion for assessing the impact of low level chemicals on human health.

6.4 SUGGESTED FURTHER READING

FORMATION OF REACTIVE METABOLITES

Anders, M.W. (ed.). Bioactivation of Foreign Compounds. Orlando, Fla: Academic Press, 1985.

Dauterman, W.C. Selective toxicity conferred by activation, In IUPAC Pesticide Chemistry, Human Welfare and the Environment, Miyamoto J. (ed.), New York: Pergamon Press, 1983, pp. 247–254.

Ioannides, C., Lum, P.Y., Parke, D.V. Cytochrome P-448 and the activation of toxic chemicals and carcinogens. Xenobiotica 1984; 14:119–137.

Jerina, D.M. Metabolism of aromatic hydrocarbons by the cytochrome P-450 system and epoxide hydrolase. Drug Metab. Disposition 1983; 11:1–4.

Nelson, S.D. Metabolic activation and drug toxicity. J. Medicinal Chem. 1982; 25:753–765.

Ravindranth, V., Burka, L.T., Boyd, M.R. Reactive metabolites from the bioactivation of toxic methylfurans. Science 1984; 224:884–886.

ACUTE TOXICITY

Arena, J.M. Poisoning: Toxicology, Symptoms, Treatments. 4th ed. Springfield, Ill.: Charles C Thomas, 1979.

Bayer, M.J., Rumach, B.H. (eds.). Poisoning and Overdose. Rockville, Md.: Aspero Systems, 1983.

Haddad, L.M., Winchester, J.F. (eds.). Clinical Management of Poisoning and Drug Overdose. Philadelphia: W.B. Saunders, 1983.

Oehme, F.W., Brown, J.F., Fowler, M.E. Toxins of animal origin. In Doull, J., Klaassen, C.D., Amdur, M.O. (eds.). Casarett and Doull's Toxicology: The Basic Science of Poisons. 2d ed. New York: Macmillan, 1980, pp. 557–577.

Ten Eyck, R.P., Schaerdel, A.D., Lynett, J.E., Marks, D.H., Patrissi, G.A., Ottinger, W.E., Stansell, M.J. Stroma-free methemoglobin as an antidote for cyanide poisoning: A preliminary study. Clin. Toxicol. 1985; 21:343–358.

CARCINOGENESIS

Bohrman, J.S. Identification and assessment of tumor-promoting and cocarcinogenic agents: State-of-the-art in vitro methods. CRC Crit. Rev. Toxicol. 1983; 11:121–167.

Boutwell, R.K. Biology and biochemistry of the two-step model of carcinogenesis. In Meyskens, F.L. (ed.). Modulation and Mediation of Cancer by Vitamins. Basel, Switzerland: S. Karger, 1983, pp. 1–8.

Cerutti, P.A. DNA Lesions: Nature and genesis. In Nicolini, C. (ed.). Chemical Carcinogenesis. New York: Plenum Press, 1982, pp. 75–92.

Cerutti, P.A. Prooxidant states and tumor promotion. Science 1985; 227:375–381.

Greim, H., Jung, R., Kramer, M., Marquardt, H., Oesch, F. (eds.). Biochemical Basis of Chemical Carcinogenesis. New York: Raven Press, 1982.

Hoffman, D., Hecht, S.S., Haley, N.J., Brunnemann, K.D., Adams, J.D., Wynder, E.L. Tobacco carcinogenesis: Metabolic studies in humans. In Harris, C.C., Autrup, H.N. (eds.). Human Carcinogenesis. New York: Academic Press, 1983, pp. 809–832.

Miller, E.C., Miller, J.A. Mechanisms of chemical carcinogenesis: Nature of proximate carcinogens and interaction with macromolecules. Pharmacol. Rev. 1966; 18:805–838.

Miller, J.A., Miller E.C. Some historical aspects of *N*-aryl carcinogens and their metabolic activation. Environ. Health Perspect. 1983; 49:3–12.

Searle, C.E. (ed.). Chemical Carcinogens. 2nd Ed. Vols. 1, 2. ACS Monograph 182, Washington: American Chemical Society, 1984.

Weisburger, J.H., Williams, G.M. Chemical carcinogens. In Doull, J., Klaassen, C.D., Amdur, M.O. (eds.). Casarett and Doull's Toxicology: The Basic Science of Poisons. 2nd Ed. New York: Macmillan, 1980, pp. 84–138.

Williams, G.M. Modulation of chemical carcinogenesis by xenobiotics. Fund. Appl. Toxicol. 1984; 4:325–344.

MUTAGENESIS

Herbold, B.A., Machemer, L.H. Evaluation of chemical agents for mutagenicity. Pflanzenschutz Nachrichten 1981; 34:152–179.

Kirsch-Volders, M. (ed.). Mutagenicity, Carcinogenicity and Teratogenicity of Industrial Pollutants. New York: Plenum Press, 1984.

Pegg, A.E. Alkylation and subsequent repair of DNA after exposure to dimethylnitrosamine and related carcinogens. In Hodgson, E., Bend, J.R., Philpot, R.M. (eds.). Annual Reviews in Biochemical Toxicology 5. New York: Elsevier, 1983, pp. 83–134.

Würgler, F.E. Genetic hazards. Experientia 1982; 38:882–886.

TERATOGENESIS

Abel, E.L. (ed.). Fetal Alcohol Syndrome and Fetal Alcohol Effects. New York: Plenum Press, 1984.

Abel, E.L. Prenatal Effects of Alcohol. Drug Alcohol Dependence 1984; 14:1–10.

Apfel, R.J., Fisher, S.M. (eds.). To Do No Harm: DES and the Dilemmas of Modern Medicine. New Haven, Conn.: Yale University Press, 1984.

Barlow, S.M., Sullivan, F.M. (eds.). Reproductive Hazards of Industrial Chemicals. New York: Academic Press, 1982.

Harbison, R.D. Teratogens. In Doull, J., Klaassen, C.D., Andur, M.O. (eds.). Casarett and Doull's Toxicology: The Basic Science of Poisons. 2nd ed. New York: Macmillan, 1980, pp. 158–178.

Juchau, M.R. (ed.). The Biochemical Basis of Chemical Teratogenesis. New York: Elsevier, 1981.

Persaud, T.V.N. (ed.). Advances in the Study of Birth Defects. Vol. 1. Teratogenic Mechanisms. Baltimore: University Park Press, 1979.

Schardein, J.L. (ed.). Drugs as Teratogens. Cleveland: CRC Press, 1976.

Wilson, J.G., Fraser, F.C. (eds.). Handbook of Teratology. Vol. 1. General Principles and Etiology; Vol. 2. Mechanisms and Pathogenesis. New York: Plenum Press, 1977.

HEPATOTOXICITY

Bridges, J.W., Benford, D.J., Hubbard, S.A. Mechanisms of Toxic Injury. Ann. NY Acad. Sci. 1983; 407:42–63.

Cheeseman, K.H. General mechanisms of toxic liver injury with special reference to free radical reactions. In Rainsford, K.D., Velo, G.P. (eds.). Advances in Inflammation Research 6. New York: Raven Press, 1984, pp. 179–188.

Gorrod, J.W. Covalent binding as an indicator of drug toxicity. In Gorrod, J.W. (ed.). Testing for toxicity. London: Taylor and Francis, 1981.

Miners, J.O., Attwood, J., Birkett, D.J. Determinants of acetoaminophen metabolism: Effect of inducers and inhibitors of drug metabolism on acetaminophen's metabolic pathways. Clin. Pharmacol. Ther. 1984; 35:480–486.

Plaa, G.L., Hewitt, W.R. (eds.). Toxicology of the Liver. New York: Raven Press, 1982.

Prescott, L.F. Reactive metabolites as a cause of hepatotoxicity. Int. J. Clin. Pharmacol. Res. 1983; 3:437–441.

NEPHROTOXICITY

Gorrod, J.W. (ed.). Drug Toxicity. London: Taylor and Francis, 1979.

Hook, J.B., McCormack, K.M., Kluwe, W.M. Biochemical mechanisms of nephrotoxicity. In Hodgson, E., Bend, J.R., Philpot, R.M. (eds.). Reviews in Biochemical Toxicology 1. New York: Elsevier, 1983, pp. 53–78.

Hook, J.B. (ed.). Toxicology of the Kidney. New York: Raven Press, 1981.

Metallothionein and Cadmium Nephrotoxicity Symposium. Environ. Health Perspect. 1984; 54:1–356.

Nieboer, E., Sanford, W.E. Essential, Toxic and Therapeutic Functions of Metals. In Hodgson, E., Bend, J.R., Philpot, R.M. (eds.). New York: Elsevier, 1985.

Porter, G.A. (ed.). Nephrotoxic Mechanisms of Drugs and Environmental Toxins. New York: Plenum Press, 1982.

Smith, J.H., Hook, J.B. Mechanism of Chloroform Nephrotoxicity. Toxicol. Appl. Pharmacol. 1984; 73:511–524.

PULMONARY TOXICITY

Brown, S.S., Davies, D.S. Organ-Directed Toxicity: Chemical Indices and Mechanisms. New York: Pergamon Press, 1981.

Hook, G. (ed.). Monograph on Pulmonary Toxicology. Environ. Health Perspect. 1984; 55:1–390.

Menzel, D.B., McClellan, R.O. Toxic responses of the respiratory system. In Doull, J., Klaassen, C.D., Andur, M.O. (eds.). Casarett and Doull's Toxicology: The Basic Science of Poisons. 2nd ed. New York: Macmillan, 1980, pp. 246–274.

Witschi, H., Nettesheim, P. (eds.). Mechanisms in Respiratory Toxicology. Boca Raton, Fla.: CRC Press, 1982.

BEHAVIORAL EFFECTS

Anger, W.K., Johnson, B.W. Chemicals affecting behavior. In O'Donoghue, J.L. (ed.). Neurotoxicity of Industrial and Commercial Chemicals. Vol. 1. Boca Raton, Fla.: CRC Press, 1985, pp. 51–148.

Brown, K., Cooper, S.J. (eds.). Chemical Influences on Behavior. New York: Academic Press, 1979.

Hutchins, D.E. Behavioral Teratology: A New Frontier. In Johnson, E.M., Kochhar, D.M. (eds.). Neurobehavioral Research in Teratogenesis and Reproductive Toxicology. New York: Springer-Verlag, 1983, pp. 207–235.

Geller, I., Stebbins, W.C., Wayner, M.J. (eds.). Test Methods for Definition of Effects of Toxic Substances on Behavior and Neuromotor Function. Fayetteville, New York: ANKHO International Inc., 1979.

Jensh, R.P. Behavioral testing procedures: A review. In Johnson, E.M., Kochhar, D.M. (eds.). Teratogenesis and Reproductive Toxicology. New York: Springer-Verlag, 1983, pp. 171–206.

Mello, N.K. Behavioral toxicology: A developing discipline. Fed. Proc. 1975; 34:1832–1834.

Norton, S. Is behavior or morphology a more sensitive indicator of central nervous system toxicity? Environ. Health Perspect. 1978; 26:21–27.

Schaeppi, W., Hess, R. What can specific behavioral testing procedures contribute to the assessment of neurotoxicity in laboratory animals? Agents Actions 1984; 14:131–138.

chapter seven

TOXICITY OF CHEMICALS

Patricia E. Levi

7.1 INTRODUCTION

Chemical toxicants may be classified in various ways depending on interest and need. In Chapter 6, toxic chemical agents were discussed in terms of their effects (acute toxicants, carcinogens, teratogens, and mutagens) or their target organs (hepatotoxicants, nephrotoxicants, and pulmonary toxicants). This chapter examines chemical toxicants according to exposure categories or specific uses. Of important concern today are toxic chemicals found in air, soil, water, food, and the workplace, as well as those encountered in specific uses such as pesticides, drugs, and solvents.

7.2 CHEMICAL POLLUTANTS IN THE AIR

7.2.1 History

Air pollution probably occurred as soon as humans started to use wood fires for heat and cooking, and for centuries fire was used in such a way that living areas were filled with smoke. After the invention of the chimney, combustion products and cooking odors were removed from living quarters and vented outside. Later, when soft coal was discovered and used for fuel, coal smoke became a problem in the cities. By the thirteenth century, records show that coal smoke had become a nuisance in London, and in 1273 Edward I made the first antipollution law, one that prohibited the burning of coal while Parliament was in session: "Be it known to all within the sound of my voice, whosoever shall be found guilty of burning coal shall suffer the loss of his head." Despite various other royal edicts, however, smoke pollution continued in London. In 1661, John Evelyn submitted a brochure to King Charles II and Parliament entitled "Fumifugium or the Inconvenience of Aer and Smoak of London Dissipated,

Together with Some Remedies Humbly Proposed." Some of his suggestions are still viable today and included moving industry to the outskirts of town and establishing green belts around the city. Unfortunately, none of his proposals were implemented. Various commissions in Britain in the 1800s made suggestions for controlling air pollution ranging from having locomotives "consume their own smoke" to having offending chimneys torn down.

Increasing domestic and industrial combustion of coal caused air pollution to get steadily worse, particularly in large cities. During the twentieth century, the most significant change was the rapid increase in the number of automobiles, from almost none at the turn of the century to millions within only a few decades. During this time, few attempts were made to control air pollution in any of the industrialized countries until after World War II. Action was then prompted, in part, by two acute pollution episodes in which human deaths were caused directly by high levels of pollutants.

One incident occurred in 1948 in Donora, a small steel-mill town in western Pennsylvania. During the last week of October, a heavy smog settled in the area, and a weather inversion prevented the movement of pollutants out of the valley. Twenty-one deaths were attributed directly to the effects of the smog. The "Donora episode" helped focus attention on air pollution in the United States.

In December 1952, the now infamous "Killer Smog" occurred in London. A dense fog at ground level coupled with smoke from coal fireplaces caused a severe smog lasting more than a week. The smog was so heavy that daylight visibility was only a few meters, and bus conductors had to walk in front of the buses to guide the drivers through the streets. Two days after the smog began, the death rate began to climb, and between December 5 and December 9, there were an estimated 4,000 deaths above normal. The chief causes of death were bronchitis, pneumonia, and associated respiratory complaints. This disaster resulted in the passage of the Clean Air Act in 1956.

In the United States, the smog problem began to appear in large cities across the country, becoming most severe in Los Angeles. In 1955, federal air pollution legislation was enacted, providing federal support for air pollution research, training, and technical assistance. Responsibility for the administration of the federal programs lies with the United States Environmental Protection Agency (EPA). Technological interest during the past 30 years has centered on automobile air pollution, pollution by oxides of sulfur and nitrogen, and the control of these emissions. Attention is also being directed toward the problems that may be caused by a possible "greenhouse effect" due to increasing concentrations of carbon dioxide in the atmosphere, possible depletion of the stratospheric ozone layer, long-range transport of pollution, and acid deposition.

7.2.2 Types of Air Pollutants

7.2.2.1 Unpolluted Air

What is clean air? Unpolluted air is a concept of what the air would be if humans and their works were not on earth, and if the air were not polluted by natural point sources such as volcanoes, forest fires, etc. We do not know the true composition of "unpolluted" air because humans had been polluting the air for thousands of years before they had the means and desire to measure its composition. In addition, there are many natural pollutants such as terpenes from plants, smoke from forest fires, fumes and smoke from volcanoes, etc. Table 7.1 lists the components that, in the absence of such pollution, would constitute clean air.

7.2.2.2 Gaseous Pollutants

Gaseous pollutants include substances that are gases at normal temperature and pressure as well as vapors of substances that are liquid or solid. Among pollutants of greatest concern are carbon monoxide, hydrocarbons, hydrogen sulfide (H_2S), nitrogen oxides (N_xO_y), ozone (O_3) and other oxidants, sulfur oxides (S_xO_y), and carbon dioxide (CO_2) (Table 7.2). Pollutant concentrations are usually expressed as micrograms per cubic meter ($\mu g/m^3$) or an older method for gaseous pollutants as parts per million by volume in which

$$1 \text{ ppm} = \frac{1 \text{ vol of pollutant}}{10^6 \text{ vol of air}} = 0.0001\% \text{ by volume}$$

7.2.2.3 Particulate Pollutants

Particulate pollutants consist of fine solids or liquid droplets suspended in air. Some of the different types of particulates are defined as follows:

1. Dust — relatively large particles about 100 μm in diameter which come directly from substances being used, eg, coal dust, ash, sawdust, cement dust, grain dust.

TABLE 7.1
Gaseous Components of Normal Dry Air

Gas	Percent by Volume of Dry Air	Concentration (ppm)
Nitrogen	78.09	780,900
Oxygen	20.94	209,400
Argon	0.93	9,300
Carbon dioxide	0.0325	325
Neon	0.0018	18.0
Helium	0.0005	5.2
Methane	0.0001	1.1
Krypton	0.0001	1.0
Nitrous oxide		0.5
Hydrogen		0.5
Xenon		0.008
Nitrogen dioxide		0.02
Ozone		0.01 – 0.04

TABLE 7.2
Gaseous Air Pollutants

Name	Properties	Significance as Pollutant
Sulfur dioxide, SO_2	Colorless, choking gas, soluble in H_2O to form sulfurous acid H_2SO_3	Main component acidic deposition; damage to vegetation, materials, health
Sulfur trioxide, SO_3	Soluble in H_2O to form sulfuric acid H_2SO_4	Very corrosive
Nitric oxide, NO	Colorless gas	Produced during high temperature combustion. Readily oxidized to NO_2.
Nitrogen dioxide, NO_2	Brown to orange gas	Important component of photochemical smog and acidic deposition.
Carbon monoxide, CO	Colorless and odorless	Product of incomplete combustion; combines with hemoglobin to form carboxyhemoglobin, poisonous
Carbon dioxide, CO_2	Colorless and odorless	Formed during complete combustion; may cause "greenhouse effect" and climate changes
Ozone, O_3	Highly reactive	Produced during formation of photochemical smog; damage to vegetation and property.
Hydrogen sulfide, H_2S	Rotten egg odor	Very poisonous
Hydrocarbons, C_xH_y	Numerous	Emitted from automobiles, industry, natural sources

2. Fumes—suspended solids < 1 μm in diameter usually released from metallurgical or chemical processes, eg, zinc and lead oxides.
3. Mist—liquid droplets suspended in air with a diameter < 2.0 μm, eg, sulfuric acid mist.
4. Smoke—solid particles $(0.05 – 1.0$ μm) resulting from incomplete combustion of fossil fuels.
5. Spray or aerosol—liquid or solid particles $(< 1.0$ μm) suspended in air or another gas.

7.2.3 Sources of Air Pollutants

7.2.3.1 Natural

Many pollutants are formed and emitted through natural processes. An erupting volcano emits particulate matter as well as gases such as SO_2, H_2S, and methane; such clouds may remain airborne for long periods of time. Forest and prairie fires produce large quantities of pollutants in the form of smoke, un-burned hydrocarbons, CO, nitrogen oxides, and ash. Dust storms are a common source of particulate matter in many parts of the world, and oceans produce aerosols in the form of salt particles. Plants and trees, which play a large part in the conversion of CO_2 to O_2, are still a major source of hydrocarbons on the planet; the blue haze that is so familiar over forested mountain areas is mainly from the atmospheric reactions of the volatile organics produced by the trees. Plants also produce pollen and spores, which cause respiratory problems and allergic reactions.

7.2.3.2 Man-Made

Man-made air pollutants, sometimes called anthropogenic pollutants, come primarily from three sources: (1) stationary combustion sources that burn fossil fuel to produce energy for heating and power, (2) exhaust emissions from transportation vehicles that use gasoline or diesel fuels, and (3) industrial processes.

The principal pollutants from stationary combustion are fly ash, smoke, sulfur, and nitrogen oxides, as well as CO and CO_2. Combustion of coal and oil, both of which contain significant amounts of sulfur, yields large quantities of sulfur oxides. One effect of the production of sulfur oxides is the formation of acidic deposition (Section 7.2.5.5) including acid rain. Normal rain has a pH of about 5.6, but the pH of acid rain can be as low as 3. Nitrogen oxides are formed by thermal oxidation of atmospheric nitrogen at high temperatures; thus, almost any combustion process will produce NO_x. Carbon monoxide is a product of incomplete combustion; thus, the amount of CO emitted from a source is a function of its combustion efficiency; the more efficient the combustion, the higher the ratio of CO_2 to CO.

Transportation sources, particularly automobiles, are a major source of air pollution and include smoke, lead particles from tetraethyl lead additives, CO, nitrogen oxides, and hydrocarbons. Significant progress has occurred in the last 20 years in reducing exhaust emissions, particularly with the use of low-lead or no-lead gasolines.

Industries may emit various pollutants relating to their manufacturing processes—sulfuric, acetic, nitric, and phosphoric acids; solvents and resins; chlorine and ammonia gas; and metals, such as copper, lead, and zinc from smelters. Sources of industrial pollution can usually be controlled by the use of existing technologies.

7.2.4 Human Health Effects

Most of our information on effects of air pollution on humans comes from acute pollution episodes such as the ones in Donora and London. Illnesses result from chemical irritation of the respiratory tract, with certain sensitive subpopulations being more affected: (1) very young children, whose respiratory and circulatory systems are poorly developed; (2) the elderly, whose cardiorespiratory systems function poorly; (3) people with cardiorespiratory diseases such as asthma, emphysema, and heart disease. Heavy smokers are also affected more adversely by air pollutants. In most cases, the health problems are attributed to the combined action of particulates and sulfur dioxides; no one pollutant appears to be responsible. Several questions must be asked in relating air pollution to human health: Is there a threshold, or critical concentration of pollutant necessary before a response occurs, ie, is there a "no response" level? What is the total body burden (accumulation) of the substance, and how much of that burden is contributed by air pollution? What is the synergistic effect of combinations of pollutants?

Sulfur dioxide and sulfuric acid are common components of polluted air that cause irritation of mucus membranes and bronchial constriction. Nitrogen dioxide, a gas found in photochemical smog, is also a pulmonary irritant and is known to lead to pulmonary edema and hemorrhage. Ozone, a highly irritating, oxidizing gas, is also formed by photochemical action in smog and can produce pulmonary congestion, edema, and hemorrhage. Carbon monoxide combines readily with hemoglobin (Hb) to form carboxyhemoglobin (COHb) preventing the transfer of oxygen to tissues. Concentrations > 100 ppm cause headaches, dizziness, nausea, and breathing difficulties, and an acute concentration of 1,000 ppm is invariably fatal. Carbon monoxide levels during acute traffic congestion have been known to be as high as 400 ppm; in addition, people who smoke elevate their total body burden of CO as compared with nonsmokers. The effects of low concentrations of CO over a long period are not known, but it is possible that heart and respiratory disorders are exacerbated.

One of the most familiar of the particulates in air pollutants is lead, with young children and fetuses being the most susceptible. Lead can impair renal function, interfere with the development of red blood cells, and impair the nervous system, leading to mental retardation and even blindness. There are two common routes of exposure to lead — inhalation and ingestion. It is estimated that approximately 20% of the total body burden of lead comes from inhalation.

Various solid particles of dust and fibers from coal, clay, glass, asbestos, and minerals can lead to scarring or fibrosis of the lung lining. Pneumoconiosis, or dust disease (silicosis), and asbestosis are all well-known industrial pollution diseases.

7.2.5 Environmental Effects

7.2.5.1 Vegetation, Crops, and Forests

Vegetation may be visibly injured by pollutants, as shown by bleaching, other color changes, and necrosis, or by more subtle changes such as alterations in growth or reproduction. Table 7.3 lists some of the more common visual effects of air pollutants on vegetation. Air pollution can also result in measurable effects on forest ecosystems, such as reduction in forest growth, change in forest species, and increased susceptibility to forest pests. High-dose exposure to pollutants, which is associated with point source emissions such as smelters, frequently results in complete destruction of trees and shrubs in the surrounding area.

TABLE 7.3
Examples of Air Pollution Injury to Vegetation

Pollutant	Symptoms
Sulfur dioxide	Bleached spots, interveinal bleaching
Ozone	Flecking, stippling, bleached spotting
PAN (peroxyacetylnitrate)	Glazing, silvering, or bronzing on lower surface of leaves
Nitrogen dioxide	Irregular white or brown collapsed lesions near leaf margins
Hydrogen fluoride	Tip and margin burns, dwarfing

7.2.5.2 Domestic Animals

Although domestic animals can be affected as humans are by air pollutants, the main concern is chronic poisoning resulting from ingestion of forage contaminated by airborne pollutants. Pollutants important in this connection are arsenic, lead, and molybdenum. Fluoride emissions from industries producing phosphate fertilizers and derivatives have damaged cattle throughout the world. The raw material, phosphate rock, can contain up to 4% fluoride, some of which is released into the air and water. Farm animals, particularly cattle, sheep, and swine, are susceptible to fluoride toxicity (fluorosis), which is characterized by mottled and soft teeth, and osteofluoritic bone lesions which lead to lameness and eventually death.

7.2.5.3 Materials and Structures

Building materials have become soiled and blackened by smoke; damage by chemical attack from acid gases in the air has led to the deterioration of many marble statues in Western Europe. Metals are also affected by air pollution; for example, sulfur dioxide causes many metals to corrode at a faster rate.

Ozone is known to oxidize rubber products, and one of the effects of Los Angeles smog is cracking of rubber tires. Fabrics are also affected by air pollution — a widely, publicized example was damage to women's nylon hose which caused them to disintegrate. This effect was probably due to a fine mist of sulfuric acid deposited on the nylon fibers. Leather and paper are also affected by SO_2 and sulfuric acid, causing them to crack, become brittle, and tear more easily.

7.2.5.4 Atmospheric Effects

The presence of fine particles (0.1 – 1.0 μm in diameter) or NO_2 in the atmosphere can result in atmospheric haze or reduced visibility due to light scattering by the particles. The major effect of atmospheric haze has been a degradation in visual air quality and is of particular concern in areas of scenic beauty, including most of the major national parks such as Grand Canyon, Yosemite, and Zion Park.

There is also concern over the increase in CO_2 concentration in the atmosphere. Because CO_2 absorbs heat energy strongly, it retards the cooling of the earth due to the loss of radiant energy. This is often referred to as the "greenhouse effect"; theoretically, an increase in CO_2 levels would result in a global increase in air temperatures.

7.2.5.5 Acidic Deposition

Acidic deposition is the combined total of wet and dry deposition, with wet acidic deposition being commonly referred to as acid rain. Normal uncontaminated rain has a pH of about 5.6, but acid rain can have a pH of ≤ 4.0. In the eastern United States, the acids in acid rain are approximately 65% sulfuric, 30% nitric, and 5% other, whereas in the western states, 80% of the acidity is due to nitric acid.

Hundreds of lakes in northeastern North America and Scandinavia have become so acidic that fish are no longer able to live in them. The low pH not only affects fish directly, but contributes to the release of potentially toxic metals such as aluminum. The maximum effect occurs when there is little buffering of the acid by soils or rock components. Maximum fish kills occur in early spring due to the "acid shock" from the melting of winter snows. Much of the acidity in rain may be neutralized by dissolving minerals in the soil, such as aluminum, calcium, magnesium, sodium, and potassium which are leached from the soil into surface waters. The ability of the soil to neutralize or buffer the acid rain is very dependent on the alkalinity of the soil. Much of the area in eastern Canada and the northeastern United States is covered by thin soils with low neutralizing capacity. In such areas, the lakes are more susceptible to the effects of acid deposition leading to a low pH and high levels of aluminum, a combination toxic to many species of fish.

A second area of concern is that of reduced tree growth in forests. The leaching of nutrients from the soil by acid deposition may cause a reduction in future growth rates or changes in the type of trees to those able to survive in the altered environment. The change in soil composition in conjunction with the direct effects on the trees from air pollutants may have very severe repercussions in the future. Recently, concern has been growing in West Germany over the death of significant number of trees in the German forests as well as reduced growth of young trees. A similar situation exists in many areas of the Appalachian mountains in the eastern United States.

7.3 CHEMICAL POLLUTANTS IN THE SOIL AND WATER

7.3.1 Introduction

With three quarters of the earth's surface covered by water and much of the remainder covered by soil, it is not surprising that water and soil serve as ultimate sinks for most anthropogenic chemicals. Until recently, the primary concern with water pollution was that of health effects due to pathogens. In the United States and other developed countries, treatment methods have largely eliminated bacterial disease organisms from the water supply and attention has been turned to chemical contaminants.

7.3.2 Sources of Chemical Pollutants

Industrial wastes probably constitute the greatest single pollution problem in soil and water. These contaminants include organic wastes, inorganic wastes, such as chromium and mercury, and many unknown chemicals. Contamination of soil and water results when by-product chemicals are not properly disposed of or conserved. In addition, industrial accidents may lead to severe local contamination.

Domestic and municipal wastes, both from sewage and from disposal of chemicals, are another major source of chemical pollutants. At the turn of the century, municipal wastes received no treatment, but were discharged directly into rivers or oceans. Even today, many older treatment plants do not provide sufficient treatment, especially plants in which both storm water and sewage are combined. In addition to organic matter, pesticides, fertilizers, detergents, and metals are significant pollutants discharged from urban areas.

Contamination of soil and water also results from the use of pesticides and fertilizers. Persistent pesticides applied directly to the soil have the potential to move from the soil into the water and thus enter the food chain from both soil and water. In a similar manner, fertilizers leach out of the soil and into the natural water systems.

Pollution from petroleum compounds has been a major concern in the last two decades. In 1967, the first major accident involving an oil tanker occurred. The Torrey Canyon ran onto rocks in the English Channel, spilling oil that washed onto the shores of England and France. It is estimated that at least 10,000 serious oil spills occur in the United States each year. In addition, flushing of oil tankers also contributes significantly to marine pollution. Other sources, such as improper disposal of used oil by private car owners and small garages, also contribute to oil pollution.

7.3.3 Pollutants and Their Effects

7.3.3.1 Metals

Toxic metals include lead, mercury, cadmium, zinc, copper, nickel, and arsenic. One of the most significant effects of metal pollution is that aquatic organisms can absorb and accumulate metals in their tissues, leading to increasing concentrations in the food chain. Concern about long-term exposure to cadmium intensified after recognition of the disease Itai-Itai (painful-painful) in certain areas of Japan. The disease is a combination of severe kidney damage and painful bone and joint disease and has occurred in areas where rice contained high levels of cadmium due to irrigation of the soil with water contaminated by cadmium from industrial sources. Cadmium toxicity in Japan also resulted from consumption of cadmium-contaminated fish taken from rivers near the smelting plants.

In Japan in the 1950s and 1960s, wastes from a chemical and plastics plant containing mercury were drained into Minamata Bay. The mercury was converted to the readily absorbed methylmercury by bacteria in the aquatic sediments. Consumption of fish and shellfish by the local population resulted in numerous cases of mercury poisoning or Minamata disease. By 1970, at least

107 deaths had been attributed to mercury poisoning, and 800 cases of Minamata disease were confirmed. Even though the mothers appeared healthy, many infants born to these mothers who had eaten contaminated fish developed cerebral palsylike symptoms and mental deficiency.

7.3.3.2 Pesticides

Pesticides are also a major source of concern as soil and water pollutants. Because of their stability and persistence, the most hazardous pesticides are the organochlorine compounds such as DDT, aldrin, dieldrin, and chlordane. Persistent pesticides can accumulate in food chains; for example, shrimp and fish can concentrate some pesticides as much as 1,000- to 10,000-fold. This bioaccumulation has been well documented with the pesticide DDT, which is now banned in many parts of the world. In contrast to the persistent insecticides, the organophosphates, such as malathion and the carbamates, such as carbaryl, are short-lived and generally persist for only a few weeks to a few months. Thus, these compounds do not usually represent a serious problem as soil and water contaminants. Herbicides, because of the large quantity used, are also of concern as potential toxic pollutants.

7.3.3.3 Inorganic Nutrients

Nitrates and phosphates are two important nutrients that have been increasing markedly in natural waters over the past 20 years. Nitrates from fertilizers readily leach from soils, and it has been estimated that up to 40% of applied nitrates enter water sources as run-off and leachate. Fertilizer phosphates, on the other hand, tend to be adsorbed or bound to soil particles, so that only 20–25% of applied phosphate is leached in water. Phosphate detergents are another source of phosphate, one that has received much media attention in recent years. The increase in these nutrients, particularly phosphates, is of concern because excess nutrients can lead to "algal blooms" in lakes and very slow moving rivers. The algal bloom reduces light penetration and restricts atmospheric reoxygenation of the water. When the dense algal growth dies, the subsequent biodegradation results in anaerobic conditions and the death of many aquatic organisms. High phosphate concentrations and algal blooms are not a problem in moving streams, since such streams are continually flushed out and algae do not accumulate. Thus, the above process, known as eutrophication, occurs only in lakes, ponds, estuaries, and very slow-moving rivers.

Ingested nitrates can be converted to nitrites by intestinal bacteria. After entering the circulatory system, nitrite ions combine with hemoglobin to form methemoglobin, thus decreasing the oxygen-carrying capacity of the blood and resulting in anemia or blue-baby disease. It is particularly severe in young babies who consume milk-formula prepared with nitrate-rich water; older children and adults possess an enzyme, methemoglobin reductase, that reverses the formation of methemoglobin, but the enzyme is not fully functional in infants.

7.3.3.4 Petroleum

Oils and petroleum, as previously mentioned, are ever-present pollutants in the modern environment, whether from the used oil of private motorists or spillage from oil tankers. At sea, oil slicks are responsible for the deaths of many birds.

The Torrey Canyon incident, for example, was estimated to be responsible for the deaths of at least 100,000 birds. Very few birds that are badly contaminated recover, even after de-oiling and hand feeding. Oil is deposited on rocks and sand as well, thus preventing the beaches being used for recreation until after costly clean-up. Shore animals, such as crabs, shrimp, mussels, and barnacles are also affected by the toxic hydrocarbons they ingest. The subtle and perhaps potentially more harmful, long-term effects on aquatic life are not yet understood.

7.3.3.5 Acids

Acids, present in rain or drainage from mines, are major pollutants in many freshwater lakes. Because of their ability to lower the pH of the water to toxic levels and release toxic metals into solution, acids were considered particularly hazardous (see Section 7.2.5.5, Acid deposition).

7.3.3.6 Other Organic Chemicals

The number of organic compounds found as soil and water contaminants continues to grow each year. They include polychlorinated biphenyls (PCBs), phenols, cyanides, plasticizers, solvents, and numerous industrial chemicals.

PCBs are by-products of the plastic, lubricant, rubber, and paper industries. They are stable, lipophilic, and break down only slowly in tissues. Because of these properties, they accumulate to high concentrations in water fowl; in 1969, PCBs were responsible for the death of thousands of birds in the Irish Sea.

Of recent concern is the formation of low-molecular-weight chlorinated hydrocarbons, which are produced during the chlorination of municipal water. The main organics detected by an EPA survey were chloroform, bromodichloromethane, dibromochloromethane, bromoform, carbon tetrachloride, and 1-2-dichloroethane. Studies in New Orleans in the mid-1970s showed that tap water in New Orleans contained more chlorinated hydrocarbons than did untreated Mississippi River water or well water. In addition, chlorinated hydrocarbons, including carbon tetrachloride, were detected in blood plasma from volunteers who drank treated tap water. Epidemiological studies indicated that the cancer death rate was 15% higher among white males who drank tap water than among those who drank well water.

Large areas of water and soil have been contaminated with the extremely toxic TCDD (2,3,7,8-tetrachlorodibenzo-*p*-dioxin) through industrial accidents and through widespread use of the herbicide 2,4,5-T, which contained small amounts of TCDD as a contaminant. The US Army used this herbicide, known as Agent Orange, extensively as a defoliant in Vietnam. Fortunately, TCDD has extremely low water solubility and binds firmly to soil particles.

7.4 CHEMICAL ADDITIVES AND POLLUTANTS IN FOOD

7.4.1 Introduction and Legal Aspects

Food additives are almost as old as humans, being first added to food by fire and smoke when meats were cooked, and as salts and spices later added to foods for flavor. The Egyptians were known to have used food colorings as early as 3,500 years ago.

The Food Additive Amendment of 1958 (an amendment to the Food, Drug and Cosmetic Act of 1938) provides that any substance added to food must be proven safe by the manufacturer before it is offered for sale, except for those additives generally recognized as safe (the GRAS list), based on past experience and conditions of intended use. The Color Additive Amendment (1960) required colorings to be reexamined and those found to cause cancer in any animal to be banned, while establishing use limits (certified colors). Colorings currently in use, however, were permitted to remain in use as "uncertified" colors until scientific tests were completed.

7.4.2 Reasons for Using Food Additives

Food additives are used by the food industry for four primary reasons: for nutrition, to maintain freshness, to enhance sensory properties, and as an aid in processing.

Nutritive additives are used to prevent or eliminate nutritional deficiencies, such as the addition of iodine to table salt to prevent goiter, or to replace nutrients lost in processing, eg, thiamin, which is lost in processing wheat and rice.

Antioxidants, preservatives, sequestrants, and stabilizers are the main types of chemicals used to extend the shelf life of food by maintaining freshness and retarding spoilage.

Sensory additives are compounds used to change or maintain aroma, flavor, texture, or the color of foods. All of these components affect the acceptability and thus the marketability of food.

Processing aids, such as bleaching agents, help make processing of food faster or simpler.

Table 7.4 gives a partial listing of the many use categories of food additives and some examples of each. Only a few of these additives will be discussed in detail.

7.4.3 Color Additives

Food colorings are added to enhance the acceptability of food products and must be either certified (synthetic) colors or on the accepted list of those exempt from certification (certain natural colors). As of December 1985, nine synthetic colors and 20 natural colors were permitted in the United States (Tables 7.5 and 7.6). The synthetic dyes currently in use are all water soluble and almost insoluble in organic solvents. FD&C lakes, derivatives of the dye, are insoluble pigments made by adsorbing the dye onto aluminum hydroxide, these pigments color the food by dispersion. The only fat-soluble colors are found among the natural dyes.

Among the natural coloring agents, the carotenoids are the most widespread, occurring in numerous fruits and vegetables such as carrots, tomatoes, apricots, and oranges. These colors are essential in situations in which oil-soluble food colors are deemed necessary. Annatto colors are extracted from the seeds of the tropical tree, *Bixa orellana;* the extract, bixin, which is oil soluble, is used to color butter, margarine, popcorn oil, and salad dressings. Titanium dioxide

TABLE 7.4
Lists of Types of Food Additives

Types of Additives	Examples
Anticaking agents	Calcium silicate, magnesium carbonate
Antioxidants	Ascorbic acid, BHT, BHA
Colors	Synthetic and natural
Curing agents	Nitrites and nitrates
Emulsifiers	Lecithin, cholic acid
Firming agents	Alum in pickles
Flavor enhancers	MSG (monosodium glutamate)
Flavorings	Natural (spices) and synthetic (aldehydes)
Bleaching agents	Benzoylperoxide
Humectants	Sorbitol, propylene glycol
Leavening	Baking powder
Nonnutritive sweeteners	Saccharin, aspartame
Nutrient supplements	Vitamins and minerals
Stabilizers	Starches and gums
Preservatives	Calcium propionate, sodium benzoate
Surfactants	Vegetable gums, monoglycerides, diglycerides
pH agents	Acids, alkalides, buffers
Texturizers	Starches
Sequestrants	Calcium acetate, sodium citrate
Propellants	Nitrogens, CO_2

TABLE 7.5
Certified Synthetic Colors Permitted in Food in the United States

Official Name	Common Name
FD&C Blue No. 1	Brilliant Blue FCF
FD&C Blue No. 2[a]	Indigo Carmine
FD&C Green No. 3[a]	Fast Green FCF
FD&C Red No. 3	Erythrosine
FD&C Red No. 40	Allura Red AC
FD&C Yellow No. 5	Tartrazine
FD&C Yellow No. 6[a]	Sunset Yellow FCF
Citrus Red No. 2[b]	Solvent Red 80
Orange B[c]	Acid Orange 137

Permitted as of December 1, 1981. FD&C, Food, Drug and Cosmetic Act.
[a] Provisional.
[b] For skins of oranges not intended for processing.
[c] For casings on surfaces of frankfurters or sausages.

TABLE 7.6
Colors Exempt from Certification Permitted in Food in the United States

Agent	Food
Annatto extract (bixin)	Fruit juice
Beet powder	Grape color extract[a]
Canthaxanthin	Grape skin extract[b]
Caramel	Paprika
β-Apo-8'-carotenal	Paprika olcoresin
β-Carotene	Riboflavin
Carrot oil	Saffron
Cochineal extract (carmine)	Titanium dioxide
Cottonseed flour	Tumeric
Ferrous gluconate[c]	Tumeric oleoresin
	Vegetable juice

Exempt as of December 1, 1981.
[a] For ripe olives only.
[b] For nonbeverage foods.
[c] For beverages only.

(TiO_2), a white pigment, is used primarily in icings or is mixed with sugar syrup as a coating for pharmaceutical tablets.

A common assumption is that the "artificial" colors, which were originally called "coal tar" dyes are more hazardous, while the "natural" or "vegetable" dyes are safe. The artificial dyes are purified synthetic compounds (and not derived from coal tar) whose toxicology has been studied in detail. On the other hand, the natural dyes are often complex mixtures whose only toxicological assessment is that humans have used them with apparent safety for many years.

Many of the synthetic dyes have been banned in the United States because of problems associated with use (for example, overuse of FD&C orange No. 1 and FD&C red No. 3 in candy and popcorn led to cases of diarrhea in children) or because of the results from chronic toxicity testing. Amaranth, FD&C Red No. 2, in use since 1907, was recently banned because the results of FDA studies suggested that it was embryotoxic in the rat.

Another controversy that has recently developed is that certain food dyes, particularly Yellow No. 5 (Tartrazine) can cause hyperactivity in children; however, animal studies failed to confirm this. A greater problem may be allergic reactions that many people have to this dye.

7.4.4 Antioxidants

Lipids in foods can undergo degradation reactions that result in off-flavors and off-odors. The use of food antioxidants are effective in preventing or retarding certain oxidation reactions, such as lipid oxidation of unsaturated fatty acids which produces a "rancid" flavor. Most of the naturally occurring antioxidants, as well as the synthetic antioxidants used in foods, are phenols (Figure 7.1).

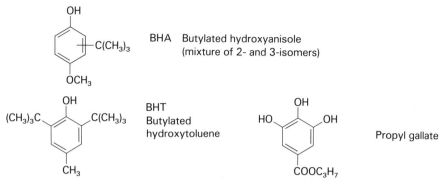

FIGURE 7.1.
Structures of some commonly used antioxidants.

Butylated hydroxyanisole (BHA) is rapidly excreted, partly in the feces as the original compound and partly in the urine in the form of glucuronides and sulfates. The metabolism of butylated hydroxytoluene (BHT) is slower; it is excreted mainly into the bile where it undergoes enterohepatic circulation. Recent interest has centered on the protective role of BHA and BHT as anticarcinogens by virtue of their role as antioxidants and free radical scavengers.

7.4.5 Preservatives

Table 7.7 lists some of the approved antimicrobial agents and uses; structures of some of the more common ones are given in Figure 7.2. Benzoic acid and sodium benzoate have been used for many years as antimicrobial agents in foods. Because they are most active at pH ≥ 4.0, they have been used widely in carbonated drinks, fruit juices, and pickles. Sodium benzoate is considered to be most active against yeasts and bacteria. Benzoate is readily excreted from the

TABLE 7.7
Some Antimicrobial Agents Used in the United States and Their Uses

Preservatives	Important Uses
Benzoic acid and sodium benzoate	Beverages, margarine, pickles
Ethyl and propyl paraben	Beverages, beer, pastries, dried fruit
Sorbates	Beverages, wine, cheese, pastries, processed meats, dried fruits
Propionates	Cheese, baked goods
Sulfides	Beverages, wines, pickles, dried fruits
Acetates, diacetates	Baked goods, salad dressings, pickles
Nitrite, nitrate	Processed meat
Ethylene and propylene oxide	Spices, nuts, glacé fruit
Diethylpyrocarbonate	Wine

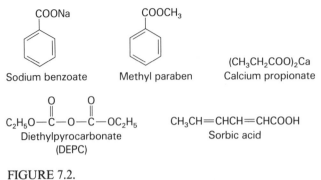

FIGURE 7.2.
Structures of some preservatives used in food.

body, being conjugated with either glycine or glucuronic acid, and eliminated through the urine.

The alkyl esters (methyl, ethyl, propyl, and butyl) of *p*-hydroxybenzoic acid (parabens) are similar in structure to benzoic acid, but are effective at a higher pH, primarily against molds and yeasts. Hydrolysis of the esters and conjugation constitute the chief route of elimination in mammals. Toxicity symptoms in mice at high doses include rapid onset ataxia and paralysis, but recovery usually occurs within 30 minutes.

Sorbic acid and its sodium and potassium salts are particularly effective against molds and yeasts, and for this reason have found extensive use in foods and on food wrappers — especially for cheese products and baked goods. Sorbic acid has very low toxicity, probably because it is metabolized in the same way as other fatty acids.

Both sodium and calcium propionates are more active against bread molds than is sodium benzoate. The calcium salt is preferred in bread because the calcium also contributes to nutritive value. The sodium salt is used in cakes and other baked goods in which the calcium ion can interfere with chemical leavening. No known mammalian toxicity is associated with the propionates.

Sulfur dioxide has been used for centuries in the wine-making industries, and the sulfides, sodium and potassium salts, are used extensively in drying of fruits and vegetables. The use of sulfides is limited by the fact that, at levels >500 ppm, the disagreeable taste becomes noticeable.

Acetic acid (vinegar) and its salts are effective antimicrobials, especially at an acidic pH when the salts are dissociated to form the free acid. Vinegar is used in such foods as catsup, mayonnaise, pickles, and salad dressings, whereas the acetate salts are used in baked goods.

Nitrates and nitrites are used in the curing of meats to develop and fix the color; the nitrites decompose to nitric oxide, NO, which then reacts with heme pigments to form nitrosomyoglobin, imparting the characteristic pink color to processed meats. Nitrites, in conjunction with the added sodium chloride, also provide antimicrobial action. Controversy in recent years has centered on the role nitrites might play in carcinogenesis. Most *N*-nitroso compounds, such as dimethylnitrosamine (DMN), are carcinogenic in a wide range of animal species. Some nitroso compounds are found in preserved meats as a result of interaction of nitrites and secondary or tertiary amines; in addition, the stomach provides favorable conditions for the generation of nitrosamines from nitrites and amines. At a low pH, nitrite is protonated to nitrous acid, a very reactive nitrosating and oxidizing agent. Although the carcinogenicity of nitroso compounds has been demonstrated in animals, epidemiological studies have not yet established a valid association between cancer and exposure to nitrates and nitrites in humans.

Ethylene and propylene oxides are used as fumigants on dry foods such as spices and nut meats. Both are broad-range microbiocides and ethylene oxide is effective against viruses.

Diethylpyrocarbonate (DEPC) permits "cold sterilization" of foods, especially wines, in which it kills yeasts. DEPC is rapidly hydrolyzed to ethanol and CO_2, leaving only trace residues and no taste or odor.

7.4.6 Flavorings

Flavor additives are a major portion of the additives used in foods, with the most commonly used ones numbering about 150. Of these, about half are natural, and the remainder are synthetic. Most of the additives are on the GRAS list; thus, their safety is subject to review. Frequently used natural flavorings are derived from spices and fruits (basil, clove, ginger, lemon, pepper, etc.) whereas many synthetic flavors are alcohols or aldehydes.

7.4.7 Artificial Sweeteners

The need for artificial sweeteners has been recognized for the control of diabetes and for others wishing to restrict sugar intake. Saccharin (Figure 7.3), accidentally discovered in 1879, has been used by diabetics for many years. Other sweeteners have been introduced by the soft-drink industry, with one of the most successful being sodium cyclamate because it does not leave the bitter aftertaste characteristic of saccharin. Chronic testing of these sweeteners has yielded conflicting results. Early tests indicated that cyclamate alone did not possess carcinogenic activity, but a subsequent test, using a combination of cyclamate and saccharin, produced bladder tumors in rats. Cyclamate was implicated and banned from use in the United States in 1969. Later studies showed that saccharin alone in very high doses could produce bladder tumors. As a result saccharin was banned in Canada, where cyclamates were still permitted, but a moratorium was placed on a proposed ban in the United States

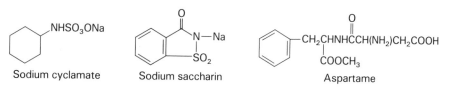

Sodium cyclamate   Sodium saccharin   Aspartame

FIGURE 7.3.
Chemical structures of three widely used artificial sweeteners.

because of public reaction and the fact that saccharin was the only artificial sweetener in use at that time.

The most recent sugar substitute is aspartame (Nutrasweet), composed of two naturally occurring amino acids, aspartic acid and phenylalanine. Extensive toxicological testing to date has not shown any carcinogenic potential. Because it does not leave a bitter aftertaste, aspartame is frequently preferred to saccharin; most diet soft drinks in the United States are now sweetened with aspartame.

There is, however, a problem with use of Nutrasweet for people with the disease phenylketonuria (PKU). This condition, caused by a mutant recessive gene, results in the absence of the enzyme phenylalanine hydroxylase which converts phenylalanine to tyrosine; about 1 in every 10,000 persons develop PKU. In the absence of phenylalanine hydroxylase, a minor pathway, little used in normal individuals, becomes prominent; this path converts phenylalanine to phenylpyruvic acid, which accumulates in the blood and is excreted in the urine. In childhood, excess circulating phenylpyruvate impairs normal brain development, causing mental retardation. PKU was among the first genetic defects of metabolism recognized in humans, and the urine of infants is routinely tested for the disease. Restriction of dietary phenylalanine reduces the blood level of phenylpyruvic acid and prevents the mental retardation. For this reason, people with PKU are advised not to use products sweetened with aspartame, and most products carry a warning label for consumers.

7.4.8 Nonintentional Additives

Nonintentional additives of food pollutants are agents that accidentally or incidentally find their way into the finished food product. These contaminants include such diverse pollutants as insect parts, pesticides, phytotoxins, mycotoxins, and antibiotics. Examples of some common types of contaminants of concern to toxicologists are listed below; many of these have been discussed previously in the sections on toxic action or classes of toxicants:

1. Metals (selenium, lead, mercury)
2. Pathogens: bacteria *(Clostridium botulinium, Salmonella)*
    mycotoxins (aflatoxins)
    viral infections (raw shellfish from waters contaminated by sewage)
3. PCBs, polybrominated biphenyls (PBBs)
4. Pesticides
5. Antibiotic residues
6. Hormone residues

7.5 CHEMICALS IN THE WORKPLACE

7.5.1 Introduction

Assessment of hazards in the workplace is a concern of occupational/industrial toxicology and has a history that dates back to ancient civilizations. The Greek historian, Strabo, who lived in the first century AD, gave a graphic description of the arsenic mines in Pantus: "The air in mines is both deadly and hard to endure on account of the grievous odor of the ore, so that the workmen are doomed to a quick death." With the coming of the industrial revolution in the nineteenth century, industrial diseases increased and new ones, such as chronic mercurialism caused by exposure to mercuric nitrate used in "felting" animal furs, were identified. Hatmakers, who were especially at risk, frequently developed characteristic tremors known as "hatters' shakes," and the expression "mad as a hatter" was coined.

In recent years, concern has developed over the carcinogenic potential of many workplace chemicals. The goal of occupational toxicology is to ensure work practices that do not entail any unnecessary health risks. To do this, it is necessary first to define suitable permissible levels of exposure, using the results of animal studies and epidemiological studies. These levels can be expressed by the following terms for allowable concentrations:

THRESHOLD-LIMIT VALUES (TLVs) refer to airborne concentrations of substances and represent conditions under which it is believed that nearly all workers may be repeatedly exposed day after day without adverse effect. Because of wide variation in individual susceptibility, a small percentage of workers may experience discomfort from some substances at or below the threshold limit; a smaller percentage may be affected more seriously by aggravation of a preexisting condition or by development of an occupational illness. Threshold limits are based on the best available information from industrial experience, from experimental human and animal studies, and, when possible, from a combination of the three. The basis on which the values are established may differ from substance to substance; protection against impairment of health may be a guiding factor for some, whereas reasonable freedom from irritation, narcosis, nuisance, or other forms of stress may form the basis for others. Three categories of TLVs are mentioned below.

THRESHOLD LIMIT VALUE — TIME-WEIGHTED AVERAGE (TLV — TWA) is the TWA concentration for a normal 8-hour work day or 40-hour work week to which nearly all workers may be repeatedly exposed, day after day, without adverse effect. Time-weighted averages allow certain permissible excursions above the limit provided they are compensated by equivalent excursions below the limit during the work day. In some instances, the average concentration is calculated for a work week rather than for a work day.

THRESHOLD LIMIT VALUE — SHORT-TERM EXPOSURE LIMIT (TLV — STEL) is the maximal concentration to which workers can be exposed for a period up to 15 minutes continuously without suffering from (1) irritation, (2) chronic or irreversible tissue change, or (3) narcosis of sufficient degree to increase accident proneness, impair self-rescue, or materially reduce work efficiency, provided that no more than four excursions per day are permitted, with at least 60 minutes between exposure periods, and provided that the daily TLV – TWA is not exceeded.

THRESHOLD LIMIT VALUE — CEILING (TLV — C) is the concentration that should not be exceeded even instantaneously. For some substances, eg, irritant gases, only one category, the TLV – ceiling, may be relevant. For other substances, two or three categories may be relevant.

BIOLOGIC LIMIT VALUES (BLVS) represent limits of amounts of substances (or their affects) to which the worker may be exposed without hazard to health or well-being as determined by measuring the worker's tissues, fluids, or exhaled breath. The biologic measurements on which the BLVs are based can furnish two kinds of information useful in the control of worker exposure: (1) measure of the worker's overall exposure, and (2) measure of the worker's individual and characteristic response. Measurements of response furnish a superior estimate of the physiologic status of the worker, and may consist of: (1) changes in amount of some critical biochemical constituent, (2) changes in activity of a critical enzyme, and (3) changes in some physiologic function. Measurement of exposure may be made by (1) determining in blood, urine, hair, nails, in body tissues and fluids, the amount of substance to which the worker was exposed; (2) determination of the amount of the metabolite(s) of the substance in tissues and fluids; and (3) determination of the amount of the substance in the exhaled breath. The biologic limits may be used as an adjunct to the TLVs for air, or in place of them.

IMMEDIATELY DANGEROUS TO LIFE OR HEALTH (IDLH). Conditions that pose an immediate threat to life or health or conditions that pose an immediate threat of severe exposure to contaminants such as radioactive materials that are likely to have adverse cumulative or delayed effects on health are termed IDLH. Two factors are considered when establishing IDLH concentrations. The worker must be able to escape: (1) without losing his life or suffering permanent health damage within 30 minutes; and (2) without severe eye or respiratory irritation or other reactions that could inhibit escape. If the concentration is above the IDLH, only highly reliable breathing apparatus is allowed.

7.5.2 Routes of Exposure

The principal routes of industrial exposure are dermal and inhalation. Occasionally, toxic agents may be ingested if food or drinking water becomes contaminated.

Exposure to the skin often leads to localized effects known as "occupation dermatosis" caused either by irritating chemicals or allergenic chemicals. Such effects include scaling, eczema, acne, pigmentation changes, ulcers, and neoplasia. Some chemicals may also pass through the skin; these include aromatic amines such as aniline and solvents such as carbon tetrachloride and benzene.

Toxic or potentially toxic agents may be inhaled in the form of gases, vapors, liquid, and solid materials into the respiratory tract, where they may cause localized effects such as irritation (eg, ammonia and chlorine gas), inflammation, necrosis, and cancer. Chemicals may also be absorbed through gas exchange in the lungs and lead to systemic toxicity (eg, CO and lead).

7.5.3 Occupational Carcinogenesis

Aside from exposure to carcinogens due to life-style, such as cigarette smoking, occupation is an important source of exposure to carcinogens. Table 7.8 lists some occupational chemical hazards and the cancers associated with them.

TABLE 7.8
Occupational Hazards and Associated Cancers

Agent	Tumor Sites	Occupation
X-rays	Bone, marrow, and skin	Medical and industrial
Radon gas, radium, and uranium	Skin, lung, bone sarcoma, and bone marrow	Medical and industrial chemists, dial painters, and miners
Ultraviolet radiation	Skin	Outdoor occupations
Polycyclic hydrocarbons in soot, tar and oil	Lung, skin, larynx, bladder, and nasal cavity	Furnaces, forges and foundaries, shale oil workers, gas workers and retort men, chimney sweeps
Benzene	Bone marrow and lymph nodes	Process workers, painters, textile workers, explosives workers
1- and 2-Naphthyl-amine, 4-biphenyl-amine, and 4-nitrobi-phenyl	Bladder	Dyestuffs makers, rubber workers and other chemical plant process workers, shoe workers, and printers
Mustard gas	Bronchial tree, lung, and larynx	Production workers
Isopropyl alcohol	Nasal cavity	Production workers
Vinyl chloride	Liver (angiosarcoma) and brain	Plastic manufacture
Chloroethers	Lung	Chemical plant, process workers
Chloroprene	Skin, lung, and liver	Neoprene production
Arsenic	Skin, lung, and liver	Insecticide workers, miners and smelters, oil refiners
Chromium	Lung, nasal cavity, and sinuses	Process and production workers, pigment workers
Cadmium	Lung, kidney, and prostate	Battery workers, smelters
Nickel	Lung and nasal sinuses	Smelters and process workers
Asbestos and similar fibers	Lung, pleura and perito-neum, larynx, stomach, and large bowel	Miners, millers, manufacturers, users, and demolition workers
Wood and leather particles	Nasal cavity	Wood and show workers
Unidentified organics	Lymph nodes	Chemists

Source: Cartwright, R.A. Cancer Epidemiology in Chemical Carcinogens. 2nd ed. Washington, D.C.: American Chemical Society, 1984. Used by permission.

7.5.4 Examples of Toxic Industrial Substances

7.5.4.1 Metals

Cadmium is a very cumulative toxicant with a biological half-life of > 10 years in humans. More than 70% of the cadmium in the blood is bound to RBCs; accumulation occurs mainly in the kidney and the liver, where it is bound to metallothionein. In humans, the critical target organ after long-term exposure to cadmium is the kidney, with the first detectable symptom of kidney toxicity being an increased excretion of specific proteins (Section 6.3.4.2b.1, Nephrotoxicity, metals).

The toxicity of chromium is due to compounds of hexavalent chromium that can be readily absorbed by the lung and gastrointestinal tract and to a lesser extent by the skin. Occupational exposure to chromium (Cr^{6+}) causes dermatitis, ulcers on hands and arms, perforation of the nasal septum (probably caused by chromic acid), inflammation of larynx and liver, and bronchitis. Chromate is a carcinogen causing bronchogenic carcinoma; the risk of chromate plant workers for lung cancer is 20 times greater than that for the general population. Compounds of trivalent chromium are poorly absorbed. Chromium is not a cumulative chemical and, once absorbed, it is rapidly excreted into the urine.

Lead is an ubiquitous toxicant in the environment; thus, the normal body concentration of lead is dependent on environmental exposure conditions. Approximately 50 % of lead deposited in the lung is absorbed, whereas usually < 10% of ingested lead passes into the circulation. Lead is not a major occupational problem today, but environmental pollution is still widespread. Lead interferes in the biosynthesis of porphyrins and heme (Figure 7.4), and several screening tests for lead poisoning make use of this by monitoring either inhibition of the enzyme δ-aminolevulinic dehydratase (ALAD) or appearance in the urine of aminolevulinic acid (ALA) and coproporphorin (UCP). The metabolism of inorganic lead is closely related to that of calcium and excess lead can be deposited in the bone, where it remains for years. Inorganic lead poisoning can produce fatigue, sleep disturbances, anemia, colic, and neuritis. Severe expo-

Succinyl CoA + Glycine

δ-aminolevulinic acid (ALA)

Porphobilinogen (PBG)

Uroporphyrinogen III

Coproporphyrinogen

Protoporphyrinogen III

Fe^{++} + Protoporphyrin IX

Heme

FIGURE 7.4.
Biosynthesis of heme: 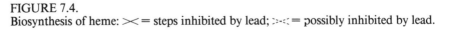 = steps inhibited by lead; = possibly inhibited by lead.

sure, mainly to children who have ingested lead, may cause encephalopathy, mental retardation and, occasionally, impaired vision. Organic lead has an affinity for brain tissue; mild poisoning may cause insomnia, restlessness, and gastrointestinal symptoms, whereas severe poisoning results in delirium, hallucinations, convulsions, coma, and even death.

Metallic mercury is widely used in scientific and electrical apparatus, with the largest industrial use of mercury being in the chlorine-alkali industry for electrolytic production of chlorine and sodium hydroxide. Worldwide, this industry has been a major source of mercury contamination. Most mercury poisoning, however, has been due to methyl mercury, particularly as a result of eating contaminated fish (see discussion of Minamata disease in Section 6.4.2 and see Section 3.3.3.4 for the mechanism of biomethylation). Inorganic and organic mercury differ in their routes of entry and absorption. Inhalation is the principal route of uptake of metallic mercury in industry, with approximately 80% of the mercury inhaled as vapor being absorbed; metallic mercury is less readily absorbed by the gastrointestinal route. The principal sites of deposition are the kidney and brain after exposure to mercury vapor and the kidney after exposure to inorganic mercury salts. Organic mercury compounds are readily absorbed by all routes. Industrial mercurialism produces features such as inflammation of the mouth, muscular tremors (hatters' shakes), psychic irritation, and a nephrotic syndrome characterized by proteinuria. Overall, however, occupational mercurialism is not a significant problem today.

7.5.4.2 Benzene

Benzene was used extensively in the latter half of the nineteenth century in the rubber industry when it was discovered that benzene, was an excellent solvent for rubber latex. The volatility of benzene, which made it so attractive to the industry, also caused high atmospheric levels of the solvent. Benzene-based rubber cements were used in the canning industry and in the shoe manufacturing industry. Although cases of benzene poisoning had been reported as early as 1897 and additional reports and warnings were issued in the 1920s, the excellent solvent properties of benzene resulted in its continued extensive use. In the 1930s, cases of benzene toxicity occurred in the printing industry where benzene was used as an ink solvent. Today benzene use exceeds 11 billion gallons per year. Benzene affects the hematopoietic tissue in the bone marrow and also appears to be an immunosuppressant. There is a gradual decrease in WBCs, RBCs, and platelets, and any combination of these signs may be seen. Continued exposure to benzene results in severe bone marrow damage and aplastic anemia. Benzene exposure has also been associated with cases of leukemia.

7.5.4.3 Asbestos and Other Fibers

Asbestos is a general name for a group of naturally occurring silicates that will separate into flexible fibers. Chrysotile ($3MgO-2SiO_2-2H_2O$) is the most important commercially and represents about 90% of the total used. Use of asbestos has been extensive, especially in roofing and insulation, asbestos cements, brake linings, electrical appliances, and coating materials. Asbestosis, a respiratory disease, is characterized by fibrosis, calcification, and lung cancer.

In humans, not only is there a long latency period between exposure and development of tumors, but other factors also influence the development of lung cancer. Cigarette smoking, for example, enhances tumor formation. Recent studies have shown that stomach and bowel cancers occur in excess in workers (such as insulation workers) exposed to asbestos. Other fibers have been shown to cause a similar disease spectrum, eg, zeolite fibers.

7.6 PESTICIDES

7.6.1 Introduction

Pesticides are unusual among environmental pollutants in that they are deliberately used for the purpose of killing some form of life. The ideal situation, of course, is that pesticides be highly selective, destroying target organisms while leaving nontarget organisms unharmed. In reality, most pesticides are not so selective.

In considering the use of pesticides, the benefits must be weighed against the risk to human health and environmental quality. Among the benefits of pesticides are control of vectorborne diseases, increased agricultural productivity, and control of urban pests. A major risk is environmental contamination, especially translocation within the environment where pesticides may enter both food chains and natural water systems. Factors to be considered in this regard are persistence in the environment and potential for bioaccumulation.

7.6.2 Classes of Pesticides

7.6.2.1 Organochlorine Insecticides

The chlorinated hydrocarbon insecticides include DDT, methoxychlor, chlordane, hepatochlor, aldrin, dieldrin, endrin, toxaphene, mirex, kepone, strobane, pentac, and lindane. The structures of several of the most familiar ones are shown in Figure 7.5.

The chlorinated hydrocarbons are neurotoxicants and cause acute effects by interfering with the transmission of nerve impulses along the axons. DDT apparently changes the transport of sodium and potassium across the axon membranes so that normal polarization is not restored.

From the 1940s through the 1960s, the organochlorines were used extensively in agriculture and mosquito control, particularly in the World Health Organization malaria control programs. Because of their persistence in the environment, potential for bioaccumulation through the food chain, injury to wildlife, contamination of the human food supply, and suspected carcinogenicity, many organochlorine insecticides are being phased out and replaced by degradable insecticides. Two organochlorine insecticides with relatively low persistence, toxaphene and methoxychlor, are still widely used.

7.6.2.2 Organophosphorus Insecticides

Organophosphates (OPs) are phosphoric acid esters or thiophosphoric acid esters (Figure 7.6). In the 1930s and 1940s in Germany, Gerhard Schrader and workers began investigating organophosphates. They realized the insecticidal

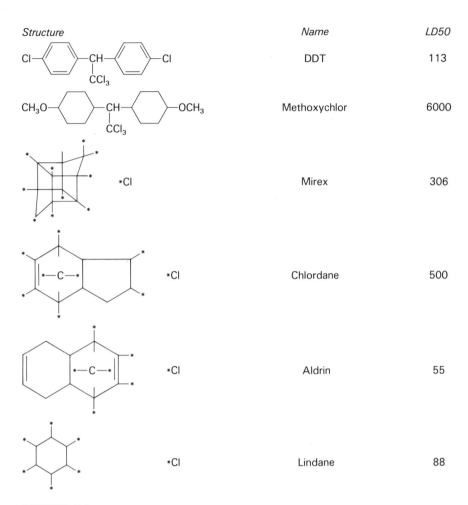

Structure	Name	LD50
	DDT	113
	Methoxychlor	6000
	Mirex	306
	Chlordane	500
	Aldrin	55
	Lindane	88

FIGURE 7.5.
Structures of some organochlorine insecticides.

properties of these compounds and by the end of the war had made many of the insecticidal phosphates in use today, such as dimefax in 1940, schradan (as it is now called, after its discoverer) in 1942; and parathion in 1944. The first organophosphate insecticide in wide use was tetraethylpyrophosphate, TEPP, which was approved in Germany in 1944 and marketed as a substitute for nicotine against aphids. Because of its high mammalian toxicity and rapid hydrolysis in water, TEPP was soon replaced by other organophosphates. Parathion soon became a widely used insecticide due to its stability in aqueous solutions and its broad range of insecticidal activity. Because it has high mammalian toxicity by all routes of exposure, however, other less hazardous compounds are now often used (Figure 7.6). Malathion, in particular, has low mammalian toxicity due to the fact that mammals possess carboxylesterases, which readily hydrolyze the carboxyester link, detoxifying the compound. Insects, by contrast, do not readily hydrolyze this ester, and the result is its selective insecticidal action.

Structure	Name	LD50
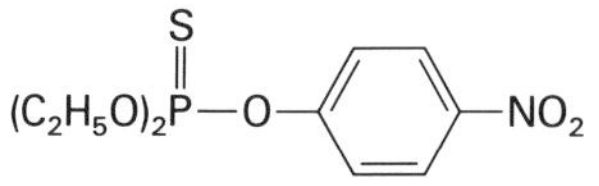 (C₂H₅O)₂P—O—⟨benzene⟩—NO₂ (S double bond on P)	Parathion	3–30
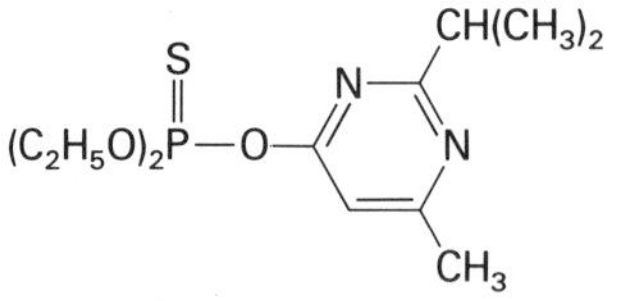 (C₂H₅O)₂P—O—⟨pyrimidine with CH(CH₃)₂ and CH₃⟩ (S double bond on P)	Diazinon	100–150
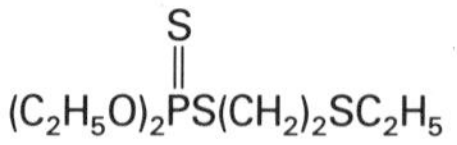 (C₂H₅O)₂PS(CH₂)₂SC₂H₅ (S double bond on P)	Disulfoton	12.5
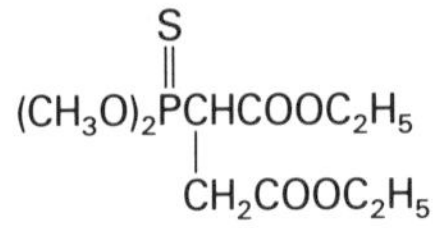 (CH₃O)₂PCHCOOC₂H₅ with CH₂COOC₂H₅ (S double bond on P)	Malathion	1000–1375

FIGURE 7.6.
Structures of some organophosphate insecticides. LD50 male rats. Analytical Reference Standards and Supplemental Data for Pesticides and Other Organic Compounds, US Environmental Protection Agency, 1981.

Organophosphates are toxic because of their inhibition of the acetylcholinesterase activity of nerve tissue (see Section 6.2.2.1, Cholinesterase inhibitors), resulting in the accumulation of acetylcholine in nerve tissue and effector organs, with the principal site of action being the peripheral nervous system. Symptoms of organophosphate poisoning from cholinesterase inhibition include tightness in the chest due to bronchoconstriction and increased bronchial secretions, increased salivation, lacrimation, sweating, nausea, vomiting, diarrhea, and constriction of the pupils. Muscular effects include fatigue, weakness and cramps. In fatal organophosphate poisoning, the immediate cause of death is respiratory failure.

The organophosphate insecticides, as well as the carbamate insecticides, are relatively nonpersistent in the environment. They are applied to the crop, or directly to the soil as systemic insecticides, and they generally persist from only a few hours to several months.

Thus, these compounds, in contrast to the organochlorine insecticides, do not represent a serious problem as contaminants of soil and water and rarely enter the human food chain. Being esters, the compounds are susceptible to hydrolysis, and their breakdown products are generally nontoxic.

7.6.2.3 Carbamate Insecticides

The carbamate insecticides are esters of *N*-methyl (or occasionally *N,N*-dimethyl) carbamic acid, with the toxicity varying according to the phenol or alcohol group (Figure 7.7). For example, aldicarb (Temik), which is extremely toxic by both oral and dermal routes, is recommended only for limited use.

Like the organophosphates, the mode of action of the carbamates is inhibition of acetylcholinesterase — although with carbamates the inhibition is more rapidly reversed than it is with organophosphates (see Section 6.2.2.1, Cholinesterase inhibitors).

Structure   *Name*   *LD50*

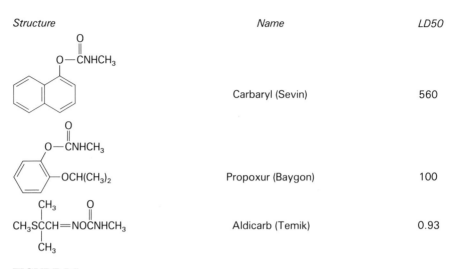

Carbaryl (Sevin)   560

Propoxur (Baygon)   100

Aldicarb (Temik)   0.93

FIGURE 7.7.
Structures of some carbamate insecticides.

7.6.2.4 Botanical (Natural) Insecticides

Pyrethrum, which is extracted from several types of chrysanthemum, is one of the oldest insecticides used by humans (Figure 7.8). Pyrethrins are used in many household insecticides because of their quick "knockdown" action but are too rapidly degraded by heat and sunlight to be useful for agricultural pest control. Mammalian toxicity to pyrethrins is very low, apparently due to the rapid breakdown by liver microsomal enzymes and esterases. The most frequent reaction to pyrethrins is contact dermatitis and allergic respiratory reactions, probably due to other constituents in the extract; about 50% of patients who are sensitive to ragweed show cross-reactivity to pyrethrum. Many of the synthetic pyrethrins, known as pyrethroids, have greater insecticidal activity and are more photostable than pyrethrum, especially those containing the α

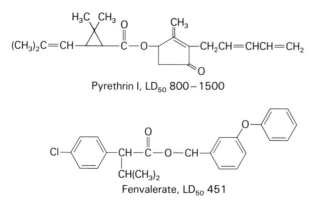

FIGURE 7.8.
Structure of pyrethrin I, one of the six pyrethrins in natural pyrethrum, and fenvalerate, one of the synthetic pyrethroids.

cyano group, such as fenvalerate (Figure 7.8). Pyrethrins affect nerve membranes by modifying the sodium and potassium channels, resulting in depolarization of the membranes.

7.6.2.5 Herbicides

Phenolic compounds, such as dinitrophenol, dinitroorthocresol, and pentachlorophenol, are used as contact herbicides; the chlorophenols are also used as fungicides, especially for the preservation of wood products. The mode of action is the uncoupling of oxidative phosphorylation, increasing O_2 consumption and heat production, leading to hyperthermia (see Section 6.2.3.2, Uncouplers of oxidative phosphorylation).

The chlorophenoxy herbicides such as 2,4-D and 2,4,5-T are systemic herbicides for broadleaf plants that act by excess stimulation of plant growth hormones. The concern over the toxicity of the chlorophenoxy herbicides is due primarily to the presence of the extremely toxic contaminant TCDD, which is present as a result of the manufacturing process (Figure 7.9). TCDD is one of the most toxic synthetic substances known for laboratory animals: LD50 for male rats, 0.022 mg/kg; LD50 for female rats, 0.045 mg/kg; LD50 for female guinea pigs, the most sensitive species tested, 0.0006 mg/kg. In addition, it is fetotoxic to pregnant rats at a dose of only $\frac{1}{400}$ of the LD50, and has been shown to cause birth defects at levels of 1–3 ng/kg. TCDD is a proven carcinogen in both mice and rats, with the liver being the primary target. A mixture of 2,4-D and 2,4,5-T, known as Agent Orange, was used by the US military as a defoliant during the Vietnam conflict, and much controversy has arisen over claims by military personnel of long-term health effects.

TCDD is a good example of species variability to a toxic chemical; although TCDD is extremely toxic to certain laboratory animals, evidence is lacking that it has any serious long-term effects on humans. None of the many epidemiological studies done on people exposed to dioxins has demonstrated that TCDD causes severe chronic human effects. Many essentially acute symptoms have been observed; they include chloracne (a skin irritation resembling acne caused by exposure to various chlorinated organic chemicals), digestive disorders, effects on some essential enzyme systems, aches and pains of muscles and joints, and effects on the nervous system. These symptoms have been transitory except for a few cases of chloracne, and no long-term effects such as birth defects, chromosomal damage, or a higher than normal mortality rate have

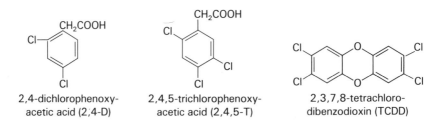

2,4-dichlorophenoxy-
acetic acid (2,4-D)

2,4,5-trichlorophenoxy-
acetic acid (2,4,5-T)

2,3,7,8-tetrachloro-
dibenzodioxin (TCDD)

FIGURE 7.9.
Chlorophenoxy herbicides and the toxic contaminant TCDD.

been identified. In light of the considerable toxicity in animals, however, the concern about its effects on human health and the environment is understandable.

Paraquat is a very water-soluble contact herbicide that is active against a broad range of plants and is used as a defoliant on many crops. Most poisoning cases, which are often fatal, are due to accidental ingestion of paraquat, ie, drinking pesticide that had been stored in a drink container. The toxic effect, even following ingestion, is due to fatal lung injury (see Section 6.3.4.3c, Pulmonary toxicity: activation of toxicants).

7.6.2.6 Fungicides

Fungicides include such compounds as mercury fungicides used to treat seed grains, pentachlorophenol used as a wood preservative (Figure 6.7), and dithiocarbamates (Maneb, Zineb, and Nabam) used widely in agriculture. The dithiocarbamates, in general, have a low acute toxicity.

7.6.2.7 Rodenticides

The main toxicological problem associated with rodenticides is due to accidental or suicidal ingestion of the compounds. Fluoroacetate (compound 1080) and fluoroacetamide (compound 1081) are highly toxic compounds, (see Section 6.2.4, Lethal synthesis) and their use is restricted to pest control operators. Other rodenticides are warfarin (an anticoagulant), red squill (cardiac poison), ANTU (α-naphthylthiourea), and strychnine.

7.6.2.8 Fumigants

Fumigants are gases used to protect stored produce, especially grains, and to kill soil nematodes. They present a special hazard due to inhalation exposure and rapid diffusion into the pulmonary blood. Most are also extremely toxic. Commonly used fumigants include methylbromide, carbon tetrachloride, acrylonitrite, carbon disulfide, ethylene dibromide, ethylene oxide, hydrogen cyanide, formaldehyde, acrolein, chloropicrin, and phosphine. The use of many of these (eg, ethylene dibromide) is now being restricted or banned, particularly in the United States.

7.7 THERAPEUTIC DRUGS

In the medical use of drugs, a narrow dose range often separates the clinically desired effect from a harmful or toxic manifestation of the drug. In addition, problems with therapeutic drugs occur due to accidental acute intoxication by children and deliberate suicidal and homicidal overdose by adults. The opportunities for these events are numerous in a drug-oriented society. Drug abuse, drug addiction, adverse drug effects, and chronic drug intoxications all contribute to serious health problems as well as increased medical costs. Several categories of therapeutic drugs that either are frequently used or are associated with toxicities are briefly discussed in the following section. The toxicities of acetaminophen and nephrotoxic antibiotics have already been discussed (Sections

6.1.5.3 and 6.3.4.1d, Acetaminophen; and Section 6.3.4.2b2, Nephrotoxic antibiotics).

7.7.1 Barbiturates (Barbitals)

Barbiturates are derivatives of barbituric acid (Figure 7.10) and, depending on the compound, have a wide range of duration of activity from < 1 hour up to 12 hours (Table 7.9). In recent years, the death rate from overuse of barbiturates has been declining due to a voluntary decrease in prescriptions by doctors together with the introduction of safer drugs such as the benzodiazepines. Many elderly patients continue to use barbiturates for their hypnotic effect, however, and they continue to be an important cause of overdose deaths. Barbiturates are legally available only on prescription, but the street use of "downers" continues. Barbiturates are administered orally and most are metabolized by the liver, with some metabolism in the kidney and other tissues. The desired central nervous system (CNS) effect is mild sedation to general anesthesia; in addition, some have anticonvulsant activity and lessen anxiety. Tolerance to barbiturates develops very rapidly, so that increasing doses are necessary to be effective, often by as much as six times. Although barbiturates induce the liver microsomal enzymes that metabolize barbiturates, the level of tolerance is more than can be accounted for by induction of the microsomal enzymes. Induction of the microsomal cytochrome P-450–dependent monooxygenase system causes a significant increase in the elimination of other drugs such as dicumarol, digoxin, tetracycline, oral contraceptives, and hormones.

Most cases of barbiturate poisoning are suicide attempts, but accidental poisoning is more common with children and street users. The characteristic signs and symptoms of barbiturate poisoning are depression of the CNS and

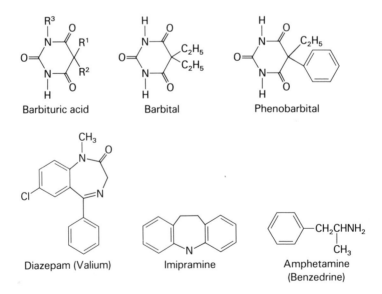

FIGURE 7.10.
Structures of some common tranquilizers, antidepressants, and stimulants.

TABLE 7.9
Some Common Barbiturates and Duration of Activity

Barbituate	Duration of Action (h)
Ultrashort-acting Thiopental Thiamylal	0.3
Short-acting Hexobarbital Pentobarbital	1–3
Intermediate-acting Amobarbital Butabarbital	3–6
Long-acting Barbital Phenobarbital Primidone	6–12

cardiovascular system. Severe intoxication produces coma and may progress to death, frequently due to cardiorespiratory arrest. The simultaneous ingestion of other drugs such as alcohol may contribute to CNS depression.

7.7.2 Benzodiazepines

The benzodiazepines (Figure 7.10 and Table 7.10) are nonbarbiturate compounds that possess CNS-depressant properties and are often described as hypnotics, sedatives, depressants, tranquilizers, or relaxants. These drugs have

TABLE 7.10
Benzodiazepines Approved for Use in the United States

Generic Name	Brand Name
Alprazolam	Xanax
Chlordiazepoxide	Librium (and others)
Clonazepam	Clonopin
Clorazepate dipotassium	Tranxene
Chlorazepate monopotassium	Azene
Diazepam	Valium Valrelease
Flurazepam	Dalmane
Halazepam	Paxipam
Lorazepam	Ativan
Oxazepam	Serax
Prazepam	Centrax, Verstan
Temazepam	Restoril

largely replaced the barbiturates. In the 1970s, diazepam (Valium) was the most widely prescribed drug in the United States. Benzodiazepines are popular because of their efficacy as well as their safety. They are relatively safe in overdose and not associated with serious addiction, abstinence syndrome, tolerance development, or microsomal enzyme induction.

The most frequent side effect of therapeutic doses is drowsiness; in some cases, dizziness and weakness occurs. The usual result of benzodiazepine overdose is sleep induction and occasionally coma; in most overdose fatalities involving benzodiazepines, other drugs were also ingested. Benzodiazepines alone rarely cause respiratory or circulatory depression. It has been suggested that there is a risk of teratogenicity when the drugs are used during the first trimester, but epidemiological studies have not confirmed this association.

7.7.3 Tricyclic Antidepressants

The tricyclic antidepressants (Figure 7.10 and Table 7.11) are the drugs preferred for use in endogenous depression. Because they are given to patients who often become suicidal, they are a major cause of toxic overdose in clinical use. The parent compound, usually a tertiary amine, and its metabolite, a secondary amine, are responsible for both the antidepressant and the toxic effects. Side effects of use are tiredness, dizziness, blurred vision, and urinary retention. The CNS effects of overdose include confusion, agitation and, finally, coma; anticholinergic effects include flushing, dry mouth, and dilated pupils. The cardiotoxic effects, arrhythmias and hypotension, are the cause of death, however.

7.7.4 Amphetamines

Amphetamine (Figure 7.10) was first synthesized in 1887 and marketed in the United States in 1932 as a nasal inhalant and decongestant. It is a CNS stimulant and during World War II was widely used to combat battle fatigue and

TABLE 7.11
Tricyclic Depressants Available in the United States

Imipramine	Nortriptyline
Tofranil	Aventy
Imavate	Pamelor
Presamine	
Janimine	Doxepin
SK-Pramine	Sinequan
Imipramine	Adapin
	Curatin
Amitriptyline	
Elavil	Protriptyline
Endep	Vivactil
Amitriptyline	
Trivil	Maprotiline
Eltrafon	Ludiomil
Limbitrol	
Desipramine	
Norpramine	
Pertofrane	

Trade names are listed under the generic name.

domestically to increase production among workers. In the 1950s, amphetamines were popular with college students for use while studying for examinations as well as with cross-country truckers. Abuse became a serious problem, however, and legal use became more tightly controlled. Until recently, amphetamines were used to treat obesity as a major component of "diet pills"; today, medical use is restricted to treatment of narcolepsy and hyperkinetic behavior in children.

Although no longer as readily available, amphetamines are easily synthesized from commercially available starting materials. Amphetamines have widespread street use; they are known by various names—bennies, mollies, jelly beans, pep pills, speed, splash, uppers, wake-ups, nuggets, and whites—to name a few.

Symptoms of overdose are restlessness, irritability, tremor, confusion, and sweating in mild cases, to delirium, arrhythmias, convulsions, coma, and occasionally death in severe overdose.

Birth defects, including limb deformities, have been associated with amphetamine use during the first trimester, and neonatal withdrawal symptoms also occur.

7.7.5 Narcotic Analgesics (Opiates)

The word narcotic comes from the Greek *narkoun,* which means to be numb or in a stupor; generally, the term narcotic is used to refer to compounds with sedative, mood-altering, analgesic properties and includes the drugs most often prescribed for relief of intense pain, such as opium and its derivatives. Opiates include drugs derived from opium, synthesized from opium, or wholly synthetic drugs (Figure 7.11 and Table 7.12).

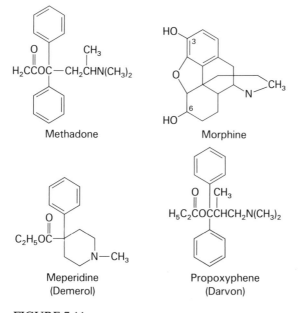

FIGURE 7.11.
Structures for several opiates and synthetic narcotic analgesics.

TABLE 7.12
Some Commonly Used Opiates

Opium Derivatives
  Codeine
  Morphine

Semisynthetic
  Heroin
  Hydromorphone (Dilaudid)
  Oxycodone (in Percodan, Percocet, Tylox)
  Oxymorphone (Numorphan)

Synthetic
  Alphaprodine (Nisentil)
  Anileridine (Leritine)
  Butorphanol (Stadol)
  Dextromethorphan
  Diphenoxylate (Lomotil)
  Fentanyl (in Sublimaze)
  Levorphanol (Levo-Dromoran)
  Meperidine (Demerol)
  Methadone (Dolophine)
  Nalbuphine (Nubain)
  Pentazocine (Talwin)
  Propoxyphene (Darvon, Darvocet)

Heroin is prepared by acetylation of the hydroxyl groups at C-3 and C-6 of morphine, resulting in the ethyl ester of both hydroxyl groups; codeine is the methyl ester of the hydroxyl at the C-3 position.

The effects of the opiates on the CNS are a combination of depression and stimulation and include increased pain tolerance, suppression of anxiety, and sedation. Higher doses result in drowsiness, mood changes, mental clouding, nausea, and respiratory depression. The major complications of chronic clinical opiate use are development of tolerance, psychological dependence, and physical dependence.

Opiate poisoning occurs most commonly following intravenous (IV) heroin administration or oral methadone overdose by addicts or nontolerant, infrequent users. Severe overdose is characterized by apnea, circulatory collapse, convulsions, cardiac arrest, and death.

7.7.6 Anticonvulsants (Phenytoin and Diphenylhydantoin)

Phenytoin (Dilantin) is the preferred drug in the treatment of epilepsy and in the control of arrhythmias from intoxication by other drugs such as digitalis and tricyclic antidepressants. There have been very few reported deaths from either acute or chronic overdoses, and most of these have been due to hypersensitivity of patients already intoxicated from other drugs.

Phenytoin, however, has been associated with a wide range of congenital abnormalities in infants of mothers taking the drug for control of epilepsy. These effects, known as the fetal hydantoin syndrome, include cleft palate, hydrocephalus, microcephalus, broad nose, digital thumbs, short neck, and various heart defects.

7.7.7 Isoniazid

Isoniazid (INH) is an antimicrobial that has been used in the treatment of tuberculosis since 1952 and has proved to be very effective with a relatively low toxicity (Figure 7.12). In the United States, however, the incidence of acute INH overdose is especially high in populations in which tuberculosis is prevalent, such as American Indians and Eskimos. Early clinical effects include nausea, dizziness, and slurred speech. Severe overdose produces brain damage. Isoniazid overdose affects the metabolism of γ-aminobutyric acid (GABA) in the brain with the subsequent decrease in GABA levels leading to seizures and coma. INH inhibits the activity of vitamin B_6, which is essential for the enzymatic formation of GABA from glutamic acid. Treatment of patients who have ingested potentially toxic amounts of INH includes IV administration of vitamin B_6 (pyridoxin hydrochloride).

Therapeutic doses of isoniazid lead to liver injury in some patients. This damage is due to a reactive intermediate formed from the isoniazid metabolite acetylisoniazid (Figure 7.12) and occurs most often in patients who are genetically fast acetylators, thus metabolizing isoniazid more rapidly than do slow acetylators. Among both black and white Americans, about 50% of the population are fast acetylators, whereas >95% of the Eskimo population are fast acetylators. The Japanese are also rapid acetylators, with about 88% of the population being rapid acetylators, whereas among Egyptians, only 18% are rapid acetylators.

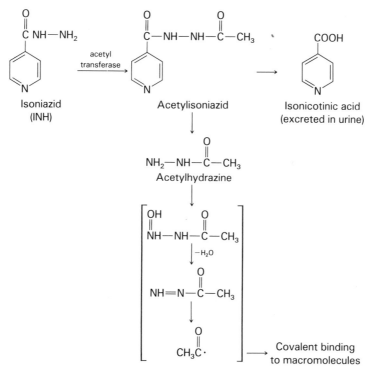

FIGURE 7.12.
Metabolism of isoniazid showing formation of a reactive metabolite that can bind covalently to macromolecules, resulting in liver necrosis.

7.7.8 Lithium

The use of lithium carbonate has become an indispensable tool in the psychiatric treatment of manic-depressive illness. Lithium was first used to treat mania in 1949; prior to that time, lithium carbonate had been used as a "salt" substitute, was added to mineral waters, such as "lithia water," and was even a major ingredient in the soft drink "7-Up" at one time.

Lithium has a narrow therapeutic window, and slight elevations of serum levels will result in toxicity. For this reason, patients on therapy must be monitored closely. A gradual onset of intoxication is more common than an acute overdose; the early symptoms include drowsiness, lethargy, slurred speech, muscle twitching, vomiting, and diarrhea. Extremely high serum lithium levels may lead to life-threatening toxicity.

7.8 OTHER DRUGS (INCLUDING DRUGS OF ABUSE)

7.8.1 Cocaine

Cocaine has probably been used for $>2,000$ years as a stimulant. Cocaine (Figure 1.1) is an alkaloid (basic, ie, alkali-like, nitrogen compound) from the plant *Erythroxylon coca,* which grows extensively in the Andes Mountains of South America; its leaves contain from $1-2\%$ cocaine. The Indians living in the region chew the leaves to offset fatigue and hunger and, as a result of the drug's stimulant effect, are able to work for long hours. People of the ancient Inca civilizaton regarded the coca plant as a gift from the gods.

In the late nineteenth and early twentieth centuries, cocaine from the coca leaves was a major ingredient in many popular beverages, such as Mariani Coca Wine. Coca-Cola was first marketed as an elixir containing cocaine from the coca leaf and caffeine from the African kola nut; hence the name Coca-Cola. In 1906, after public pressure, Coca-Cola agreed to use decocainized coca leaves. Cocaine came under strict control with the passage of the Harrison Narcotics Act of 1914, and was seen by many legislators as the major drug problem at that time. Use of cocaine diminished and became insignificant from the 1930s to the 1950s. Starting in the 1960s, however, an explosion in use occurred. Cocaine use increased more rapidly during the 1970s than that of any other drug, and it is considered by many users to be the "champagne of drugs," appealing especially to many wealthy, professional users.

In clinical use, cocaine is an excellent local anaesthetic and vasoconstrictor of mucous membranes. For these reasons, it is used widely in nasal surgery, rhinoplasty, and emergency nasotracheal intubation.

Cocaine is brought into this country illegally from South America—mainly from Peru, Bolivia, and Ecuador—where it is extracted and refined to form the hydrochloride salt. The cocaine is then "cut" with mannitol, lactose, glucose, or cornstarch. Some common street names for cocaine are coke, snow, flake, lady, she, girl, C, leaf, flake, white lady, and nose candy. The most common route of use is intranasal, or "snorting." The cocaine is chopped with a razor blade into lines or columns on a piece of glass, and the line is then inhaled through a straw or a rolled dollar bill. "Freebase," a form of purified street cocaine, is occasionally used. After it is "snorted," the onset of action is rapid, occurring within $5-10$ minutes, and has a duration of about 60 minutes.

Cocaine is a powerful CNS stimulant, and occasional users experience euphoria, stimulation, reduced fatigue, garrulousness, a joyous feeling, increased energy, confidence, and a sensation of mastery and competence. The cocaine high is extremely pleasurable; laboratory animals will give up food for self-administered doses of cocaine and will even starve to death to continue receiving the drug. Heavy regular use generates a number of unpleasant side effects, however: insomnia, anxiety, paranoia, and hallucinations. A common occurrence is "cocaine bugs"—the sensation of bugs crawling under the skin. The chronic user may be prone to violence, particularly due to delusions of persecution. Cocaine does not produce physical addiction but does become psychologically addictive. Acute overdoses are most common when users inject cocaine intravenously (IV) or use freebase; toxicological symptoms include seizures, cardiac arrhythmias, and respiratory arrest.

7.8.2 Phencyclidine (PCP)

Phencyclidine (PCP) was marketed in 1958 for experimental use in humans as a general anaesthetic under the trade-name Sernyl (Figure 7.13). It was a superior anaesthetic in that it was non-narcotic and did not depress repiration, but its use was discontinued because of adverse side effects, including extreme agitation, delirium, disorientation, and hallucinations. In 1967, it was reintroduced as a veterinary anesthetic, Sernylan, and was used until 1978 when it was voluntarily withdrawn. In 1967, illegal use started in the Haight-Ashbury district of San Francisco, where it was called the "Peace Pill"; because of "bad

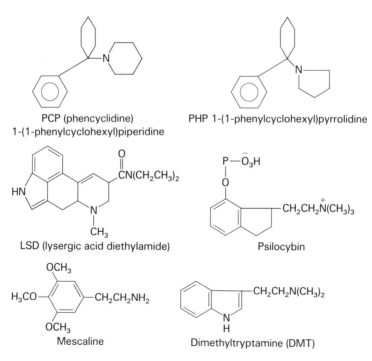

PCP (phencyclidine)
1-(1-phenylcyclohexyl)piperidine

PHP 1-(1-phenylcyclohexyl)pyrrolidine

LSD (lysergic acid diethylamide)

Psilocybin

Mescaline

Dimethyltryptamine (DMT)

FIGURE 7.13.
Structures of some common hallucinogens.

trips," however, PCP disappeared within a year. The next year, it appeared briefly on the East Coast as "hog," but it also had a short street life there. By the early and mid-1970s, it again appeared on the streets. Because it was so easily and cheaply synthesized in "kitchen" laboratories, it was frequently disguised and sold as THC, cannabinol, LSD, mescaline, or other psychedelics. In addition to these uses, PCP also became the drug preferred by many users.

Phencyclidine has various street names such as angel dust, angel hair, crystal, dust, hog, hog dust, magic mist, monkey dust, peace, stardust, and others. PCP can be taken by mouth, inhalation (smoking), or snorting; rarely is it used IV. PCP is often smoked by being sprinkled on marijuana — giving rise to the name "supergrass."

Phencyclidine has > 30 chemical analogs, many of which produce similar effects. PHP, a PCP analog (Figure 7.13) has come into very prevalent use not only because it is difficult to detect but also because there are no sales restrictions on its pyrrolidine precursor, whereas piperidine, a PCP-precursor, is now a controlled substance. Much of the motivation for producing and using new PCP analogs is because they are not yet classified as controlled drugs; thus, possession and use is not considered a crime.

Users of low doses of PCP frequently feel inebriated and disoriented and experience a kind of "numbness," progressing to inability to feel pain. True hallucinations are uncommon, but illusions and delusions leading to bizarre behavior are common, eg, the delusion of superhuman strength or loss of fear. Violent acts may also be committed, such as assaults on friends or strangers, or self-mutilation. Nystagmus, or involuntary movement of the eyeballs, is frequently seen with PCP use and is characteristic of that drug.

Moderate to high doses usually result in the user becoming comatose — most often for only a few hours, but occasionally as long as 6 – 10 days. Deaths from PCP intoxication are usually the result of accidents related to delirium of the user, eg, drownings, automobile accidents, fires, street fights, and other dangers; PCP itself is relatively nontoxic.

7.8.3 Lysergic Acid Diethylamide (LSD)

Lysergic acid diethylamide (LSD) (Figure 7.13) is a very potent and widely used hallucinogen. LSD was synthesized by the Swiss chemist Albert Hoffman in 1938 (LSD is an abbreviation of the German lyserg saure diethylamid). Its potent psychoactive properties were discovered by Hoffman in 1943 when he accidentally inhaled a minute quantity of the drug. He described his experience: ". . . fantastic visions of extraordinary vividness accompanied by a kaleidoscopic play of intense coloration continuously swirled around me. After two hours this condition subsided."

In the middle to late 1950s, LSD was used widely by psychiatrists in diverse clinical investigations, most frequently to increase insight and resurrect repressed material. Because efficacy was inconsistent and it was not superior to other forms of psychotherapy, however, its use declined.

Because of its extremely high potency, an ounce of uncut LSD will provide up to 150,000 doses of 200 μg each. LSD is available in tablet or powder;

occasionally it is placed on sugar cubes, chewing gum, crackers, thin squares of gelatin ("window panes"), colored dots of LSD on aspirin ("blue dots") and others. Some common street names for LSD are acid, blotter acid, crackers, orange wedges, pink dots, and yellow dots. LSD is almost always taken orally, rather than IV or by smoking.

LSD is rapidly absorbed from the GI tract, producing effects within 30 minutes with peak activity in 1–2 hours. At times, the psychic effects last for 10–12 hours. The effects of visual illusions and altered perceptions of color and distances are frequent. Time sense is lost, and concentration is attenuated; many users believe that they can think "more deeply" and may become engrossed in philosophical or ethical issues which to an "outsider" make little or no sense.

The most common adverse reactions to LSD results from a bad trip associated with frightening illusions, and the user develops a panic state, fearing insanity. Other phenomena of LSD use are flashbacks, or spontaneous recurrences of the trip; these may occur several times a day and sometimes up to 18 months after use. These flashbacks occur most frequently in chronic LSD users and may be pleasant or unpleasant.

LSD is most often implicated in accidental deaths (for example, users who believe they can fly) and suicides. Several investigations of the ability of LSD to cause teratogenesis or chromosome breaks have proven inconclusive.

7.8.4 Mescaline/Peyote

Mescaline (Figure 7.13), named after the Mascalero, an Apache tribe, is the major active psychedelic alkaloid in the peyote cactus, which grows in Mexico and the Southwestern United States. Mescaline was first isolated in 1896 and was successfully synthesized in 1918. Today, it is available for street use as either peyote extracts or from synthesis. Frequently, drugs sold under the guise of mescaline are actually LSD or PCP, sometimes diluted with amphetamines.

The term peyote refers to the unmodified cactus, usually chewed in the form of a dried "button," which may contain as much as 6% mescaline. Peyote was used in Mexico by the Aztecs in religious ceremonies for centuries, and peyote cults became established in this country in the late nineteenth century as a result of raids into Mexico. Peyote use in Indian religious ceremonies became widespread, and the Native American Church was founded in 1918 as a defense against antipeyote legislation. In this church, peyote use is a religious sacrament, a practice that is legal in the United States.

7.8.5 Psilocybin

The ancient Aztec rituals included not only the use of peyote cactus, but also morning glory seeds (which have psychedelic properties) and the "sacred" mushroom, teonanacatl, containing at least 20 hallucinogenic mushroom species. The active ingredient is psilocybin (Figure 7.13), a derivative of dimethyltryptamine. Psilocybin is shorter-acting, but with similar effects to LSD.

7.8.6 Dimethytryptamine (DMT)

Dimethyltryptamine (DMT) (Figure 7.13), is representative of many of the hallucinogenic tryptamine derivatives. DMT was first isolated from hallucinogenic snuffs used by the native Indians of the Caribbean and South America. DMT is inactive when ingested orally, so it is usually inhaled either by sniffing the powder or by smoking tobacco or marijuana previously soaked in it. DMT and DET (diethyl-tryptamine) have effects similar to those of LSD, but the "high" lasts for only 30–60 minutes. For this reason, they have been called the "businessman's" or "lunchtime" psychedelics.

7.8.7 Marijuana

Marijuana is by far the most commonly used illegal drug in America. Although there are fads in illegal drug use, the use of marijuana has remained consistently high. *Cannabis sativa* is a hemp plant that has been used for centuries not only for its psychoactive resin but also for production of hemp fiber and rope. The cannaboid Δ-9-tetrahydrocannabinol (THC) is the principal active ingredient in the plant (Figure 1.1). Depending on cultivation, the concentration of THC can range from 0.4% to 5%. Marijuana generally refers to tobaccolike preparations of leaves and flowers, whereas hashish is the resin extracted from the tops of the flowering plants and may contain up to 10% THC.

Smoking the cigarette or "joint" is the most common method of use of marijuana in the United States, and effective brain levels are rapidly achieved. Users of low to moderate doses generally report a feeling of well-being, a state of pleasant relaxation, a heightening of their senses (for example, clearer perception of music), and an alteration of time and space perception. Most describe their use in favorable terms and enjoy their experiences. However, while intoxicated, users may have poor cognitive functions and difficulty with motor functions. Due to widespread use, there has been much concern that these effects may have a significant impact on the performance of students, individuals in work situations, or persons driving automobiles if they perform these tasks while intoxicated.

The chronic effects of marijuana remain controversial; although there is no direct evidence that smoking marijuana correlates with lung cancer, evidence does indicate that daily use of marijuana can lead to lung damage similar to that seen in cigarette smokers. Studies on reproductive effects have also been inconclusive. Although decreases in sperm count and motility have been found, there is usually a return to normal when marijuana use is discontinued.

7.9 SOLVENTS

Organic solvents and their vapors are commonly encountered in our modern environment—in industries in which large quantities may be used in manufacturing and processing and in the home as a result of exposure to materials such as gasoline vapors, aerosol sprays, and paint removers.

7.9.1 Aliphatic Hydrocarbons

Methane and ethane are the gases present in natural gas; they are not usually associated with systemic effects, but are asphyxiants when the concentration is high enough to reduce oxygen levels in inhaled air. Propane and butane (bottled gas) are highly volatile liquids, and inhalation of the vapors produces CNS depression, resulting in dizziness and incoordination.

Many commercial products and solvents contain mixtures of the higher molecular weight hydrocarbons — pentane, hexane, heptane, and octane, including both straight-chain and branched-chain compounds. Inhalation of vapors from products containing these hydrocarbons produces CNS depression. Gasoline and kerosene are mixtures of hydrocarbons that contain both aromatic and aliphatic hydrocarbons. In normal exposure, such as the vapors encountered by gas station attendants, toxic effects do not normally occur.

A significant source of poison deaths, however, is ingestion of petroleum products by children, especially under the age of 5 years; such ingestion accounts for up to 25% of all poison deaths in this age group. The most commonly ingested hydrocarbons, in order of frequency, are kerosene, mineral seal oil preparations, turpentine, gasoline, lighter fluids, and pesticides with a petroleum base. An important factor in ingestion by children is that these compounds, such as kerosene, are often placed in soft drink bottles or other unlabeled containers and left within easy access of children. The acute toxicity of these compounds is quite low, but significant damage can occur due to small quantities entering the lung, where a thin layer spreads rapidly over the moist lung surfaces, resulting in edema and hemorrhage due to damage of the pulmonary membranes. For this reason, it is wise not to induce vomiting.

7.9.2 Aliphatic Halogenated Hydrocarbons

Among the compounds most widely used as industrial solvents are the aliphatic halogenated hydrocarbons, due to their excellent solvent properties and generally low flammability. A common physiological property associated with these compounds is their anesthetic effect.

7.9.2.1 Chloroform

Chloroform ($CHCl_3$) was once used extensively as a clinical anaesthetic but, because of liver injury, and to a lesser extent cardiac sensitization, it is no longer used for this purpose. It is widely used in industry and in the laboratory as a chemical intermediate and solvent. Because chloroform has been established as a carcinogen in laboratory animals, its use is no longer permitted as a component in drugs. High concentrations of chloroform or repeated exposure may lead to liver and kidney damage. Chloroform is metabolized by cytochrome P-450 isozymes to produce chloromethanol (Figure 7.14), which rapidly and spontaneously dechlorinates to yield HCl and the toxic compound phosgene, $COCl_2$. Normally, phosgene forms a nontoxic conjugate with glutathione, but when hepatic and renal levels of glutathione fall below a critical level, covalent

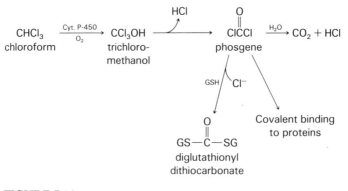

FIGURE 7.14.
Metabolism of chloroform.

binding to tissue macromolecules occurs, resulting in hepatic and renal necrosis.

7.9.2.2 Carbon Tetrachloride

Carbon tetrachloride (CCl_4) was once widely used as a drycleaning chemical, degreasing agent, and fire extinguisher. Recent FDA regulations have now restricted its use to industry and laboratories. Carbon tetrachloride has anesthetic properties similar to those of chloroform, but is less potent. In addition, it causes marked hepatic and renal toxicity, and even low concentrations cause fatty degeneration in the liver (see Section 6.3.4.1b Mechanisms of toxicity).

7.9.2.3 Methylene Chloride

Methylene chloride (CH_2Cl_2) is a common ingredient in paint removers and is a solvent in aerosol products. Due to its extreme volatility, high concentrations may occur readily in poorly ventilated areas. Following inhalation, methylene chloride is metabolized by the cytochrome P-450 monooxygenase system to CO_2 and CO. Significant levels of carboxyhemoglobin may occur due to carbon monoxide binding to hemoglobin in the blood. In common with other low-molecular-weight halogenated hydrocarbons, methylene chloride is a CNS depressant. Initial signs of inhalation are dizziness and numbness; other symptoms that have been reported are tingling of the extremities, fatigue, and nausea. Severe or prolonged exposure may lead to respiratory depression and death. If high carboxyhemoglobin levels are present, the symptoms of acute CO poisoning will also occur.

7.9.2.4 Methyl Chloride

Methyl chloride (CH_3Cl) is a colorless gas used as a chemical intermediate, particularly in methylating reactions. Occasionally it is used as a blowing agent in molding polystyrene and polyurethane. Following acute exposure, patients feel inebriated and develop nausea, abdominal pains, and diarrhea. Chronic industrial exposure has led to confusion, blurring of vision, slurred speech, and staggering gait.

7.9.2.5 Trichloroethylene

Trichloroethylene (Cl_2C=$CHCl$) and tetrachloroethylene (CCl_2=CCl_2) are both used widely as industrial degreasing solvents and in the drycleaning industry. Overexposure by inhalation results in depression of the CNS, confusion, incoordination, nausea, and irritation of the eyes and nose. At high concentrations, these compounds may be fatal.

7.9.2.6 Vinyl Chloride

Vinyl chloride (CH_2=$CHCl$, monochloroethylene) (Figure 7.15) is a colorless gas that is highly flammable and explosive and is usually handled as a liquid under pressure. In this form, it polymerizes readily at temperatures between 40 and 70 °C to form polyvinylchloride (PVC). Vinyl chloride was considered for use as an anesthetic agent but was abandoned because it was found to induce cardiac arrhythmias. Epidemiological studies of autoclave cleaners in PVC plants showed high occurrences of a rare tumor, angiosarcoma of the liver.

The main route of absorption of vinyl chloride is through the lungs, although some skin penetration does occur. Metabolism of vinyl chloride to the reactive metabolite occurs through the hepatic cytochrome P-450 monooxygenase system (Figure 7.15). The epoxide has been shown to bind covalently to DNA, RNA, and protein, whereas chloroacetaldehyde is a known mutagen. Detoxication of these metabolites occurs mainly by conjugation with glutathione. If glutathione levels are depleted beyond a certain critical point, the liver is no longer protected against the toxic metabolites.

7.9.3 Alcohols

The aliphatic alcohols have wide application as industrial solvents, and, of this series, only ethanol has the physiological effects and low toxicity that has

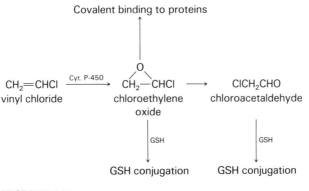

FIGURE 7.15.
Metabolism of vinyl chloride.

resulted in use as an alcoholic beverage. The other alcohols, especially methanol, are characterized by considerable toxicity.

7.9.3.1 Methanol

Methanol (CH_3OH, methyl alcohol or wood alcohol) is a widely used commercial solvent, and is a solvent in paints, varnishes, and shellacs. It is commonly used in windshield wiping fluids and in formulations as a liquid fuel for small engines. Methanol, since it resembles ethanol in odor and taste and is tax-free and less expensive than ethanol, has caused considerable problems as an adulterant in alcoholic beverages, and "epidemics" of methanol poisoning are not uncommon.

Although toxicity may occur from skin absorption or inhalation, the main route of uptake is ingestion. In poisoning, about 30% of the dose is excreted as methanol by the respiratory tract (the main mode of excretion of unchanged methanol); the remainder of the methanol is converted, principally in the liver, by alcohol dehydrogenase to formaldehyde and then to formic acid by aldehyde dehydrogenase. The local production of formaldehyde in the retina is thought to be responsible for the production of the retinal edema and blindness characteristic of methanol poisoning.

Symptoms of methanol poisoning may be delayed for 6 – 18 hours due to the delayed metabolism of methanol to the toxic products, formaldehyde and formic acid, resulting in acidosis. The initial symptoms are a minor CNS intoxication similar to ethyl alcohol followed by a mild drowsiness. This is followed by an asymptomatic period (6 – 30 hours) and then the characteristic symptoms and signs of methanol poisoning (Table 7.13). In severe cases, delirium may be a marked feature, and death may be either rapid or occur many hours after the onset of the coma. Ethanol is administered immediately to act as a competitive substrate for alcohol dehydrogenase to inhibit the conversion of methanol to formaldehyde. This is followed by hemodialysis to remove the methanol, formic acid, and formaldehyde.

7.9.3.2 Isopropyl Alcohol

Isopropyl alcohol is an important alcohol used in industry and in medicine as rubbing alcohol. In the home, isopropyl alcohol may be found in rubbing

TABLE 7.13
Major Symptoms/Signs of Methanol Intoxication

Early
Inebriation
Drowsiness
Delayed (6 – 30 h)
Dizziness
Abdominal pain, vomiting
Breathing difficulty
Blurred vision
Dilated pupils
Blindness
Urinary formaldehyde smell

alcohol, aftershave lotions, and window-cleaning solutions. As with methanol, isopropyl alcohol is sometimes ingested mixed with or in place of ethanol. Isopropyl alcohol is more toxic than ethanol but less toxic then methanol. The signs and symptoms are similar to those of ethanol toxicity; acute ingestion may be followed by a deep coma and respiratory arrest, all occurring within a few hours.

7.9.3.3 Higher Saturated Alcohols

The higher saturated alcohols have some toxicity. The butyl alcohols are generally less toxic than the amyl alcohols, but are more toxic than isopropanol. *N*-butanol vapors have produced conjunctivitis and keratitis, and inhalation may produce pulmonary injury. In general, however, toxicity is not a problem with the higher alcohols.

7.9.4 Glycols and Derivatives

Glycols (Figure 7.16) have general use as heat exchangers, antifreeze formulations, hydraulic fluids, chemical intermediates, solvents for pharmaceuticals, food additives, and cosmetics. Due to their low volatility, the glycols have little vapor hazard at ordinary temperatures.

7.9.4.1 Ethylene Glycol

Ethylene glycol ingestion results in serious and dramatic poisoning. As with methanol and isopropanol, ethylene glycol has been ingested in place of or mixed with ethanol. Ethylene glycol itself appears to be nontoxic, and the toxicity results from its four major breakdown products: aldehydes, glycolate, oxalate, and lactate. Initially, the user appears to be drunk, but without an alcohol smell on the breath; this is followed by nausea, coma, seizure, respira-

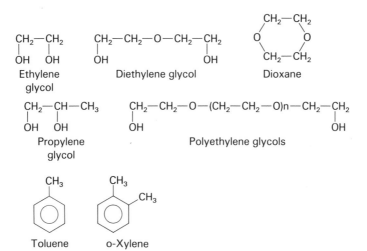

FIGURE 7.16.
Structures of some glycols and aromatic hydrocarbons.

tory failure, and cardiovascular collapse. Survivors of the acute phase experience renal failure caused by deposition of calcium oxalate crystals in the renal tubules and severe acidosis due to aldehyde, glycolate, and lactate production. These changes also occur in the liver, blood vessels, brain meninges, and heart. Hypocalcemia also occurs due to chelation of calcium ions by oxalate.

The metabolism of ethylene glycol depends on hepatic alcohol dehydrogenase and, as in methanol poisoning, ethanol is administered to act as a preferential substrate for the enzyme. During subsequent hemodialysis, ethanol is commonly added to the dialysate to maintain plasma levels of ethanol.

7.9.4.2 Propylene Glycol

Propylene glycol is relatively nontoxic and is used in cosmetics, foods, and as a solvent for certain drugs; eg, it is a major part of the solvent composition for the IV preparation of phenyltoin and on its own can cause cardiac arrhythmias when injected IV too rapidly. Most of the higher-molecular-weight glycols are also of very low toxicity.

7.9.4.3 Glycol Ethers

Glycol ethers are both water soluble and soluble in organic solvents, and thus are used in many oil–water combinations. Toxicity from these compounds generally occurs by inhalation of the vapors, which have been known to cause bone marrow depression and kidney damage.

7.9.5 Aromatic Hydrocarbons

7.9.5.1 Benzene

Benzene, the simplest of the aromatic hydrocarbons, has excellent solvent properties and high volatility, and dries rapidly, which accounts for its use in certain industries such as printing. In addition, it has widespread use as starting material for the synthesis of various aromatic products. The toxicity of benzene has been discussed in detail in Section 6.4.4.4b.

7.9.5.2 Toluene

Toluene (Figure 7.16) is a colorless liquid used extensively as a solvent in the chemical, rubber, paint, and pharmaceutical industries, but with much lower volatility than benzene. Toluene is a narcotic; acute symptoms from inhalation include euphoria, excitement, dizziness, headache, and nausea. Extreme acute exposure can result in coma and even death. Because toluene is a solvent for glue, it is frequently one of the solvents associated with "glue sniffing." Chronic exposure to toluene does not involve the hematologic effects that characterize benzene exposure.

7.9.5.3 Xylene

Xylene (Figure 7.16) is another aromatic hydrocarbon that is widely used as a solvent in paints, lacquers, pesticides, adhesives, and paper-coating industry.

Inhalation may lead to dizziness, excitement, drowsiness, and lack of coordination.

7.10 SUGGESTED FURTHER READING

AIR, SOIL AND WATER POLLUTANTS

Amdur, M.O. Air pollutants. In Doull, J., Klaassen, C.D., Amdur, M.O. (eds.). Casarett and Doull's Toxicology: The Basic Science of Poisons. 2nd ed. New York: Macmillan, 1980, pp. 608–631.

Dix, H.M. Environmental Pollution. New York: Wiley, 1981.

Health Effects of Toxic Wastes. Environ. Health Perspect. 1983; 48:1–145.

Hodgson, E. (ed.). Reviews in Environmental Toxicology 1, 2. Elsevier Biomedical Press, New York, 1984, 1986.

Menzer, R.E., Nelson, J.O. Water and soil pollutants. In Doull, J., Klaassen, C.D., Amdur, M.O. (eds.). Casarett and Doull's Toxicology: The Basic Science of Poisons. 2nd ed. New York: Macmillan, 1980, pp. 632–660.

Mutagenicity and carcinogenicity of air pollutants. Environ. Health Perspect. 1983; 47:1–345.

Stern, A.C., Bonbel, R.W., Turner, D.B., Fox, D.L. Fundamentals of Air Pollution. 2nd ed. Orlando, Fl.: Academic Press, 1984.

Vesilind, P.A., Pierce, J.J. Environmental Pollution and Control. 2nd ed. Ann Arbor, Mich. Ann Arbor Science Publishers, 1983.

FOOD ADDITIVES

Arnold, D.L. Toxicology of saccharin. Fund. Appl. Toxicol. 1985; 4:674–685.

Conning, D.M., Lansdown A.B.G., (ed.). Toxic Hazards in Food. Raven Press, New York, 1983.

Furia, T.E. (ed.). CRC Handbook of Food Additives. Cleveland: Chemical Rubber Co., 1968.

Hathcock, J.N. (ed.). Nutritional Toxicology. Vol. 1. New York: Academic Press, 1982.

Health Effects of Nitrate, Nitrite and N-Nitroso Compounds. National Academy of Sciences, National Academy Press, Washington, D.C., 1981.

Kilgore, W.W., Li, M.Y. Food additives and contaminants. In Doull, J., Klaassen, C.D., Amdur, M.O. (eds.). Casarett and Doull's Toxicology: The Basic Science of Poisons. 2nd ed. New York: Macmillan, 1980, pp. 593–607.

OCCUPATIONAL TOXICANTS

Barlow, S.M., Sullivan, F.M. (eds.). Reproductive Hazards of Industrial Chemicals. New York: Academic Press, 1982.

Documentation of the Threshold Limit Values. 4th ed. Cincinnati: American Conference of Governmental Industrial Hygienists, Inc., 1981.

Lauwerys, R.R. Industrial Chemical Exposure: Guidelines for Biological Monitoring. Davis, Cal.: Biomedical Publications, 1983.

O'Donoghue, J.L. (ed.). Neurotoxicity of Industrial and Commercial Chemicals. Vols. 1, 2. Boca Raton, Fla.: CRC Press, 1985.

Searle, C.E. (ed.). Chemical Carcinogens. 2nd ed. Washington, D.C.: American Chemical Society, 1984.

Snyder, R. The benzene problem in historial perspective. Fund. Appl. Toxicol. 1984; 4:692–699.

PESTICIDES

Analytical Reference Standards and Supplemental Data for Pesticides and Other Organic Compounds. U.S. Environmental Protection Agency, 1981.

Guthrie, F.E., Perry, J.J. (eds.) Introduction to Environmental Toxicology. New York: Elsevier, 1980.

Matsumura, F. Toxicology of Insecticides. New York: Plenum Press, 1975.

Murphy, S.D. Pesticides. In Doull, J., Klaassen, C.D., Amdur, M.O. (eds.). Casarett and Doull's Toxicology: The Basic Science of Poisons. 2nd ed. New York: Macmillan, 1980, pp. 357–408.

DRUGS

Bayer, M.J., Rumack, B.H. Poisoning and Overdose. Rockville, Md.: Aspen Systems, 1983.

Brecher, E.M. (ed.). Licit and Illicit Drugs, the Consumer's Union Report on Narcotics, Stimulants, Depressants, Inhalants, Hallucinogens, and Marijuana Including Caffeine, Nicotine, and Alcohol. Boston; Little, Brown, 1972.

Davis, D.M. (ed.). Textbook of Adverse Drug Reactions. New York: Oxford University Press, 1981.

Goode, E. Drugs in American Society. 2nd ed. New York: Alfred A. Knopf, 1984.

Gorrod, J.W. Drug Toxicity. London: Taylor and Francis, 1979.

Haddad, L.M., Winchester, J.F. (eds.). Clinical Management of Poisoning and Drug Overdose. Philadelphia: W.B. Saunders, 1983.

Harris, R.T., McIsaac, W.R., Schuster, C.R. (eds.). Drug Dependence. Austin: University of Texas Press, Capital Printing, 1970.

Lieber, C.E. Ethanol metabolism and toxicity. In Hodgson, E., Bend, J.R., Philpot, R.M. (eds.). Reviews in Biochemical Toxicology 5. Elsevier, New York, 1983, pp. 267–312.

Mitchell, J.R., Snodgrass, W.R., Gillette, J.R. The role of biotransformation in chemical-induced liver injury. Environ. Health Perspect. 1976; 15:27–38.

Skoutakis, V.A. (ed.). Clinical Toxicology of Drugs: Principles and Practice. Philadelphia: Lea & Febiger, 1982.

SOLVENTS

Cornish, H.H. Solvents and vapors. In Doull, J., Klaassen, C.D., Amdur, M.O. (eds.). Casarett and Doull's Toxicology: The Basic Science of Poisons. 2nd ed. New York: Macmillan, 1980, pp. 468–496.

Haddad, L.M., Winchester, J.F. (ed.). Clinical Management of Poisoning and Drug Overdose. Philadelphia: W.B. Saunders, 1983.

Pohl, L.R. Biochemical toxicology of chloroform. In Hodgson, E., Bend, J.R., Philpot, R.M. (eds.). Reviews in Biochemical Toxicology 1. New York: Elsevier, 1979, pp. 79–107.

Toxic Effects of Glycol Ethers. Environ Health Perspect. 1984; 57:1–278.

chapter eight

MEASUREMENT OF TOXICITY

Ernest Hodgson

8.1 INTRODUCTION

Although testing for toxicity might be expected to be one of the more routine aspects of toxicology, it is actually one of the more controversial. Among the many areas of controversy are the use of animals for testing and the welfare of the animals used, extrapolation from experimental animals to humans (risk analysis), extrapolation from high-dose to low-dose effects, choice of animals and genetic strains, and the increasing cost and complexity of testing protocols relative to the benefits expected. New tests are constantly being devised and are usually added to testing requirements already in existence.

Most testing can be subdivided into in vivo tests for acute, subchronic or chronic effects and in vitro tests for genotoxicity or cell transformation, although other tests are used and will be described.

Any chemical that has been introduced into commerce or is being developed for possible introduction into commerce is subject to toxicity testing to satisfy the regulations of one or more regulatory agencies. Furthermore, compounds contained in the waste products of industrial processes (combustion products, etc.) are also subject to testing.

Toxicity assessment is the determination of the potential of any substance to act as a poison, the conditions under which this potential will be realized, and the characterization of its action. Risk assessment, on the other hand, is a quantitative assessment of the probability of deleterious effects under given conditions. Both of these are involved in the regulation of toxic chemicals. This is the control, by statute, of the manufacture, transportation, sale or disposal of chemicals deemed, after testing procedures or according to criteria laid down in the law in question, to be toxic.

Testing in the United States is carried out by many groups: industrial, governmental, academic, and others (Table 8.1). Regulation, on the other hand, is carried out by a narrow range of governmental agencies each charged with the formulation of regulations under a particular law or laws and the administration of those regulations. Those for the United States are shown in Table 8.2. Other industrialized countries have counterpart laws and agencies for the regulation of toxic chemicals.

Although the objective of much but by no means all toxicity testing is the elimination of potential risks to humans, most of the testing is carried out on experimental animals. This is necessary because our current knowledge of quantitative structure–activity relationships (QSAR) does not permit accurate extrapolation to new compounds. Human data is difficult to obtain experimentally for ethical reasons but is necessary for such deleterious effects as irritation, nausea, allergies, odor evaluation, and some higher nervous system functions. Some insight may be obtained in certain cases from occupational exposure data, although this tends to be irregular in time and not clearly defined as to the composition of the toxicant or the exposure levels, since multiple exposure is common. Clearly, any experiments involving humans must be carried out under carefully defined conditions after other testing is complete.

Although extrapolation from experimental animals to humans presents problems due to differences in metabolic pathways, penetration, mode of action, etc., experimental animals present numerous advantages in testing procedures. These advantages include the possibility of clearly defined genetic constitution and their amenity to controlled exposure, controlled duration of exposure, and the possibility of detailed examination of all tissues following necropsy.

Although not all tests are required for all potentially toxic chemicals, any of the tests shown in Table 8.3 may be required by the regulations imposed under a

TABLE 8.1
Some Examples of Organizations Involved in Testing for Toxicity in the United States

Industry (in-house or through contract laboratories)

Nongovernment institutes
   Chemical Industries Institute for Toxicology (CIIT)

Contract laboratories
   Hazleton Laboratories
   Research Triangle Institute
   SRI International

Federal agencies (often through contract laboratories)
   Environmental Protection Agency (EPA)
   National Toxicology Program (NTP)
   National Cancer Institute (NCI)
   Food and Drug Agency (FDA)
   National Institute for Occupational Safety and Health (OSHA)
   National Center for Toxicological Research (NCTR)

Academic institutions (usually involved only specific parts of the overall testing program or in methods development)

TABLE 8.2
Agencies and Statutes Involved in the Regulation of Toxic Chemicals in the United States

FDA
Food and Drug Cosmetic Act
Labor Department
Occupational Safety and Health Act
Consumer Products Safety Commission
EPA
Federal Insecticide, Fungicide and Rodenticide Act
Clean Air Act
Federal Water Pollution Control Act
Safe Drinking Water Act
Toxic Substances Control Act
Resource Conservation and Recovery Act
State governments
Various state and local laws
Enforcement of certain aspects of federal law delegated to the states

FDA, Food and Drug Administration; EPA, Environmental Protection Agency.

particular law. The particular set of tests required depends on the predicted or actual use of the chemical, the predicted or actual route of exposure, and the chemical and physical properties of the chemical.

8.2 EXPERIMENTAL ADMINISTRATION OF TOXICANTS

Regardless of the chemical tested and whether the test is for acute or chronic toxicity, all in vivo testing requires the administration of a known dose of the chemical under test, applied in a reproducible manner, which is generally related to the expected route of exposure of humans to the chemical in question. The nature and degree of toxic effect may or may not be affected by the route of administration (eg, Table 8.4). This may be related to differences at the portals of entry or to effects on pharmacokinetic processes. In the latter case, one route may give rise to a concentration high enough to saturate some rate-limiting process, whereas another may distribute the dose over a longer time and avoid such saturation. Another key question is that of appropriate experimental controls. To identify effects of handling and other stress as well as the effects of the solvents or other carriers, it is usually better to compare treated animals with both solvent-treated and untreated or possibly sham-treated controls.

ORAL.   Oral administration is often referred to as administration per os (PO). Compounds can be administered either mixed in the diet, dissolved in drinking water, by gastric gavage, by controlled release capsules, or by gelatin capsules. In the first two cases, either a measured amount can be provided or access can be ad libitum, with the dose estimated from consumption measurements. In the last case controls should be pair-fed, ie, permitted only the amount of food consumed by treated animals, and, in either case, it is essential to consider

TABLE 8.3
A Summary of Tests for Toxicity

1. Chemical and physical properties
   For the compound in question, probable contaminants from the industrial synthesis as well as intermediates (and waste products) in the synthetic process.

2. Exposure and environmental fate
   A. Degradation studies—hydrolysis, photodegradation, etc.
   B. Degradation in soil, water, etc., under various conditions
   C. Mobility and dissipation in soil, water and air
   D. Accumulation in plants, aquatic animals, wild terrestrial animals, food plants and animals, etc.

3. In vivo tests
   A. Acute
      LD50 and/or LC50—oral, dermal, or inhaled
      Eye irritation
      Dermal irritation
      Dermal sensitization
   B. Subchronic
      90-day feeding
      30 to 90-day dermal or inhalation exposure
   C. Chronic
      Chronic feeding (including oncogenicity tests)
      Teratogenicity
      Reproduction (more than one generation)
   D. Special tests
      Neurotoxicity (delayed neuropathy)
      Potentiation
      Metabolism
      Pharmacodynamics
      Behavioral

4. In vitro tests
   Mutagenicity—prokaryote (Ames test)
   Mutagenicity—eukaryote (Drosophila, mouse, etc.)
   Chromosome aberration (Drosophila, sister chromatid exchange, etc.)

5. Effects on wildlife
   Selected species of wild mammals, birds, fish, and invertebrates—acute toxicity, accumulation, and reproduction in laboratory simulated field conditions, or actual field conditions

possible nutritional effects caused by reduction of food intake due to distasteful or repellent test materials. In the case of gastric gavage, the test material is administered through a stomach tube or gavage needle; if a solvent is necessary, it is administered also to control animals.

DERMAL. Dermal administration is required for estimation of toxicity of chemicals that may be taken up through the skin, as well as for estimation of skin irritation and photosensitization. Compounds are applied, either directly or in a suitable solvent, to the shaved skin of experimental animals. Frequently, the animals must be under restraint to prevent licking, and hence oral uptake,

TABLE 8.4
Variation in Toxicity by Route of Exposure

Chemical	Species/Sex	Route	LD50 (mg/kg)
N-Methyl-N-(1-naphthyl) fluoroacetamide[a]	Mouse/M	Oral, dermal, subcutaneous	371 402 250
N-Methyl-N-(1-naphthyl) fluoroacetamide[a]	Rat/M	Oral, dermal, subcutaneous	115 300 78
Chlordane[b]	Rat/M	Oral, dermal	335 840
Endrin[b]	Rat/M	Oral, dermal	18 18

[a] Data from Hashimoto, Y. et al. Toxicol. Appl. Pharmacol. 1968; 12:536–547.
[b] Data from Allen, J.R., et al. Pharmacol. Ther. 1979; 7:513–547.

of the material. Solvent and restraint controls are necessary since considerable stress is involved. Skin irritancy tests may be conducted on humans, using volunteer test panels.

INHALATION.   The respiratory system is an important portal of entry and, for evaluation purposes, animals must be exposed to atmospheres containing potential toxicants. The generation and control of the physical characteristics of such contaminated atmospheres is technically complex and expensive in practice. The alternative, direct instillation into the lung through the trachea, presents problems of reproducibility and stress and for these reasons is generally unsatisfactory.

Inhalation toxicity studies are conducted in inhalation chambers. The complete system contains an apparatus for the generation of aerosol particles, dusts or gas mixtures of defined composition and particle size, a chamber for the exposure of experimental animals, and a sampling apparatus for the determination of the actual concentration within the chamber. All these devices present technical problems that are difficult to resolve.

Animals are normally exposed for a fixed number of hours each day and a fixed number of days each week. Exposure may be head only, in which the head of the animal, wearing an airtight collar, is inserted into the chamber, or whole body, in which the animal is placed inside the chamber. In the latter case, variations due to unequal distribution are minimized by rotation of the position of the cages in the chamber during subsequent exposures. Figure 8.1 shows a typical inhalation system and supporting equipment.

INJECTION.   Except in the case of certain pharmaceuticals and drugs of abuse, injection (parenteral administration) does not correspond to any of the expected modes of exposure. It may be useful, however, in studies of mechanism or in QSAR studies in order to bypass absorption and permit rapid action. Methods of injection include intravenous (IV), intramuscular (IM), intraperi-

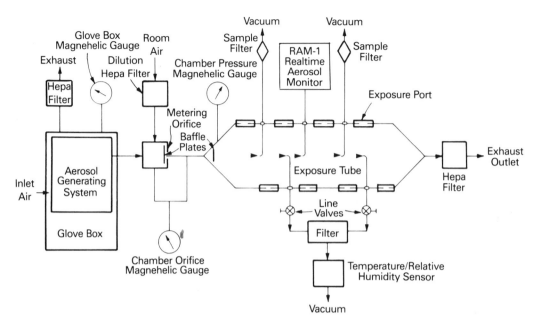

FIGURE 8.1.
An inhalation exposure system. Source: Modified from Adkins et al. Am. Int. Hyg. Assoc. J. 1980; 41:494.

toneal (IP), and subcutaneous (SC); infusion of toxicants over an extended period is also possible. Again, both solvent controls and untreated controls are necessary for proper interpretation of the results.

8.3 CHEMICAL AND PHYSICAL PROPERTIES

Although the determination of chemical and physical properties of known or potential toxicants does not constitute a test for toxicity, it is an essential preliminary for such tests. The information obtained can be used as follows:

1. For structure activity comparisons with other known toxicants, which may indicate the most probable hazards.
2. As an aid in identification in subsequent poisoning episodes.
3. In determining stability to light, oxidizing or reducing agents, heat, etc., which may enable preliminary estimates of persistence in the environment as well as indicate the most likely breakdown products, that themselves may require testing for toxicity.
4. In establishing such properties as the lipid solubility or octanol/water partition coefficient, which may enable preliminary estimates of rate of uptake and persistence in living organisms. Vapor pressure may indicate whether the respiratory system is a probable route of entry.
5. In acquiring knowledge of the chemical and physical properties needed to develop analytical methods for the measurement of the compound and its degradation products.

If the chemical is being produced for commercial use, similar information is needed on intermediates in the synthesis or by-products of the process since both are possible contaminants in the final product.

8.4 EXPOSURE AND ENVIRONMENTAL FATE

Data on exposure and environmental fate are needed not to determine toxicity but to provide information that may be useful in the prediction of possible exposure in the event that the chemical is toxic. Primarily useful for chemicals released into the environment such as pesticides, these tests include the rate of breakdown under aerobic and anaerobic conditions in soils of various types, the rates of leaching into surface water from soils of various types, or the rate of movement toward ground water. The effect of physical factors on degradation through photolysis and hydrolysis studies and the identification of the products formed can indicate the rate of loss of the hazardous chemical or the possible formation of hazardous degradation products.

Tests for accumulation in plants and animals and movement within the ecosystem are considered in Section 8.7.

8.5 IN VIVO TESTS

Traditionally, the basis for the determination of toxicity has been administration of the suspected compound, in vivo, to one or more species of experimental animal, followed by examination for mortality in acute tests, or by pathological examination for tissue abnormalities in chronic tests. Such results are then used, by a variety of extrapolation techniques, to estimate hazard to humans. These techniques, which still offer many advantages and are widely used, are summarized in the remainder of Section 8.5. They suffer from a number of disadvantages: they require large numbers of animals, numbers deemed unnecessary by both animal rights and animal welfare advocates; they are extremely expensive to conduct; and they are time-consuming. As a result they have been supplemented by many specialized in vitro tests, some of which are summarized in Section 8.6.

8.5.1 Acute Toxicity

Acute toxicity is usually concerned with lethality through the estimation of LD50 or LC50, although other acute effects, such as eye or skin irritation, are also subject to such tests.

8.5.1.1 LD50 and LC50

The LD50 is the estimated dose that, when the toxicant is administered directly to experimental test animals, results in the death of 50% of the population so exposed under the defined conditions of the test.

The LC50 is the estimated concentration, in the environment to which animals are exposed, that will kill 50% of the population so exposed under the defined conditions of the test.

The LD50 concept was developed by Trevan in 1927. The values are usually presented as an estimate with confidence limits, derived from treating several groups of animals with different doses.

The simplest method for the determination of LD50 and LC50, with confidence limits, is a graphical one and is based on the assumption that the effect is a quantal one (all or none), that the percentage responding in an experimental group is dose related and that the cumulative effect follows a normal distribution.

Data from a typical example (Figure 8.2) can be plotted against the log dose to give either a normal distribution (frequency or mortality of one dose minus that of the lower dose) or a sigmoid curve (percentage of mortality at each dose). If the distribution is normal, the point of inflection is the LD50 and the extrapolated doses at 16% and 84% mortality are equal to ± 1 SD. The sigmoid curve causes problems of extrapolation and slope determination, however, and methods were developed to linearize mortality plots. The one described is used almost exclusively and involves the transformation of the percentage of mortality figure to probits, units based on normal distribution statistics. This is done graphically by plotting the data on log/probit graph paper on which the mortality scale is derived so that the divisions marked as percentages are in fact probit units (Figure 8.2); thus, percentage data are plotted directly as probits. Similarly, the dose scale is a logarithmic scale; by plotting the raw data on such a scale, a log transformation is obtained without calculation.

The LD50 test has been the subject of much recent controversy, being criticized on various grounds, including:

1. Used uncritically, it is an expression of lethality only, not reflecting other acute effects.
2. It requires large numbers of experimental animals to obtain statistically acceptable values. Moreover, the results of LD50 tests are known to vary with species, strain, sex, age, etc. (Table 8.5); thus, the values are seldom closely similar from one laboratory to another, despite the numbers used.
3. Because the most important information needed, for regulatory purposes, concerns chronic toxicity, little useful information is derived from the LD50 test. The small amount of information that is acquired could as well be acquired from an approximation requiring only a small number of animals.
4. Extrapolation to humans is difficult.

TABLE 8.5
Factors Causing Variation in LD50 Values

Species	Health	Temperature
Strain	Nutrition	Time of day
Age	Gut contents	Season
Weight	Route of administration	Human error
Sex	Housing	

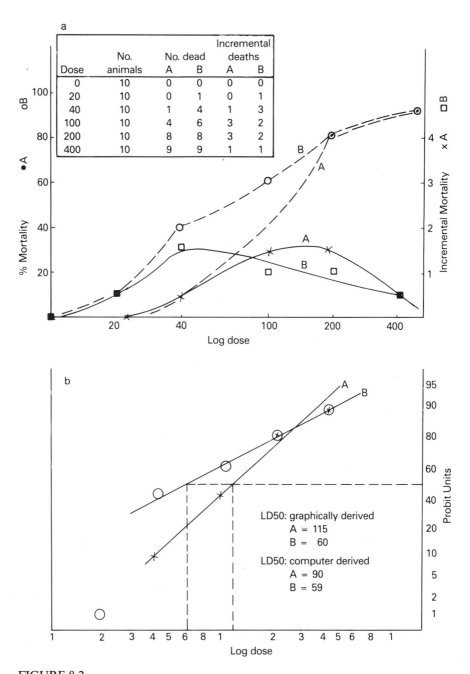

FIGURE 8.2.
Data from an LD50 experiment plotted as percentage of mortality at each dose (graph a) or with the percentages expressed as probit units (graph b).

Continued use of the test has been advocated, however, on the grounds that it is of use in the following ways:

1. Properly conducted, acute toxicity tests yield not only the LD50, but also information on other acute effects such as cause of death, time of death, symptomatology, nonlethal acute effects, organs affected, and reversibility of nonlethal effects.
2. Information concerning mode of action and metabolic detoxication can be inferred from the slope of the mortality curve.
3. The results can form the basis for the design of subsequent subchronic studies.
4. The test is useful as a first approximation of hazards to workers.
5. The test is rapidly completed.

For the above reasons, there has been a concerted effort in recent years to modify the concept of acute toxicity testing as it is embodied in the regulations of many countries and to substitute more meaningful methods that use fewer experimental animals. The article entitled "Significance of the LD50 Test for the Toxicological Evaluation of Chemical Substances" by Zbinden and Flury-Reversi is an excellent summary of the factors affecting LD50 determinations, the advantages and disadvantages of requiring such tests, and the nature and value of the information derived. It concludes that:

> The acute toxicity test (single dose toxicity) is still of considerable importance for the assessment of risk posed by new chemical substances, and for a better control of natural and synthetic agents in the human environment. It is not permissible, however, to regard a routine determination of the LD50 in various animal species as a valid substitute for an acute toxicity study.

The summary of suggested alternatives which follows owes much to the above cited review:

1. All regulations and guidelines should make clear that the classical LD50 test is not identical to the modern acute toxicity test.
2. LD50 tests on large animals should be abandoned, and comprehensive acute toxicity tests using small numbers of animals should be substituted. These tests should include detailed observations of symptoms, physiological measurements such as blood pressure, body temperature, reflex activity, electrocardiogram (ECG), electroencephalogram (EEG), food and water intake, respiration, behavior, etc. Chemical determinations such as blood chemistry and urinalysis should also be made as well as measurement of excretion of the parent compounds and its possible metabolites. Finally, gross and microscopic pathology should be determined.
3. Alternatives to the classic LD50 tests, even in those cases in which a numerical value is essential, should be used. They include the approximate lethal dose method of Deichman and Le Blanc, the moving average method of Thompson, the up and down method of Dixon and Mood, or the method recently proposed by Molinengo based on the relationship between dose and survival time. All these methods use small numbers of animals; the details of their use may be found in Hayes (see Section 8.10).
4. For many regulatory purposes, it is valuable to classify chemicals into

toxicity classes (Table 8.6). This can be done by treating small numbers with doses that represent the upper limit of the class, starting with the lowest dose and stopping the test with the dose at which $\geq 50\%$ of the animals die.

5. LD50 tests should never be carried out on pharmacologically inert compounds. It is sufficient to know that a single oral dose of 5 g/kg or a single parenteral dose of 2 g/kg causes neither death nor acute symptoms.

8.5.1.2 Eye Irritation

Because of the prospect of permanent blindness, ocular toxicity has long been a subject of both interest and concern. Although all regions of the eye are subject to systemic toxicity, usually chronic but sometimes acute, the tests of concern in this section are tests for irritancy of compounds applied topically to the eye. The tests used are all variations of the Draize test, and the preferred experimental animal is the albino rabbit.

The test consists of adding the material to be tested directly into the conjunctival sac of one eye of each of several albino rabbits, with the other eye serving as the control. The lids are held together for a few seconds, and the material is left in the eye for at least 24 hours. After that time, it may be rinsed out, but in any case, the eye is graded after 1, 2, and 3 days. Grading is subjective and based on the appearance of the cornea, particularly as regards opacity; the iris, as regards both appearance and reaction to light; the conjunctiva, as regards redness and effects on blood vessels; and the eyelids, as regards swelling. Fluorescein may be used to assist visual examination since the dye is more readily absorbed by damaged tissues, which then fluoresce when the eye is illuminated. Each item in the evaluation is scored on a numerical scale and chemicals are compared on this basis. Although each regulatory agency may require a slightly different evaluation protocol, all are variations of the above.

This test is probably the most criticized by advocates of animal rights and animal welfare, primarily on the grounds that it is inhumane. It has also been criticized on narrower scientific grounds in that both concentration and volumes used are unrealistically high, and that the results, because of high variability and the greater sensitivity of the rabbit eye, may not be applicable to

TABLE 8.6
Toxicity Classes

Class		LD50 (mg/kg)	Example*
I	Super toxic	5	TCDD
II	Extremely toxic	5–50	Pictrotoxin
III	Very toxic	50–500	Phenobarbital
IV	Moderately toxic	500–5,000	Morphine sulfate
V	Slightly toxic	5,000–15,000	Ethanol

Source: Toxicity classes. Modified after Zbinden, G., and Flury-Reversi, M. Arch. Toxicol. 1981; 47:77–99. Based on Loomis, T.A. Essentials of Toxicology, 2nd ed. 1978.

humans. It is clear, however, that because of great significance of visual impairment, tests for ocular toxicity will continue.

Attempts to solve the dilemma have taken two forms: to find substitute in vitro tests and to modify the Draize test so that it becomes not only more humane but also more predictive for humans. Substitute tests consist of attempts to use cultured cells or eyes from slaughtered food animals, but neither method is yet acceptable as a routine test. Modifications consist primarily of using smaller volumes and concentrations of test materials. This appears to reduce variability and should probably be adopted.

8.5.1.3 Dermal Irritation and Sensitization

There are tests for dermal irritation caused by topical application of chemicals. These fall into four general categories: primary irritation, cutaneous sensitization, phototoxicity, photosensitization. Because many foreign chemicals come into direct contact with the skin, including cosmetics, detergents, bleaches, and many others, these tests are considered essential to the proper regulation of such products. Less commonly dermal effects may be caused by systemic toxicants.

In the typical primary irritation test, the backs of albino rabbits are clipped free of hair and two areas of about 5 cm^2 on each rabbit are used in the test. One such area is lightly abraded; both areas are then treated with eithr 0.5 mL or 0.5 g of the compounds to be tested and are covered with a gauze pad. The entire trunk of the rabbit is wrapped with an impervious material held in place with adhesive tape. After 23 hours, the tape and gauze are removed; after another hour, the treated areas are evaluated for erythematous lesions (redness of the skin produced by congestion of the capillaries) and edematous lesions (accumulation of excess fluid in SC tissue), each of which is expressed on a numerical scale. After an additional 48 hours, the treated areas are again evaluated.

Some tests are simply variants of the above and are the most frequently used tests for evaluation of primary skin irritation. Other tests such as the mouse ear test and the guinea pig immersion test are also available but are used much less frequently.

Skin sensitization tests are designed to test the ability of chemicals to affect the immune system in such a way that a second contact causes a more severe reaction. This latter may be elicited at a much lower concentration and in areas beyond the area of initial contact. The antigen involved is presumed to be formed by the binding of the chemical to body proteins, the ligand – protein complex then being recognized as a foreign protein to which antibodies can be formed. Subsequent exposure may then give rise to an allergic reaction.

The test animal commonly used in skin sensitization tests is the guinea pig; animals are treated either with the test compound in a suitable vehicle, with the vehicle alone, or with a positive control such as 2,4-dinitrochlorobenzene in the same vehicle. During the induction phase, the animals are treated for each of three days evenly spaced during a two-week period. This is followed by a two-week rest period, followed by the challenge phase of the test. This consists of a 24-hour topical treatment carried out as described for primary skin irritation tests. The lesions are scored on the basis of severity and the number of animals responding (incidence).

Other test methods include those in which the induction phase is conducted by intradermal injection together with Freund's adjuvant (a chemical mixture that enhances the antigenic response) and the challenge by dermal application, or tests in which both induction and challenge doses are topical but the former is accompanied by intradermal injections of Freund's adjuvant. It is important that compounds that cause primary skin irritation be tested for skin sensitization at concentrations low enough that the two effects are not confused.

Phototoxicity tests are designed to evaluate the combined dermal effects of light (primarily ultra violet [UV] light) and the chemical in question. Tests have been described for both phototoxicity and photoallergy. In both cases, the light energy is believed to cause a transient excitation of the toxicant molecule which, on returning to the lower energy state, generates a reactive, free radical intermediate. In phototoxicity, these organic radicals act directly on the cells to cause lesions, whereas in photoallergy they bind to body proteins. These modified proteins then stimulate the immune system to produce antibodies, since the modifications cause them to be recognized as foreign or "non-self" proteins. These tests are basically modifications of the tests for primary irritation and sensitization except that, following application of the test chemical, the treated area is irradiated with UV light. The differences between the animals treated and irradiated and those treated and not irradiated is a measure of the photo effect.

These dermal tests have all been criticized on various grounds. They can cause discomfort and are, to some extent, inhumane. The data generated are hard to extrapolate to humans; some tests (for example, those involving intradermal injection) are considered unrealistic. None of the in vitro tests investigated as alternatives have yet proven applicable, however, nor have they been accepted by regulatory agencies.

Much knowledge in these areas was previously obtained using human test panels. Objections to this on ethical grounds have been almost as numerous as objections to animal studies. At the same time, in view of the large number of chemicals to which human skin is exposed, it is difficult to foresee a time when some form of testing for dermal toxicity will not be required.

8.5.2 Subchronic Tests

Subchronic tests examine toxicity caused by repeated dosing over an extended period, but not one that is so long as to constitute a significant portion of the expected life span of the species tested. A 90-day oral study in the rat or dog would be typical of this type of study, as would a 30-day dermal application study or a 30-day to 90-day inhalation study. Such tests provide information on essentially all types of chronic toxicity other than carcinogenicity and are usually believed essential for establishing the dose regimens for prolonged chronic studies. They are frequently used as the basis for the determination of the no-observable-effect level (NOEL). This value is often defined as the highest dose level at which no deleterious or abnormal effect can be measured, and is often used in risk assessment calculations. Subchronic tests are also useful in providing information on target organs and on the potential of the test chemical to accumulate in the organism.

8.5.2.1 Ninety-Day Feeding Tests

Chemicals are usually tested by administration in the diet, less commonly in the drinking water, and only when absolutely necessary by gavage, since the last process involves much handling and subsequent stress. The complexity of these tests is such that absolute care and attention must be paid at all times. Numerous experimental variables must be controlled and biological variables evaluated. In addition, the number of endpoints that can be measured is also large and, as a consequence, record keeping and data analysis present problems. If all is done with care, however, much may be learned from such tests.

8.5.2.1a Experimental (Nonbiological) Variables

Several environmental variables may affect toxicity evaluations, some directly and others by their effects on animal health. Major deviations from the optimum temperature and humidity for the species in question can cause stress reactions. Stress can also be caused by housing more than one species of experimental animal in the same room. Many toxic or metabolic effects show diurnal variations that are related to photoperiod. Cage design and the nature of the bedding have also been shown to affect the toxic response.

Thus, the optimum housing conditions are clean rooms, each containing a single species, with the temperature, humidity and photoperiod being constant and optimized for the species in question. Cages should be the optimum design for the species, bedding should be inert (not cause enzyme induction or other metabolic effect), and cages should not be overcrowded, with individual caging whenever possible.

Dose selection, preparation, and administration are all important variables. Subchronic studies are usually conducted using three (less often, four) dose levels. The highest should produce obvious toxicity but not high mortality and the lowest only slight or no mortality, whereas the intermediate dose(s) should give effects clearly intermediate between these two extremes. Although the doses can be extrapolated from acute tests, such extrapolation is difficult, particularly in the case of compounds that accumulate in the body; frequently, a 14-day range finding study is made. Although the route of administration should ideally mimic the expected route of exposure in humans, in practice the chemical is usually administered ad libitum in the diet, since this is, on average, most appropriate. Measurement of food consumption and pair-feeding with controls is recommended. In cases in which accurate measurement of consumption is an important factor in the experimental design, the animals may be fed by gavage or with capsules containing the toxicant.

To avoid effects from nonspecific variations on the diet, enough feed from the same batch should be obtained for the entire study. Part is set aside for the controls, and the remainder is mixed with the test chemical at the various dose levels. Care should be taken to store all food in such a way that not only does the test chemical remain stable but the nutritional value is also maintained. The identity and concentration of the test chemical should be checked periodically by chemical analysis.

Subchronic studies are usually conducted with 10–20 males and 10–20 females of a rodent species at each dose level and 4–8 of each sex of a larger species, such as the dog, at each dose level. Animals should be drawn from a larger group and assigned to control or treatment groups by some random process, but the larger group should not vary so much that the mean weights and ages of the subgroups vary significantly from each other at the beginning of the experiment.

8.5.2.1b Biological Variables

Subchronic studies should be conducted on two species, ideally a rodent and a nonrodent. Although the species chosen should be those with the greatest pharmacokinetic and metabolic similarity to humans for the compound in question, this information is seldom available. In practice, the most common rodent used is the rat, and the most common nonrodent used is the dog. It has long been held that inbred rodent strains should be used to reduce variability. This, and the search for strains that were sensitive to chemical carcinogenesis but did not have an unacceptably high spontaneous tumor rate, led to widespread use of the F344 rat and the B6C3F$_1$ mouse.

Although the age should be matched to the expected exposure period in terms of the stage of human development, this is not often done. Young adult or adolescent animals that are still growing are preferred in almost all cases, and both sexes are routinely used.

Good animal care is critical at all times, since toxicity has been shown to vary with diet, disease, and environmental factors. Animals should be quarantined for some time before being admitted to the test area, their diet should be optimum for the test species, and the facility should be kept clean at all times. Regular inspection by a veterinarian is essential, and any animals showing unusual symptoms not related to the treatment, eg, in controls or in low-dose but not high-dose animals, should be removed from the test and autopsied.

8.5.2.1c Results

Although the information required from subchronic tests varies somewhat from one regulatory agency to another, the requirements are basically similar (Table 8.7). Although in practice, the data collected may be limited to those required for regulatory purposes, a great deal of additional information can be obtained from a complete test. In either case, the data are of two types, that which can be obtained from living animals during the course of the test and that which is obtained from animals sacrificed either during or at the end of the test period. Many of the tests performed on living animals can be carried out first before the test period begins to provide a baseline for comparison to subsequent measurement. A group of treated animals should be removed from the treated food at the end of the test period and returned to the control diet for 21 – 28 days while the various endpoints are followed. This is necessary to establish whether or not any effects noted are reversible. Autopsies should be performed on all animals found dead or moribund during the course of the test.

The following is a list of tests that may be carried out during a 90-day oral toxicity study.

Interim Tests. Interim tests are carried out at intervals before the study, to establish baselines at intervals during the study, and at the end of the study, prior to killing the animals.

TABLE 8.7
Summary of Subchronic Test Guidelines

Test Characteristics	Regulatory Agency					
	EPA Pesticide Assessment Guidelines (1982)	FDA "Red Book" (1982)	FDA IND/NDA Pharmacology Review Guidelines (1981)	OECD (1981)	EPA Health Effects Test Guidelines (1982)	NTP (1976)
Purpose	Pesticide registration support	Food additives and color additives; safety assessment	IND/NDA pharmacology review guidelines (1981)	Assessment and evaluation of toxic characteristics	Select chronic dose levels	Predict dose range for chronic study
	No-observed-effect level	No observed adverse effects, no-effect level	Characterize pharmacology, toxicology, pharmacokinetics, and metabolism of drugs for precautionary clinical decisions	Select chronic dose levels; Useful information and permissible human exposure	Establish safety criteria for human exposure; No-observed-effect level	
Species	Rat (20)[a], Dog (8)	Rat (40), dog (8)	Rat, mouse, other rodents; Dog, monkey, other non-rodents	Rat (20), dog (8)	Rats (20), dogs (8)	Fischer 344 Rats (100), B6C3F1 Mice (120)
Doses	Three dose levels	Three dose levels	Three dose levels	Three dose levels	Three dose levels	Five dose levels
Endpoints	Ophthalmology Hematology; Clinical chemistry; Histopathology (29)[b] Rat (30), dog (33)	Ophthalmology Hematology; Clinical chemistry; Histopathology Rat (41)	Ophthalmology Hematology; Clinical chemistry; Histopathology	Ophthalmology Hematology; Clinical chemistry; Histopathology (41)	Ophthalmology Hematology; Clinical chemistry; Histology (41)	Weight loss, histopathology
	Target organs	Target organs	Target organs, behavioral and pharmacological effects	Target organs	Target organs	Target organs

Source: From the Report of the NTP Ad Hoc Panel on Chemical Carcinogenesis Testing and Evaluation, USPHS, 1984.
[a] (X) Number of animals per test group.
[b] (X) Number of tissues per animal.

Appearance—Mortality and morbidity as well as the condition of the skin, fur, mucous membranes, and orifices should be checked at least daily. Presence of palpable masses or external lesions should be noted.

Eyes—Ophthalmologic examination of both cornea and retina should be carried out at the beginning and end of the study.

Food consumption.

Body weight.

Neurologic response.

Behavioral abnormalities.

Respiration—Rate, regularity, etc., should be assessed.

ECG—Particularly with larger animals.

EEG—Particularly with larger animals.

Hematology—Assessment should be made prior to chemical administration (pretest) and monthly thereafter. Hemoglobin, hematocrit, RBC and WBC and differential counts, platelets, reticulocytes and clotting parameters should be assessed.

Blood Chemistry—Pretest and monthly tests should be done. Electrolytes and electrolyte balance, acid/base balance, glucose, urea nitrogen, serum lipids, serum proteins (albumin/globulin ratio), enzymes indicative of organ damage such as transaminases and phosphatases, also plasma and RBC cholinesterase. Toxicant and metabolite levels.

Urinalysis—Pretest and monthly tests should be done. Microscopic appearance (sediment, cells, stones, etc.), pH, specific gravity, chemical analysis for reducing sugars, proteins, ketones, bilirubin, etc., toxicant and metabolite levels.

Fecal Analysis—Occult blood, fluid content, and toxicant and metabolite levels should be assessed.

Termination Tests. Because the number of tissues that may be sampled is large (Table 8.8) and the number of microscopic methods is also large, it is necessary to consider all previous results before carrying out the pathological examination. For example, clinical tests or blood chemistry analyses may implicate a particular target organ that can then be examined in greater detail. All control and high dose animals are examined in detail. If lesions are found, the next lowest dose group is examined for these lesions and this is continued until a no-effect group is reached.

Because pathology is largely a descriptive science with a complex terminology that varies from one practitioner to another, it is critical that the terminology be defined at the beginning of the study and that the same pathologist examine the slides from both treated and control animals. Pathologists are not in agreement on the necessity or the wisdom of coding slides so that the assessor is not aware of the treatment given the animal from which a particular slide is derived. Such coding will, however, eliminate unintentional bias, a hazard in a procedure that depends on subjective evaluation. Other items of utmost importance are quality control, slide identification, and data recording. Many tissues may be examined; consequently, an

TABLE 8.8
Tissues and Organs to Be Examined Histologically in Chronic and Subchronic
Toxicity Tests

Adrenals
Bone, including bone marrow
Brain
Cecum
Colon
Cartilage
Duodenum
Esophagus
Eyes
Gall bladder
Heart
Ileum
Jejunum
Kidneys
Larynx
Liver
Lungs and bronchi
Lymph nodes
Mammary glands
Mandibular lymph node
Mesenteric lymph node
Nasal cavity
Ovaries
Pancreas
Parathyroids
Pituitary
Prostate
Rectum
Salivary gland
Sciatic nerve
Seminal vesicles
Skin
Spleen
Spinal cord
Stomach
Testes
Thigh muscle
Thyroid
Thymus
Urinary bladder
Uterus

even larger number of tissue blocks must be prepared. Because each of these
may yield many slides to be stained, comparable quality of staining and the
accurate correlation of a particular slide with its parent block, tissue, and
animal is critical.

Necropsy—This must be conducted with care to avoid postmortem damage
to the specimens. Tissues are removed, weighed and examined closely for
gross lesions, masses, etc. Tissues are then fixed for subsequent histological

examination in neutral buffered formalin or Millonigs phosphate-buffered formalin.

Histology—The tissues listed in Table 8.8 plus any lesions, masses, or abnormal tissues are embedded, sectioned, and stained for light microscopy. Parafin embedding and stained with hemotoxylin and eosin are the preferred routine methods, but special stains may be used for particular tissues or for a more specific examination of certain lesions. Electron microscopy is also used for more specific examination of lesions or cellular changes after their initial localization by more routine methods.

8.5.2.2 Thirty-Day Dermal Tests

Thirty-day dermal tests are particularly important when the expected route of human exposure is by contact with the skin, as is the case with many industrial chemicals, pesticides, etc. Compounds to be tested are usually applied weekly to shaved or clipped areas on the back of the animal, either undiluted or in a suitable solvent. In the latter case, the solvent is applied alone to the controls. Selection of a suitable solvent is difficult since many affect the skin, causing either drying or irritation, whereas others may markedly affect the rate of penetration of the test chemical. Corn oil, ethanol, or carboxylmethyl cellulose are preferred to dimethyl sulfoxide (DMSO) or acetone. It should also be considered that some of the test chemical may be ingested as a result of grooming by the animal, although this can be controlled to some extent by use of restraining collars.

The criteria for environment, dose selection, species selection, etc., are not greatly different to those used for 90-day feeding tests nor are the endpoints to be examined. It is necessary, however, to pay close attention to the skin at the point of application, since local effects may be as important as systemic ones.

8.5.2.3 Thirty-Day to Ninety-Day Inhalation Tests

Inhalation studies are indicated whenever the expected route of exposure is expected to be through the lungs. Animals are commonly exposed for 6–8 hours each day, 5 days each week, in chambers of the type previously discussed. Even in those cases in which the animals are maintained in the inhalation chambers during nonexposure hours, food is always removed during exposure. Despite this, exposure tends to be in part dermal and, due to grooming of the fur, in part oral. Environmental and biological parameters are the same as for other subchronic tests, as are the routine endpoints to be measured before, during, and after the test period. Particular attention must be paid, however, to effects on the tissues of the nasal cavity and the lungs, since these are the areas of maximum exposure.

8.5.3 Chronic Tests

Chronic tests are those conducted over the greater part of the life span of the test animal or, in some cases, over more than one generation. The most important tests of this type are chronic toxicity, carcinogenicity, teratogenicity, and reproduction.

8.5.3.1 Chronic Toxicity and Carcinogenicity

Tests for both chronic toxicity and carcinogenicity are included here since the design is similar, so similar in fact that they can be combined into one test, although this is not usually done. If they were combined, the length of time and the number of animals involved, as well as the many endpoints to be examined, would require a complex and difficult protocol. This is avoided, to some extent, by conducting the tests separately. In the latter case, differences between the test protocols can also be permitted.

Chronic toxicity tests are designed to discover any of numerous toxic effects and to define safety margins to be used in the regulation of chemicals. As with subchronic tests, two species are usually used, one of which is either a rat or a mouse strain, in which case the tests are run for 2–2.5 years or 1.5–2.0 years, respectively. The nonrodent species, if used, may be the dog, a non-human primate, or a small carnivore such as the ferret. Chronic toxicity tests may involve administration in the food, in the drinking water, by gavage or by inhalation, the first being the most common. The dose used is the maximum tolerated dose (MTD) and usually two lower doses, 0.25 MTD and 0.125 MTD. The MTD has been defined for testing purposes by the US Environmental Protection Agency (EPA) as:

> The highest dose that causes no more than a 10% weight decrement, as compared to the appropriate control groups; and does not produce mortality, clinical signs of toxicity, or pathologic lesions (other than those that may be related to a neoplastic response) that would be predicted to shorten the animals' natural life span.

It is determined by extrapolation from subchronic studies.

The requirements for animal facilities, housing, and environmental conditions are as described for subchronic studies. Special attention must be paid to diet formulation, since it is impractical to formulate all of the diets for ≥ 2-year study from a single batch. In general, semisynthetic diets of specified components should be formulated regularly and analyzed before use.

The endpoints used in these studies are those described for the subchronic study: appearance, ophthalmology, food consumption, body weight, clinical signs, behavioral signs, hematology, blood chemistry, urinalysis, fecal analysis, organ weights, and histology. Some animals may be killed at fixed intervals during the test (eg, 6, 12, or 18 months) for histological examination. Particular attention is paid to any organs or tests that showed compound-related changes in the subchronic tests.

Carcinogenicity tests have many requirements in common (physical facilities, diets, etc.) with both chronic and subchronic toxicity tests as previously described above; these will not be repeated. Because of the numbers and time required, most tests are carried out using rats and/or mice, but in some cases an additional nonrodent species may also be used. The chemical under test may be administered in the food, the drinking water, by gavage, by dermal application, or by inhalation, the first and third methods being the most common. Because the oncogenic potency of chemicals varies through extreme limits, the purity of the test chemical is of great concern. A 1% contaminant need only be 100 times as potent as the test chemical to have an equivalent effect, and differences of this magnitude and greater are not uncommon.

Dosing is carried out over the major part of the life span (1.5–2.0 years for mice and ≥ 2.0 years or more for rats) starting at weaning. The highest dose used is the MTD, together with one lower dose, usually 0.5 MTD.

The principal endpoint is tumor incidence as determined by histological examination. The statistical problem of distinguishing between spontaneous tumor occurrence in the controls and chemical-related tumor incidence in the treated animals is great; for that reason, large numbers of animals are used. A typical test involves ≥ 50 rats or mice of each sex in each treatment group. Thus, a typical one-species test will include 300 animals: 50 males and 50 females at the MTD, 50 males and 50 females at 0.5 MTD; and 50 males and 50 females as controls. Some animals are necropsied at intermediate stages of the test, eg, at 12 months, as are any animals found dead or moribund; all surviving animals are necropsied at the end of the test.

Tissues to be examined are listed in Table 8.8, with particular attention being paid to abnormal masses, lesions, etc.

8.5.3.2 Reproductive Toxicity and Teratogenicity

The task of presenting a brief but instructive account of toxicity testing in this area is difficult, primarily because there appears to be little unanimity between either experts in the area or between regulatory agencies. The result is that many complex protocols exist, with little available objective criteria to facilitate a preference for any one over the others. Additional problems exist in that the terminology used in teratology is extensive, highly specialized and varies from one research group to another. The following description represents an attempt to embody the general features of the most common protocols and, where necessary, to comment on additional features of protocols not described. The subject is divided into four areas:

1. Fertility and general reproductive performance — single generation studies;
2. Fertility and general reproductive performance — multigeneration studies;
3. Teratology;
4. Effect of chemicals in late pregnancy and lactation.

In all these descriptions, the principles of animal husbandry as they apply to facilities, cages, environmental controls, diet, etc., should be closely adhered to, as mentioned in the previous sections on acute, subchronic and chronic testing.

8.5.3.2a Fertility and General Reproductive Performance: Single-Generation Tests
Single-generation tests for fertility and general reproductive performance are usually carried out on rats (Figure 8.3); in typical tests, 20 males are treated with the test compound for 60 days prior to mating, and 20 females are treated for 14 days prior to mating. These treatment times are selected to coincide with the times during which spermatogenesis and ovulation occur. After mating, treatment of the females is continued through pregnancy and until the pups are weaned.

F_0 females treated for 14 days	Mating	Gestation 50% of females sacrificed at day 15	F_1 Lactation pups sacrificed at weaning
F_0 males treated for 60 days			

FIGURE 8.3.
Abbreviated protocol for a one-generation reproductive toxicity test.

The test compound is administered either in the feed, in the drinking water, or by gavage. The high dose is variously described as that which causes some, but not excessive, maternal toxicity or that which just fails to cause maternal toxicity. The low dose should either be that to which humans are expected to be exposed or a dose that gives measurable tissue levels but no measurable toxicity. Because the effects in question generally vary linearly when plotted against the logarithm of the dose, the intermediate dose(s) should be evenly spaced, on a logarithmic scale, between the low and high doses.

The rats are placed in cohabitation, with one male and one female caged together. Mating is confirmed by the appearance of spermatozoa in the daily vaginal smear for rats or by the appearance of a copulatory (vaginal) plug in mice. Day 1 of gestation is the day insemination is confirmed. Half of the females are killed at mid-gestation and examined for preimplantation and postimplantation lethality, the other half are permitted to bear and nurse their pups, the litters being culled to a constant number, usually 10, after 3–4 days. At weaning, the pups are killed and autopsied for gross and internal abnormalities.

Because both males and females are treated, it is not possible to distinguish between maternal and paternal effects in the subsequent performance. To permit this separation, it is necessary to treat additional animals to the stage of mating and then to outcross them to untreated members of the opposite sex. Subsequent examination of the females may be carried out as in the combined tests. Similarly, with effects seen at weaning, it is not possible to distinguish between effects mediated in utero or mediated by lactation. Thus distinction can be made by "cross-fostering" the offspring of treated females to untreated females and vice versa.

The endpoints observed are as follows:

1. Preimplantation death. The number of corpora lutea in the ovaries relative to the number of implantation sites;
2. Postimplantation deaths. The number of resorption sites in the uterus relative to the number of implantation sites;
3. Gross effects on male or female reproductive system;
4. Duration of gestation;
5. Litter size and condition, number of dead and live pups, weight of pups, gender of pups, gross morphological variation in pups;
6. Subsequent survival and performance of dam and pups, weight gain, mortality, etc;
7. Gross and visceral abnormalities in weanlings.

Detailed examination of the pups is possible, but is better done under the protocol described for teratology testing. A number of variations of this test have been proposed. For example, it has been suggested that a number of weanlings be left to develop and be tested later for behavioral and/or physiological defects.

8.5.3.2b Fertility and General Reproductive Performance: Multigeneration Tests

Multigeneration tests for fertility and general reproductive performance (Figure 8.4) are also carried out with rodents, usually rats. The test compound is administered to males and females from weaning of the F_0 generation and throughout the test, which is carried out for up to three generations. The test compound is administered in the food or drinking water, usually at three levels. The high level is approximately one-tenth of the LD50, the low dose is one that subchronic studies indicate should not cause toxic effects in either dams or fetuses of the F_1 generation and the intermediate dose (or doses) should be equally spaced on a logarithmic scale between the low and high doses. Enough

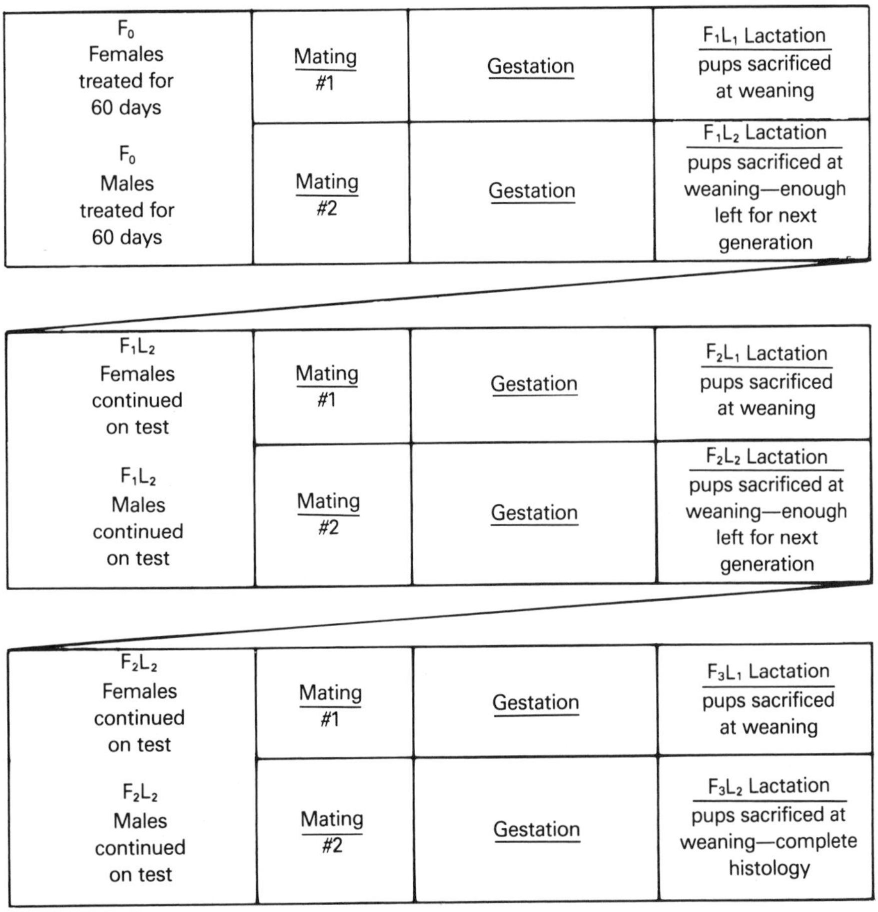

| F_0 Females treated for 60 days | Mating #1 | Gestation | F_1L_1 Lactation pups sacrificed at weaning |
| F_0 Males treated for 60 days | Mating #2 | Gestation | F_1L_2 Lactation pups sacrificed at weaning—enough left for next generation |

| F_1L_2 Females continued on test | Mating #1 | Gestation | F_2L_1 Lactation pups sacrificed at weaning |
| F_1L_2 Males continued on test | Mating #2 | Gestation | F_2L_2 Lactation pups sacrificed at weaning—enough left for next generation |

| F_2L_2 Females continued on test | Mating #1 | Gestation | F_3L_1 Lactation pups sacrificed at weaning |
| F_2L_2 Males continued on test | Mating #2 | Gestation | F_3L_2 Lactation pups sacrificed at weaning—complete histology |

FIGURE 8.4.
Abbreviated protocol for a multigeneration reproductive toxicity test.

females from the F_0 group and enough survivors of the F_1 and F_2 group are provided so that each generation has 20 pregnant females per dose level (including controls).

After males and females of the initial group have been treated for 60 days, they are mated to produce the first F_1 litter (F_1L_1). After birth, the pups are weighed, differentiated by sex, and examined for external abnormalities, after which the litters are culled to a constant number of pups (usually ten). Pup weight and survival are followed to weaning; the pups are killed and necropsied to detect internal abnormalities, obtain organ weights, etc. The parents are permitted to mate again after the first litter is weaned, to produce the second litter (F_1L_2). The pups of the second litter are treated in the same way as the first except that enough are permitted to survive to produce the 20 or more males and females for the next generation. Again each pair is allowed to produce two litters (F_2L_1 and F_2L_2), which are treated in the same way as those of the first generation, setting aside enough animals to produce the two litters of the third generation (F_3L_1 and F_3L_2). Because this is the final generation, all weanlings are examined as previously described except that a selected number are used in a complete histological examination. As with other tests, all animals that die or become moribund during the course of the test are given a complete necropsy.

The following endpoints are evaluated:

1. Fertility index, the number of pregnancies relative to the number of matings;
2. The number of live births, relative to the number of total births;
3. Gender and initial weight of pups;
4. Growth rate of pups;
5. Survival of pups relative to number born (or relative to the number to which litters are culled);
6. Gross deformities at birth;
7. Internal abnormalities at weaning;
8. Histological changes at weaning (third generation only).

With this test, as with the single-generation test, males or females of any question can be mated to unmated individuals of the opposite sex to determine the sex specificity of any effect observed. It has been suggested that modification of the test would permit delayed effects on physiological or behavioral parameters to be assessed. This may be useful for low-dose studies of these parameters but high-dose studies would have to be carried out as separate one-generation studies. Similarly, modifications to permit detailed teratological evaluation have been proposed but, again, these would be optimal if conducted as separate one-generation studies including higher dose levels.

8.5.3.2c Teratology

Teratology is the study of abnormal fetal development. In teratogenic testing, exposure to the test chemical may be from implantation to parturition, although it is usually restricted to the period of major organogenesis, the most sensitive period for inducing structural malformations (see Section 6.3.2.2.b). Observations may be extended throughout life, but usually they are made immediately prior to birth. The endpoints currently observed are mainly morphologic (structural changes and malformations), although embryo-fetal mortality is also used as an endpoint. Although many protocols have been used, a description of the most straightforward follows (Figure 8.5), with others being commented on as necessary.

Teratogenic studies are carried out in a rodent species, usually the rat, sometimes also in another species, such as the rabbit, but only rarely in species such as nonhuman primates or dogs. Enough females should be used so that, given normal fertility for the strain, there are 20 pregnant females in each dosage group of rodents or ten pregnant females per dosage group of nonrodents. The test chemical is administered in the diet, in the drinking water, or by gavage, the latter being required by some regulatory agencies. The high-dose level is one at which some maternal toxicity is known to occur, but only that which will cause < 10% mortality. The low dose should be one at which no maternal toxicity is apparent, and the intermediate dose(s) should be spaced evenly, on a logarithmic scale, between the low and high doses.

The timing of compound administration is usually such that the dam is exposed during the period of major organogenesis, ie. days 6 – 15 of gestation in the case if the rat or mouse and days 6 – 18 in the case of the rabbit. Day 1 is the day spermatozoa appear in the vagina or a vaginal plug appears in the case of rats and mice, or the day of mating in the rabbit.

The test is terminated by killing and dissection of the dams on the day before normal delivery is expected. The uterus is examined for implantation and resorption sites and for live and dead fetuses and the ovaries for corpora lutea. In rodent studies, one-third of the fetuses are examined for soft tissue malformations, and the remaining two-thirds are examined for skeletal malformations. In nonrodents, all fetuses are examined for both soft tissue and skeletal malformations. The various endpoints that may be examined include maternal toxicity, embryo-fetal toxicity, external malformations, and soft tissue and skeletal malformations. A brief discussion of each of these follows.

Maternal toxicity is evaluated from a relatively small number of parameters and is useful in assessing the validity of the high-dose level and the possibility that maternal toxicity is involved in subsequent events. The parameters used

Teratology

Untreated females	Mating	Gestation Pregnant females treated on days 6-15. Pups and dams sacrificed day 20
Untreated males		

Perinatal/Postnatal

Untreated females	Mating	Gestation Pregnant females treated on days 15-21	Lactation Females treated to weaning. Pups and dams sacrificed at weaning
Untreated males			

FIGURE 8.5.
Abbreviated protocol for a teratology test and for a perinatal/postnatal toxicity test.

include body weight, food consumption, clinical signs, and necroscopy data such as organ weights.

Because exposure starts after implantation, conception and implantation rates should be the same in controls and all treatment levels. If not, the test is suspect, with a possible error in the timing of the dose.

Embryo-fetal toxicity is determined from the number of dead fetuses and resorption sites relative to the number of implantation sites. In addition to the possibility of lethal malformations, such toxicity can be due to maternal toxicity, stress, or direct toxicity to the embryo or fetus that is not related to developmental malformations. A high level of embryo-fetal toxicity may also obscure teratological effects that could have occurred at a lower dose. In that case, the next lower dose level should be evaluated with care and, if necessary, the study

TABLE 8.9
External Malformation Commonly Seen in Teratogenicity Tests

Brain, cranium, spinal cord
  Encephalocele (EN) — protrusion of the brain through an opening of the skull. The cerebrum is well formed and covered by transparent connective tissue.
  Exencephaly (EX) — lack of skull with disorganized outward growth of the brain.
  Microcephaly (M) — small head on normal-sized body.
  Hydrocephaly (H) — marked enlargement of the ventricles of the cerebrum.
  Craniorachischisis (CR) — exposed brain and spinal cord.
  Spina bifida (B) — Nonfusion of spinal processes. Usually the covering ectoderm is missing, and the spinal cord is evident.

Nose
  Enlarged naris (EN) — enlarged nasal cavities.
  Single naris (SN) — a single naris, usually median.

Eye
  Microphthalmia (M) — small eye.
  Anophthalmia (A) — lack of eye.
  Open eye (O) — no apparent eyelid; eye is open.

Ear
  Anotia (A) — absence of the external ear.
  Microtia (M) — small ear.

Jaw
  Micrognathia (M) — small lower jaw.
  Agnathia (A) — absence of lower jaw.
  Aglossia (AG) — lack of tongue.
  Astomia (AS) — lack of mouth opening.
  Bifid tongue (BT) — forked tongue.
  Cleft lip (CL) — may be either unilateral or bilateral cleft of the upper lip.

Palate
  Cleft palate (CP) — a cleft or separation of the median portion of the palate.

Limbs
  Clubfoot (C) — a foot that has grown in a twisted manner, resulting in an abnormal shape or position. It is possible to have a malposition of the whole limb.
  Micromelia (M) — abnormal shortness of the limb.
  Hemimelia (H) — absence of any of the long bones, resulting in a shortened limb.
  Phocomelia (P) — absence of all the long bones of a limb; the feet are attached directly to the body.

should be repeated with additional dose levels. Fetal weight and fetal size may also be a measure of toxicity but should not be confused with the variations seen as a result of differences in the number of pups per litter.

Anomalies may be regarded either as variations that may not adversely affect the fetus and not have a fetal outcome, or as malformations that are considered to have adverse effects on the fetus. There is little agreement on a precise definition of which anomalies fall in which class and the distinction may be academic, since a dose-related increase, even in a variation known to occur in controls, is still regarded as evidence of teratogenic potential. An example of such a variation is the number of ribs in the rabbit.

Common external anomalies (Table 8.9) are determined by examination of fetuses fixed in Bouin's fixative or by the method of Staples and by hand sectioning by the method of Wilson. Some common visceral anomalies are listed in Table 8.10.

Skeletal anomalies are examined by first fixing the fetus and then staining the cartilage with Alizarin Red. Numerous skeletal variations occur in controls and may not have an adverse effect on the fetus (Table 8.11). Their frequency of occurrence may, however, be dose related and should be evaluated.

Almost all chemically induced malformations have been observed in control animals, and essentially all such malformations are known to be produced by more than one cause. Thus, it is obvious that great care and a conservative approach are necessary in the interpretation of teratogenic studies.

Many variations in teratogenic tests have been suggested, some trivial, others impractical, but some worthy of serious consideration. It has been suggested that dosing be extended to the end of pregnancy, and at least one regulatory

TABLE 8.10
Some Common Visceral Anomalies Seen in Teratogenicity Tests

Intestines
Umbilical hernia (UH)—protrusion of the intestines into the umbilical cord.
Ectopic intestines (EI)—extrusion of the intestines outside the body wall.

Heart
Dextrocardia (D)—rotation of the heart axis to the right.
Enlarged heart (E)—either the atrium or the ventricle may be enlarged.

Lung
Enlarged lung (L)—all lobes are usually enlarged.
Small lung (S)—all lobes are usually small. Lobes may have immature appearance.

Sex, uterus, testes
Undescended testes (U)—testes are located anterior to the bladder instead of lateral; may be bilateral or unilateral.
Agenesis of testes (AT)—one or both testes may be missing.
Agenesis of uterus (AU)—one or both horns of the uterus may be missing.

Kidney
Hydronephrosis (H)—fluid-filled kidney, often grossly enlarged. This condition may be accompanied by hydroureter (enlarged fluid-filled ureter).
Fused (F)—kidneys fused, appearing as one misshapen kidney with two ureters.
Agenesis (A)—one or both kidneys missing.
Misshapen (M)—small, enlarged (normal internally), spherical, or odd-shaped kidneys.

TABLE 8.11
Skeletal Abnormalities Commonly Seen in Teratogenicity Tests

Digits
Polydactyly (P) — presence of extra digits. Because five is the normal number in the mouse, a polydactylous fetus would have six or more.
Syndactyly (S) — fusion of two or more digits.
Oligodactyly (O) — absence of one or more digits.
Brachydactyly (B) — smallness of one or more digits.

Ribs
Wavy ribs (W) — ribs may be any aberrant shape.
Extra ribs (E) — may have extra ribs on either side.
Missing ribs (M) — may be missing on either side.
Fused ribs (F) — may be fused anywhere along length of rib.
Branched ribs (B) — single base and branched.

Tail
Short tail (S) — short tail, usually lack of vertebrae.
Missing tail (A) — absence of tail.
Corkscrew (C) — corkscrew-shaped tail.

agency requires such a protocol, even though this type of procedure may be counterproductive. Of more importance is the suggestion that some of the offspring born to dams treated for teratogenic evaluation should be allowed to survive and be subjected to a variety of behavioral tests as they develop. Such tests would have the potential to detect functional defects that are either not apparent morphologically or that appear later in development. Physiological functions could also be tested postnatally, including growth rate, kidney function, liver function, EEG, and EKG. Such testing is advisable.

8.5.3.2d Effect of Chemicals in Late Pregnancy and Lactation (Perinatal/Postnatal Effects)

These tests are usually carried out on rats, and 20 pregnant females per dosage group are treated during the final third of gestation and through lactation to weaning (day 15 of pregnancy through day 21 postpartum) (Figure 8.5). The duration of gestation, parturition problems, and the number and size of pups in the naturally delivered litter are observed, as is the growth performance of the offspring. Variations of this test are the inclusion of groups treated only to parturition and only postpartum in order to separate prenatal and postnatal effects. Cross-fostering of pups to untreated dams may also be used to the same end. Behavioral testing of the pups has been suggested, and this and other physiological testing is to be recommended.

8.5.4 Special Tests

This general heading is used to include brief assessments of tests that are not usually required but that may be required in particular cases or have been suggested as useful adjuncts to current testing protocols. Many are in areas of toxicology that are developing rapidly; as a result, no consensus has yet evolved as to the best tests or sequence of tests, only an understanding that such evaluations may shed light on previously undefined aspects of chemical toxicity.

8.5.4.1 Neurotoxicity (Including Delayed Neuropathy)

The nervous system is complex, both structurally and functionally, and toxicants can affect one or more units of the system in selective fashion. It is necessary, therefore, to devise tests or sequences of tests that measure not only changes in overall function but that also indicate which basic unit is affected and how the toxicant interacts with its target. This is complicated by the fact that the nervous system has a considerable functional reserve, and specific observable damage may not affect overall function until it becomes even more extensive. Types of damage to the nervous system are classified in various ways but include neuronal toxicity, axonopathy, toxic interruption of impulse transmission, myelinopathy, and synaptic alterations in transmittor release or receptor function. With the exception of tests for the delayed neuropathy associated with certain organophosphates, specific tests for neurotoxicity are seldom required by regulatory agencies since neurotoxicity is frequently revealed by the acute, subchronic, chronic, behavioral, and other tests that are required. Neurotoxicity is of great significance in toxicology, however, and tests have been devised to supplement those routinely required.

1. Behavioral and pharmacological tests involve the observation of clinical signs and behavior. These include signs of changes in awareness, mood, motor activity, CNS excitation, posture, motor incoordination, muscle tone, reflexes, and autonomic functions. If these tests so indicate, more specialized tests can be carried out that evaluate spontaneous motor activity, conditioned avoidance responses, operant conditioning, as well as tests for motor incoordination such as the inclined plane or rotarod tests. Such a sequence of tests was described by Irwin in 1964.

Tests for specific classes of compounds include the measurement of transmitter stimulated adenyl cyclase and Na^+K^+-ATPase for compounds which affect receptor function, or cholinesterase inhibition for organophosphates or carbamates. Electrophysiological techniques may detect compounds such as DDT or pyrethroids which affect impulse transmission.

2. Neuropathological methods. It is difficult to carry out routine pathological examination of all parts of a structure as complex as the nervous system, and the routine methods of pathology can, in any case, detect only fairly extensive damage. Recently, however, it has been suggested that, using more sensitive methods and sampling at only two sites—the medulla oblongata and the tibial nerve—can permit detection of distal axonopathies, neuronopathies, and myelinopathies. This technique, said to be sensitive enough to detect early damage, consists of fixation with buffered glutaraldehyde, postfixation with osmium tetroxide, preparation of thin plastic sections, and staining with a variety of routine stains.

3. Biochemical methods include the appearance of cholesterol esters and the increase in β-glucuronidase and β-galactosidase characteristic of Wallerian degeneration. The latter two enzymes are easily measured and this technique may prove to be generally applicable to a wide range of toxicants. The measurement of cholinesterase (plasma, red blood corpuscle or brain) is a well-established and easily performed test for cholinesterase inhibitors and is routinely carried with some categories of pesticides.

The delayed neurotoxic potential of certain organophosphates such as tri-*o-*

cresyl phosphate (TOCP) is usually tested for by clinical signs (paralysis of leg muscles in hens) or pathology (degeneration of the motor nerves in hens), but a biochemical test involving the ratio between the ability to inhibit cholinesterase relative to the ability to inhibit an enzyme that has been referred to as the neurotoxic esterase, or NTE, has been suggested. The ability of chemicals to cause delayed neuropathy is generally correlated with their ability to inhibit this nonspecific esterase, found in various tissue, although the role, if any, of the enzyme in the sequence of events leading to nerve degeneration is not known. The preferred test organism is the mature hen, since the clinical signs are similar to those in humans and such symptoms cannot be readily elicited in the common laboratory rodents.

Although in vitro cultivation of nerve cells has been possible for some time, none of the in vitro tests of nerve function have yet been developed to the point at which they may be of practical use in routine toxicity testing.

8.5.4.2 Potentiation

Potentiation and synergism represent interactions between toxicants that are potential sources of hazard, since neither humans or other species are exposed to one chemical at a time. The enormous number of possible combinations of chemicals makes routine screening for all such effects not only impractical, however, but impossible.

One of the classic cases is the potentiation of the insecticide malathion by another insecticide, EPN, the LD50 of the mixture being dramatically lower than that of either compound alone. This potentiation can also be seen between malathion and certain contaminants which are formed during synthesis, such as isomalathion. For this reason, quality control during manufacture is essential. This example of potentiation involves inhibition, by EPN or isomalathion, of the carboxylesterase responsible for the detoxication of malathion in mammals.

It is practical to test for potentiation only when there has been some preliminary indication that it might occur or when either or both of the compounds belong to chemical classes previously known to cause potentiation. Such a test can be conducted by comparing the LD50, or any other appropriate toxic endpoint, of a mixture of equitoxic doses of the chemicals in question with the same endpoint measured with the two chemicals administered alone.

In the case of synergism, in which one of the compounds is relatively nontoxic when given alone, the toxicity of the toxic compound can be measured when administered alone or after a relatively large dose of the nontoxic compound.

8.5.4.3 Toxicokinetics and Metabolism

Routine toxicity testing without regard to the mechanisms involved is likely to be wasteful of time and of human, animal and financial resources. A knowledge of toxicokinetics and metabolism can give valuable insights and provide for testing that is both more efficient and more informative. Such knowledge provides the necessary background to make the most appropriate selection of test animal species and of dose levels, and the most appropriate method for extrapolating from animal studies to the assessment of human hazard. Moreover, they may provide information on possible reactive intermediates as well as information on induction or inhibition of the enzymes of xenobiotic metabolism, the latter being critical to an assessment of possible interactions.

The nature of metabolic reactions and their variations between species is detailed in Chapters 3 and 4, with some elementary aspects of toxicokinetics in Chapter 2. The methods used for the measurement of toxicants and their metabolites are detailed in Chapter 9. The present section will not be concerned with these aspects but with the general principles, use, and need for metabolic and toxicokinetic studies in toxicity testing.

Toxicokinetic studies are designed to measure the amount and rate of the absorption, distribution, metabolism, and excretion of a xenobiotic. These data are used to construct predictive mathematical models so that the distribution and excretion of other doses can be simulated. Such studies are carried out using radiolabeled compounds to facilitate measurement and total recovery of the administered dose. This can be done entirely in vivo by measuring levels in blood, expired air, feces, and urine; these procedures can be done relatively noninvasively and continuously in the same animal. Tissue levels can be measured by sequential killing and analysis of organ levels. It is important to measure not only the compound administered but also its metabolites, since simple radioactivity counting does not differentiate between them.

The metabolic study, considered separately, consists of treatment of the animal with the labeled compound followed by chemical analysis of all metabolites formed in vivo and excreted via the lungs, kidneys, or bile. Although reactive intermediates are unlikely to be isolated, the chemical structure of the end-products may provide vital clues to the nature of the intermediates involved in their formation. The use of tissue homogenates, subcellular fractions, and purified enzymes may serve to clarify events occurring during metabolic sequences leading to the end-products.

Information of importance in test animal selection is the similarity in toxicodynamics and metabolism to that of humans. Although all of the necessary information may not be available for humans, it can often be inferred with reference to metabolism and excretion of related compounds, but it is clearly ill-advised to use an animal that differs from most others in the toxicokinetics or metabolism of the compound in question or that differs from humans in the nature of the end-products. Dose selection is influenced by a knowledge of whether a particular dose saturates a physiological process such as excretion or whether it is likely to accumulate in a particular tissue, since these factors are likely to become increasingly important the longer a chronic study continues.

8.5.4.4 Behavior

Although the primary emphasis in toxicity testing has long been the estimation of morphologic changes, with particular reference to carcinogenesis, much recent interest has focused on more fundamental evaluations. One such aspect has been the evaluation of chemical effects on behavior. For a number of years, behavioral tests have been incorporated as part of the regulatory process in the USSR, but not in the United States or Western Europe, and the claim has often been made that behavioral tests are more sensitive than pathological tests. This latter is difficult to document but, it is clear that behavior is the functional integration of all of the various activities of the nervous system and even, in part, of some other systems such as the endocrine glands, whose activity affects the nervous system. For this reason alone, behavioral tests are necessary to evaluate toxicity fully.

Many behavioral tests exist, and no particular set or sequence has been prescribed for regulatory purposes. The categories of methods used in behavioral toxicology have been classified by Norton, however. They fall into two principal classes, stimulus-oriented behavior and internally generated behavior. The former includes two types of conditioned behavior: operant, in which animals are trained to perform a task in order to obtain a reward or avoid a punishment, and classical conditioning, in which an animal learns to associate a conditioning stimulus with a reflex action. Stimulus-oriented behavior also involves unconditioned responses in which the animal's response to a particular stimulus is recorded. Internally generated behavior includes observation of animal behavior in response to various experimental situations, and includes exploratory behavior, circadian activity, social behavior, etc. The performance of animals treated with a particular chemical is compared with that of untreated controls as a measure of the effect of the chemical.

Many of the variables associated with other types of testing must also be controlled in behavioral tests: sex, age, species, environment, diet, and animal husbandry. Behavior may vary with all of these.

Norton describes a series of four tests that may form an appropriate series inasmuch as they represent four different types of behavior; the series should therefore reflect different types of nervous system activity. They are as follows:

1. Passive avoidance. This test involves the use of a shuttle box in which animals can move between a light and dark side. After an acclimatization period in which the animal can move freely between the two sides, it receives an electric shock while in the dark side. During subsequent trials, the time spent in the "safe side" is recorded.
2. Auditory startle. This test involves the response (movement) to a sound stimulus either without, or preceded by, a light flash stimulus.
3. Residential maze. Movements of animals in a residential maze are automatically recorded during both light and dark photoperiods.
4. Walking patterns. Gait is measured in walking animals, including such characteristics as the length and width of stride and the angles formed by the placement of the feet.

Problems associated with behavioral toxicology include the functional reserve and adaptability of the nervous system. Frequently, behavior is maintained despite clearly observable injury. Other problems are the statistical ones associated with multiple tests, multiple measurements, and the inherently large variability in behavior.

The use of human subjects occupationally exposed to chemicals is often attempted, but such tests are complicated by the subjective nature of the endpoints (dizziness, etc.).

8.5.4.5 Covalent Binding

Toxicity has been associated with covalent binding in a number of ways. Organ-specific toxicants administered in vivo bind covalently to macromolecules, usually at a higher level in the target tissues than in nontarget tissues. Examples include acetaminophen in the liver, carbon tetrachloride in the liver, p-aminophenol in the kidney, and ipomeanol in the lung. Similarly, many carcinogens are known to give rise to DNA adducts. In general, covalent binding occurs as a result of metabolism of the toxicant to highly reactive intermediates, usually, but not always, by cytochrome P-450. Because they are highly reactive electrophiles, the intermediates bind to many nucleophilic sites on DNA, RNA or protein molecules, not just the site of toxic action. Thus, measurement of covalent binding may be a measure of toxic potential rather than a specific measurement, directly related to a mechanism of action. The occurrence of covalent binding at the same time as toxicity is so common an occurrence, however, that a measurement of covalent binding of a chemical may be regarded as an excellent though perhaps not infallible indication of potential for toxicity. Although such tests are not routine, considerable interest has been shown in their development.

The measurement of DNA adducts is an indirect indication of genotoxic (carcinogenic) potential, and DNA adducts in the urine are an indication, obtained by a noninvasive technique, of recent exposure. Protein adducts give an integrated measure of exposure since they accumulate over the life span of the protein and, at the same time, indicate possible organ toxicity.

Tissue protein adducts are usually demonstrated in experimental animals following injection of radiolabeled chemicals and, after a period of time, the organs are removed, homogenized and, by rigorous extraction, all the noncovalently bound material is removed. Extraction methods include lipid solvents, acids and bases, concentrated urea solutions, and solubilization and precipitation of the proteins. They tend to underestimate the extent of covalent binding since even covalent bonds may be broken by the rigorous procedures used. Newer methods involving dialysis against detergents will probably prove more appropriate.

Blood proteins, such as hemoglobin, may be used in tests of human exposure since blood is readily and safely accessible. For example, the exposure of mice to ethylene oxide or dimethylnitrosamine was estimated by measuring alkylated residues in hemoglobin. The method was subsequently extended to people occupationally exposed to ethylene oxide by measuring N-3-(2-hydroxyethyl) histamine residues in hemoglobin. Similarly, methyl cysteine residues in hemoglobin can be used as a measure of methylation.

DNA/RNA adducts can also be measured in various ways, including rigorous extraction, separation and precipitation following administration of labeled compounds in vivo, or use of antibodies raised to chemically modified DNA or RNA. Attempts have also been made to measure adducts of DNA degradation products in the urine, a method that should prove valuable in human studies.

Although many compounds of different chemical classes have been shown to bind covalently when activated by microsomal preparations in vitro (eg, aflatoxin, ipomeanol, stilbene, vinyl chloride), these observations have not been developed into routine testing procedures. Clearly, such procedures would be useful in predicting toxic potential.

8.5.4.6 Immunotoxicity

Immunotoxicology comprises two distinct types of toxic effects: the involvement of the immune system in mediating the toxic effect of a chemical and the toxic effects of chemicals on the immune system. The former is shown, for example, in tests for cutaneous sensitization, the latter in impairment of the ability to resist infection.

Tests for immunotoxicity are not yet required by all regulatory agencies, but it is an area of great interest, both in the fundamental mechanisms of immune function and in the design of tests to measure impairment of immune function. As a result of the recent rapid expansion of knowledge in this area, there is no uniform agreement on a test or series of tests. Moreover, there is considerable functional reserve in the immune system, so that the demonstration in vitro of impairment of a particular facet of the system may not be reflected in an impairment of in vivo function.

As indicated previously, many compounds can elicit immune reactions even though they may not be proteins or other macromolecules normally associated with antibody formation. Presumably this occurs because they, or their metabolites, interact with endogenous macromolecules to modify them in such a way that the immune system then sees them as "foreign" or "non-self." The result may be allergies, delayed hypersensitivity, etc. This aspect will not be considered further; the remainder of the section is devoted to impairment of immune function.

The humoral and cell-mediated systems represent the two major parts of the overall immune system (Figure 8.6), the former involving primarily the B lymphocytes and the latter the T lymphocytes. The humoral system is involved in the production of antibodies that react with foreign material (antigens), whereas the latter involves primarily the mobilization of phagocytic leucocytes to ingest such foreign organisms as bacteria. The two systems function together by complex feedback mechanisms. One of the key characteristics in immune function is the rapid amplification of the number of cells capable of specific reaction to an antigen. This derives from memory cells that were specifically adapted to the antigen at the time of initial exposure.

Tests of the immune system may be divided into three classes:

1. Weight and morphology of the lymphoid organs;
2. Capacity to respond to challenges such as those of mitogens, ie, compounds that induce mitosis (phytohemagglutinin, concavalin A, lipopolysaccharide, pokeweed mitogen) or antigens (Candida, typhoid).
3. Specific in vitro tests of components of the immune system designed to elicit the mechanism of changes shown in tests in 1 and 2.

The initial examination consists of routine hematology, since changes in blood cells, particularly in the differential WBC count, may be indicative of effects on the immune system. Examination of the weight and pathology of the

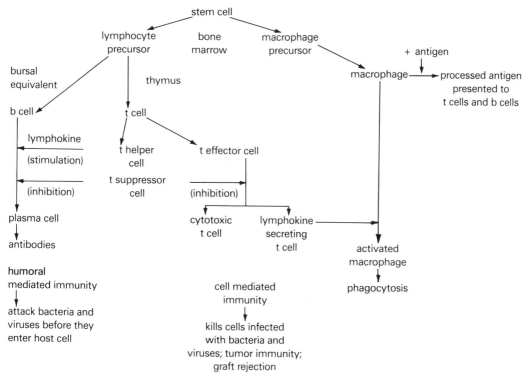

FIGURE 8.6.
Diagrammatic representation of the mammalian immune system.

thymus and spleen are considerably more important, however, since effects noted therein are more specific (though not infallible) indications of immune impairment. For example, atrophy of the thymus usually indicates immuno-suppression, although some nonimmunosuppressive chemicals can cause thymus atrophy. Similarly, changes in the bone marrow, lymph nodes, spleen, and thymus may, after treatment with a particular chemical, indicate changes in the immune system such as B or T cell deficiency. B cells and T cells are either formed or reside in particular locations in these organs and their presence or absence may be indicative of dysfunction.

The second category of tests, those for overall immunocompetence, includes skin tests for antibody-mediated responses and for delayed hypersensitivity. It also includes tests that determine the predisposition of animals for disease, such as infections with *Streptococcus pneumoniae,* and increased susceptibility to cancer and autoallergic effects or autoimmune diseases.

The third category consists of a constantly growing body of tests, each of which examines some narrow aspect of the immune system in great detail. It includes tests for the production of different classes of antibodies as well as tests of leukocyte function and differentiation: macrophage aggregation, inhibition of macrophage migration, lymphocyte transformation by antigens and mito-gens, and many others.

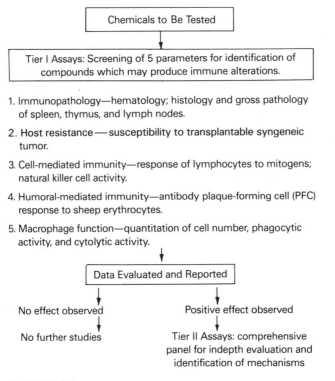

FIGURE 8.7.
Screening tests for potential immunotoxicity.

It is not yet clear how best to select from the tests available or how these tests can be integrated to provide a coherent picture of immunotoxic effects. It is clear, however, that this is important, and one such attempt is shown in Figure 8.7.

8.6 IN VITRO AND OTHER SHORT-TERM TESTS

8.6.1 Introduction

The toxicity tests that follow are tests conducted largely in vitro with isolated cell systems. Some are short-term tests carried out in vivo or are combinations of in vivo and in vitro systems. The latter are included because of similarities in approach, mechanism, or intent. In general, these tests measure effects on the genome or on cell transformation; their importance lies in the relationship between such effects and the mechanism of chemical carcinogenesis. Mutagenicity of cells in the germ line is itself an expression of toxicity, however, and the mutant genes can be inherited and expressed in the next or subsequent generations.

The theory that the initiating step of chemical carcinogenesis is a somatic mutation is well recognized, and considerable evidence shows that mutagenic potential is correlated with carcinogenic potential. Thus, the intent of much of this type of testing is to provide early warning of carcinogenic potential without the delay involved in conducting lifetime chronic feeding studies in experimental animals. Despite the numerous tests that have been devised, regulatory agencies have not yet seen fit to substitute any of them, or any combination of them, for chronic feeding studies. Instead, they have been added as additional testing requirements. One function of such tests should be to identify those compounds with the greatest potential for toxicity and enable the amount of chronic testing to be reduced to more manageable proportions.

8.6.2 Prokaryote Mutagenicity

8.6.2.1 Ames Test

The Ames test, developed by Bruce Ames and his coworkers of the University of California at Berkeley, depends on the ability of mutagenic chemicals to bring about reverse mutations in mutant *Salmonella typhimurium* strains which have defects in the histidine biosynthesis pathway. These strains will not grow in the absence of histidine but can be caused to mutate back to the wild type, which can synthesize histidine and hence can grow in its absence. The postmitochondrial supernatant (S-9 fraction), obtained from homogenates of livers of rats previously treated with PCBs in order to induce the cytochrome P-450 monooxygenase system, is also included to provide the activating enzymes involved in the production of the potent electrophiles often involved in the toxicity of chemicals to animals.

Bacterial tester strains have been developed that can test for either base-pair (eg, strain TA-1531) or frameshift (eg, strains TA-1537, TA-1538) mutations. Other, more sensitive strains such as TA-98 and TA-100 are also used, although they may be less specific with regard to the type of mutation caused.

In brief, the test is carried out (Figure 8.8) by mixing a suspension of bacterial cells with molten top agar. This also contains cofactors, S-9 fraction, and the material to be tested. The mixture is poured onto Petri plates containing hardened minimal agar. The number of bacteria that revert and acquire the wild type ability to grow in the absence of histidine can be estimated by counting the colonies that develop on incubation. To provide a valid test, a number of concentrations are tested, and positive controls with known mutagens are included along with negative controls that lack only the test compound. The entire test is replicated often enough to satisfy appropriate statistical tests for significance. Parallel tests without the S-9 fraction may help distinguish between chemicals with intrinsic mutagenic potential and those that require metabolic activation.

Although several hundred chemicals have been tested by this method, according to McCann et al, only about one third of these tests were adequate for quantitative analysis. It is clear, however, that the Ames test, if properly conducted, is reproducible and accurate.

The question of correlation between mutagenicity and carcinogenicity is crucial in any consideration of the utility of this or similar tests. In general, this appears to be high, although a small proportion of both false negatives and false positives occurs. For example, certain base analogs, and inorganics such as

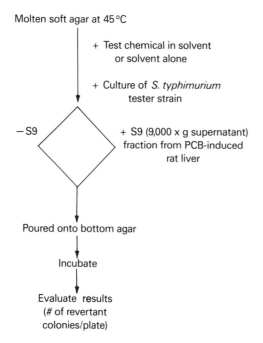

Molten soft agar at 45°C

+ Test chemical in solvent
or solvent alone

+ Culture of *S. typhimurium*
tester strain

−S9   + S9 (9,000 x g supernatant)
fraction from PCB-induced
rat liver

Poured onto bottom agar

Incubate

Evaluate results
(# of revertant
colonies/plate)

FIGURE 8.8.
Protocol for the Ames test for mutagenesis.

manganese, are not carcinogens but are mutagens in the Ames test, whereas diethylstilbestrol (DES) is a carcinogen but not a bacterial mutagen.

8.6.2.2 Related Tests

Related tests include tests based on reverse mutations, as is the Ames test, as well as tests based on forward mutations. Examples include:

1. Reverse mutations in *Escherichia coli*. This test is similar to the Ames test and depends on reversion of tryptophan mutants, which cannot synthesize this amino acid, to the wild type which can. The S-9 fraction from the liver of induced rats can also be used as an activating system in this test. Other *E coli* reverse-mutation tests utilize nicotinic acid and arginine mutants.

2. Forward mutations in *S typhimurium*. One such assay, dependent on the appearance of a mutation conferring resistance to 8-azaguanine in a histidine revertant strain, has been developed and is said to be as sensitive as the reverse-mutation tests.

3. Forward mutations in *E coli*. These mutations depend on the mutation of galactose-nonfermenting *E coli* to galactose-fermenting *E coli* or the change from 5-methyl tryphtophane sensitivity to 5-methyltryptophane resistance.

4. DNA repair. Polymerase-deficient, and thus DNA repair-deficient, *E coli* has provided the basis for a test that depends on the fact that the growth of a deficient strain is inhibited more by a DNA-damaging agent than is that of a repair-competent strain. The recombinant assay using *Bacillus subtilis* is

conducted in much the same way, since recombinant deficient strains are more sensitive to DNA-damaging agents.

8.6.3 Eukaryote Mutagenicity

8.6.3.1 Mammalian Cell Mutation

The development of cell culture techniques that permit both survival and replication have led to many advances in cell biology, including the use of certain of these cell lines for detection of mutagens. Although such cells, if derived from mammals, would seem ideal for testing for toxicity towards mammals, there are several problems. Primary cells, which generally resemble those of the tissue of origin, are difficult to culture and have poor cloning ability. Because of these difficulties, certain established cell lines are usually used. These cells, such as Chinese hamster ovary cells and mouse lymphoma cells, clone readily and do not become senescent with passage through many cell generations. Unfortunately, they have little metabolic activity toward xenobiotics and thus do not readily activate toxicants. Moreover, they usually show chromosome changes, such as aneuploidy, ie, more or fewer than the usual diploid number of chromosomes.

The characteristics usually involved in these assays are resistance to 8-azaguanine or 6-thioguanine (the hypoxanthine guanine phosphoribosyl transferase or HGPRT locus), resistance to bromodeoxyuridine or trifluorothymidine (the thymidine kinase or TK locus) or resistance to ouabain (the OU or Na/K-ATPase locus). HGPRT is responsible for incorporation of purines from the medium into the nucleic acid synthesis pathway. Its loss prevents uptake of normal purines and also of toxic purines such as 8-azaguanine or 6-thioguanine, which would kill the cell. Thus, mutation at this locus confers resistance to these toxic purine analogs. Similarly, TK permits pyrimidine transport, and its loss prevents uptake of toxic pyrimidine analogs and confers resistance to them. In the absence of HPGRT or TK, the cells can grow by de novo synthesis of purines and pyrimidines. Ouabain kills cells by combining with the Na/K ATPase. Mutation at the OU locus alters the ouabain binding site in a way that prevents inhibition and thus confers resistance.

A typical test system is the analysis of the TK locus in mouse lymphoma cells for mutations that confer resistance to bromodeoxyuracil. The tests are conducted with and without the S-9 fraction from induced rat liver since the lymphoma cells have little activating ability. Both positive and negative controls are included, and the parameter measured is the number of cells formed that are capable of forming colonies in the presence of bromodeoxyuridine.

8.6.3.2 Drosophila Sex-Linked Recessive Lethal Test

The advantages of *Drosophila* (fruitfly) tests are that they involve an intact eukaryotic organism with all of its interrelated organ systems and activation mechanisms but, at the same time, are fast, relatively easy to perform, and do not involve mammals as test animals. The most obvious disadvantages are that the hormonal and immune systems of insects are significantly different from those of mammals and that the nature, specificity, and inducibility of cytochrome P-450s are not as well understood in insects as they are in mammals.

In a typical test, males that are 2 days postpuparium and that were raised from eggs laid within a short time period (usually 24 hours) are treated with the test compound in water, with sucrose added to increase palatability. Males from a strain carrying a gene for yellow body on the X chromosome are used. Preliminary tests determine that the number of offspring of the survivors of the treatment doses (usually 0.25 LD50 and 0.5 LD50) are adequate for future crosses. Appropriate controls, including a solvent control (with emulsifier if one was necessary to prepare the test solution), and a positive control, such as ethyl methane sulfonate, are routinely included with each test. Individual crosses of each surviving treated male with a series of three females are made on a 0 to 2-, 3 to 5-, and 6 to 8-day schedule. The progeny of each female is reared separately, and the males and females of the F_1 generation are mated in brother–sister matings. If there are no males with yellow bodies in a particular set of progeny, it should be assumed that a lethal mutation was present on the treated X chromosome. A comparison of the F_2 progeny derived from females inseminated by males at different times after treatment allows a distinction to be made between effects on spermatozoa, spermatids, and spermatocytes.

In the Basc (Muller-5) test shown in Figure 8.9, the strain used for the females in the F_1 cross is a multiple-marked strain that carries a dominant gene for bar eyes and recessive genes for apricot eyes and a reduction of bristles on the thorax (scute gene). Basc is an acronym for bar, apricot, and scute.

8.6.3.3 Related Tests

Many tests related to the two types of eukaryote-mutation tests are discussed in Sections 8.6.3.1 and 8.6.3.2, and many of them are simply variations of the tests

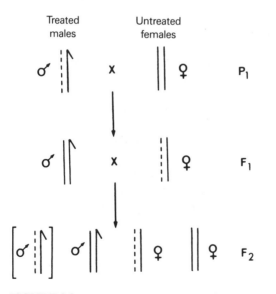

FIGURE 8.9.
The Basc (Muller-5) mating scheme. Dashed lines represent the treated X chromosome of males. Brackets indicate males with yellow bodies, which would be absent if a lethal mutation occurred on the X chromosome of the treated male.

described. Two distinct classes are worthy of mention: the first uses yeasts as the test organisms, and the second is the spot test for mutations in mice.

One group of tests using yeasts includes tests for gene mutations and strains that can be used to detect forward mutations in genes that code for enzymes in the purine biosynthetic pathway; other strains can be used to detect reversions. Yeasts can also be used to test for recombinant events such as reciprocal mitotic recombination (mitotic crossing over) and nonreciprocal mitotic recombination. *Saccharomyces cerevisiae* is the preferred organism in almost all these tests. Although yeasts possess cytochrome P-450s capable of metabolizing xenobiotics, their specificity and sensitivity are limited as compared with those of mammals, and an S-9 fraction is often included, as in the Ames test, to enhance activation.

The gene mutation test systems in mice include the specific locus test in which wild-type treated males are crossed with females carrying recessive mutations for visible phenotypic effects. The F_1 progeny have the same phenotype as the wild-type parent unless a mutation, corresponding to a recessive mutant marker, has occurred. Such tests are accurate, and the spontaneous (background) mutation rate is very low, making them sound tests that are predictive for other mammals. Unfortunately, the large number of animals required has prevented extensive use. Similar tests involving the activity and electrophoretic mobility of various enzymes in the blood or other tissues in the F_1 progeny from treated males and untreated females have been developed. In the above tests, as with many others, sequential mating of males with different females can provide information about the stage of sperm development at which the mutational event occurred.

8.6.4 DNA Damage and Repair

Many of the endpoints for tests described in this chapter, including gene mutation, chromosome damage, and oncogenicity, develop as a consequence of damage to or chemical modification of DNA. Most of these tests, however, also involve metabolic events that occur both prior to and subsequent to the modification of DNA. Some tests, however, use events at the DNA level as endpoints. One of these, the unscheduled synthesis of DNA in mammalian cells will be described in some detail; the others will be briefly summarized.

8.6.4.1 Unscheduled DNA Synthesis in Mammalian Cells

The principle of this test is that it measures the repair that follows DNA damage and is thus a reflection of the damage itself. It depends on the autoradiographic measurement of the incorporation of tritiated thymidine into the nuclei of cells previously treated with the test chemical.

The preferred cells are usually primary hepatocytes in cultures derived from adult male rats, the cells of which are dispersed and allowed to attach themselves to glass coverslips. From this point on, the test is carried out on the attached cells. Both positive controls with agents known to stimulate unscheduled DNA synthesis, such as the carcinogen aflatoxin B_1 or 2-acetylaminofluorene, and negative controls, which are processed through all procedures except exposure to the test compound, are routinely performed with every test. Cells are exposed by replacing the medium for a short time with one containing the test chemical. The dose levels are determined by a preliminary cell viability test (trypan blue exclusion test) and consist of several concentrations that span the range from no apparent loss of viability to almost complete loss of viability. Following exposure, the medium is removed, and the cells are washed by several changes of fresh medium and finally placed in a medium containing tritiated thymidine. The cells are fixed and dried, and the coverslip with the cells attached is coated with photographic emulsion. After a suitable exposure period, usually several weeks, the emulsion is developed and the cells are stained with hemotoxylin and eosin. The number of grains in the nuclear region is corrected by subtracting non-nuclear grains, and the net grain count in the nuclear area is compared between treated and untreated cells.

This test has several advantages in that primary liver cells have considerable activation capacity and the test measures an event at the DNA level. It does not, however, distinguish between error-free repair and error-prone repair, the latter being itself a mutagenic process. Thus, it cannot distinguish between events that might lead to toxic sequelae and those that do not. A modification of this test measures in vivo unscheduled DNA synthesis. In this modification, animals are first treated in vivo, and primary hepatocytes are then prepared and treated as already described.

8.6.4.2 Related Tests

Tests for the measurement of binding of the test material to DNA have already been discussed under covalent binding (Section 8.5.4.5). Another method of assessing DNA damage is the estimation of DNA breakage following exposure to the test chemical; the DNA-strand length is estimated by using alkaline elution or sucrose density gradient centrifugation. This has been done with a number of cell lines and with freshly prepared hepatocytes, in the latter case following treatment either in vivo or in vitro. It may be regarded as promising but not yet fully validated. The polymerase-deficient *E coli* tests as well as recombinant tests using yeasts are also related to DNA repair.

8.6.5 Chromosome Aberrations

Tests for chromosome aberrations involve the estimation of effects on extended regions of whole chromosomes rather than on single or small numbers of genes. Primarily, they concern chromosome breaks and exchange of material between chromosomes.

8.6.5.1 Sister Chromatid Exchange (SCE)

Sister chromatid exchange occurs between the sister chromatids which together make up a chromosome. It occurs at the same locus in each chromatid and is thus a symmetrical exchange of chromosome material. In this regard, it is not strictly an aberration since the products do not differ in morphology from normal chromosomes. Sister chromatid exchange (SCE), however, is susceptible to chemical induction and appears to be correlated with the genotoxic potential of chemicals as well as with their oncogenic potential. The exchange is visualized by permitting the treated cells to pass through two DNA replication cycles in the presence of 5-bromo-2′-deoxyuridine, which is incorporated in the replicated DNA. The cells are then stained with a fluorescent dye and irradiated with UV light, which permits differentiation between chromatids that contain bromodeoxyuridine and those that do not (Figure 8.10).

The test can be carried out on cultured cells or on cells from animals treated in vivo. In the former case, the test chemical is usually evaluated in the presence and absence of the S-9 activating system from rat liver. Typically, cells from a Chinese hamster ovary cell line are incubated in a liquid medium and exposed to several concentrations of the test chemical, either with or without the S-9 fraction, for about 2 hours. Positive controls such as ethyl methane sulfonate (a direct-acting compound) or dimethylnitrosamine (one that requires activation), as well as negative controls, are also included. Test concentrations are based on cell toxicity levels determined by prior experiment and are selected in such a way that even at the highest dose excess growth inhibition does not occur. At the end of the treatment period, the cells are washed, bromodeoxyuridine is added, and the cells are incubated for ≥24 hours. The cells are then fixed, stained with a fluorescent dye, and irradiated with UV light. Second division cells are then scored under the microscope for SCEs (Figure 8.10).

The test can also be carried out on cells treated in vivo, and analyses have been made of SCEs in lymphocytes from cancer patients, cancer patients treated with chemotherapeutic drugs, smokers, and occupationally exposed workers. In several cases, increased incidence of SCEs has been noted. This is a sensitive test for compounds that alkylate DNA, with few false positives. It may also be useful for detecting promoters such as phorbol esters.

8.6.5.2 Micronucleus Test

The micronucleus test is an in vivo test usually carried out in mice. The animals are treated in vivo, and the erythrocyte stem cells from the bone marrow are

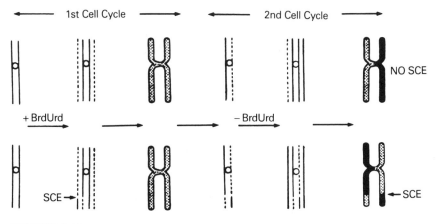

FIGURE 8.10.
Visualization of sister chromatid exchange.

stained and examined for micronuclei. Micronuclei represent chromosome fragments or chromosomes left behind at anaphase. It is basically a test for compounds that cause chromosome breaks (clastogenic agents) and compounds that interfere with normal mitotic cell division, including those that affect spindle fiber function.

Male and female mice from an outbred strain are handled by the best animal husbandry techniques, as described for acute, subchronic and chronic tests, and are treated either with the solvent, 0.5 LD50, or 0.1 LD50 of the test chemical. Animals are killed at several time intervals up to 2 days; the bone marrow is extracted, placed on microscope slides, dried, and stained. The presence of micronuclei is scored visually under the microscope.

Although the test is relatively simple and treatment is carried out on the intact animal, it is not as sensitive as many other tests, for example, the SCE test.

8.6.5.3 Dominant Lethal Test in Rodents

The dominant lethal test, which is performed using rats, mice, or hamsters, is an in vivo test to determine the germ cell risk from a suspected mutagen. The test consists of treating males with the test compound for several days followed by mating to different females each week for enough weeks to cover the period required for a complete spermatogenesis sequence. Animals are maintained under optimal conditions of animal husbandry and are dosed, usually by gavage, with several doses <0.1 LD50. The females are killed after 2 weeks of gestation and dissected; corpora lutea and living and dead implantations are counted. The endpoints used to determine the occurrence of dominant lethal mutations in the treated males are the fertility index (ratio of pregnant females to mated females), preimplantation losses (the number of implantations relative to the number of corpora lutea), the number of females with dead implantations relative to the total number of pregnant females, and the number of dead implantations relative to the total number of implantations.

8.6.5.4 Related Tests

Many cells exposed to test chemicals can be scored for chromosome aberrations by staining procedures followed by visual examination with the aid of the microscope. These include Chinese hamster ovary cells in culture treated in a protocol very similar to that used in the test for SCEs, bone marrow cells from animals treated in vivo, or lymphocytes from animals treated in vivo. The types of aberrations evaluated include: chromatid gaps, breaks, and deletions; chromosome gaps, breaks, and deletions; chromosome fragments; translocations; and ploidy.

Heritable translocations can be detected by direct examination of cells from male or female offspring in various stages of development or by crossing the treated animals to untreated animals and evaluating fertility, with males with reduced fertility being examined for translocations, etc. Progeny from this or other tests, such as those for dominant lethals, can be permitted to survive and then examined for translocations and other abnormalities.

8.6.6 Mammalian Cell Transformation

Most cell transformation assays utilize fibroblast cultures derived from embryonic tissue. The original studies showed that cells from C3H mouse fibroblast cultures developed morphologic changes and changes in growth patterns when treated with carcinogens. Later, similar studies were made with Syrian hamster embryo cells. The direct relationship of these changes to carcinogenesis was demonstrated by transplantation of the cells into a host animal and the subsequent development of tumors. The recent development of practical assay procedures involves two cell lines from mouse embryos, Balb/3T3 and C3H/10T$_{\frac{1}{2}}$, in which transformation is easily recognized and scored.

In a typical assay situation, cells, such as Balb/3T3 mouse fibroblasts, will multiply in culture until a monolayer is formed. At this point, they cease dividing unless transformed. Chemicals that are transforming agents will, however, cause growth to occur in thicker layers above the monolayer. These clumps of transformed cells are known as foci. Despite many recommended controls, the assay is only semiquantitative. The doses are selected from the results of a preliminary experiment and range from a high dose that reduces colony formation (but not by $> 50\%$) to a low dose that has no measurable effect on colony formation. After exposure for $1 - 3$ days to the test chemical, the cells are washed and incubation is continued for up to 4 weeks. At that time, the monolayers are fixed, stained, and scored for transformed foci.

Although transformation assays have not been developed to the point of being quantitative, they nevertheless have several distinct advantages. Because transplanted foci give rise to tumors in congenic hosts (those from the same inbred strain from which the cells were derived) whereas untransformed cells do not, it is believed to be illustrative of the overall expression of carcinogenesis in mammalian tissues. The two cell types used most (Balb/3T3 and C3H/10T$_{\frac{1}{2}}$) respond to promoters in the manner predicted by the multistage model for carcinogenesis in vivo and may eventually be useful in the development of assays for promotion. Unfortunately, a large number of false-negative results are obtained, since these cell lines do not show much activation capacity; it has not proven practical to combine them with the S-9 activation system. Furthermore, the cells are aneuploid and may be preneoplastic in the untreated state. Syrian hamster cells, which do have considerable activation capacity, have proven difficult to use in test procedures and are difficult to score. Other transforming systems are known but have not yet been reduced to practical assay status.

8.6.7 General Considerations and Testing Sequences

Considering all of the tests for acute and chronic toxicity, long and short term, in vivo and in vitro, it is clearly impractical to apply a complete series of tests to all commercial chemicals and all their derivatives in food, water, and the environment. The challenge of toxicity testing is to identify the most effective set or sequence of tests necessary to describe the apparent and potential toxicity of a particular chemical or mixture of chemicals. The enormous emphasis on in

TABLE 8.12
A Three-Tier Decision Point Protocol For Evaluating Chemicals for Mutagenesis and
Carcinogenesis

A. Structure of chemical

B. In vitro tests
    1. Bacterial mutagenesis (Ames test)
    2. Mammalian mutagenesis
    3. DNA repair
    4. Chromosome tests (SCE, micronucleus, etc.)
    5. Cell transformation

Decision Point 1: Evaluation of tests from A and B and selection of appropriate tests for C.

C. In vivo testing—limited bioassays
    1. Skin tumor induction in mice
    2. Pulmonary tumor induction in mice
    3. Breast cancer induction in female rats
    4. Altered foci induction in rodent liver
    5. Assays for promoters

Decision Point 2: Evaluation of data from tests A–C.

D. Long-term bioassay

Decision Point 3: Final evaluation of all the results.

Source: Weisburger, J.H., and Williams, G.M. Science 214, 401–407, 1981.

vitro or short-term tests that has occurred in the last decade had its roots in the need to find substitutes for lifetime feeding studies in experimental animals or, at the very least, to suggest a sequence of tests that would enable priorities to be set for which chemicals should be subjected to chronic tests. Such tests might also be used to eliminate the need for chronic testing for chemicals that either clearly possessed the potential for toxicity or clearly did not. Although there has been much success in test development, the challenge outlined here has not been met, primarily because of the failure of scientists and regulatory agencies, world-wide, to agree on test sequences or on the circumstances in which short-term tests may substitute for chronic ones. Thus, not only are short-term tests often required, but they are required in addition to all the other tests required before their development. As an example, the US EPA requirements for FIFRA (Federal Insecticide, Fungicide, and Rodenticide Act) include, in addition to a full battery of acute, subchronic and chronic tests, tests to address the following three categories: gene mutations, structural chromosome aberrations, and other genotoxic tests as appropriate (such as DNA damage and repair and chromosome aberrations).

It is important, however, that test sequences have been suggested and considered by regulatory agencies. One such sequence is shown in Table 8.12.

8.7 ECOLOGICAL EFFECTS

Tests for ecological effects include those designed to address the potential of chemicals to affect the environment and the occurrence of toxic chemicals in the environment. In addition to potential effects on humans and domestic animals such tests are designed to estimate the possibility of effects on field populations of vertebrates, invertebrates, and plants.

8.7.1 Laboratory Tests

There are two types of laboratory tests: toxicity determinations on wildlife and aquatic organisms and the use of model ecosystems to measure bioaccumulation and transport of toxicants and their degradation products.

Among the tests included in the first category are the avian oral LD50, the avian dietary LC50, wild mammal toxicity, and avian reproduction. The avian tests are usually carried out on bobwhite quail or mallard ducks, whereas the wild mammals may be species such as the pine mouse, *Paramyscus.* The tests are similar to those described under acute and chronic testing procedures but suffer from some drawbacks; the standards of animal husbandry used with rats and mice are probably unattainable with birds or wild mammals even though bobwhite quail and mallards are easily reared in captivity. The genetics of the birds and mammals used are much more variable than those of the traditional laboratory rodent strains.

Similar tests can be carried out with aquatic organisms, eg, the LC50 for freshwater fish such as rainbow trout and bluegills, the LC50 for estuarine and marine organisms, the LC50 for invertebrates such as *Daphnia,* and the effect of chemicals on the early stages of fish and various invertebrates.

Model systems, first developed by ecologists to study basic ecological processes, have been adapted to toxicological testing. The models developed by Metcalf have been the most important. These models were developed to determine the movement and concentration of pesticides. Typically, the model has a water phase containing vertebrates and invertebrates, and a terrestrial phase containing at least one plant species and one herbivore species (Figure 8.11). The ^{14}C-labeled pesticide or other environmental contaminant is applied to the

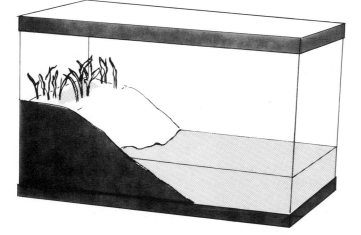

FIGURE 8.11.
Metcalf model ecosystem.

leaves of the terrestrial plant, sorghum *(Sorgum halpense);* salt marsh caterpillars *(Estigmene acrea)* are then placed on the plants. The larvae eat the plants and contaminate the water with feces and their dead bodies. The aquatic food chain is simulated with plankton, (diatoms, rotefers, etc.), water fleas *(Daphnia),* mosquito larvae *(Culex pipiens),* and fish *(Gambusia affinis).* From an analysis of the plants, animals, and substrates for the ^{14}C-labeled compound and its degradation products, the biological magnification or rate of degradation can be calculated.

More complex models involving several compartments, simulated rain, simulated soil drainage, simulated tidal flow, etc., have been constructed and their properties investigated, but none have been brought to the stage of use in routine testing. Similarly, aquatic models using static, recirculating, and continuous flow have also been used, as have entirely terrestrial models; again, none have been developed for routine testing. The most important feature of any model ecosystem designed for routine testing of environmental contaminants is the ability to measure biological magnification or the rate of degradation so as to predict the possible fate of the chemical in the environment.

8.7.2 Simulated Field Tests

Simulated field tests may be quite simple, consisting of feeding treated prey to predators and studying the toxic effects on the predator, enabling some predictions concerning effects to nontarget organisms. In general, however, the term is used for greenhouse, small plot, small artificial pond, or small natural pond tests. These serve to test biological accumulation and degradation under conditions somewhat more natural than the artificial ecosystem and the test compounds are exposed to environmental as well as biological degradation. Population effects may be noted, but these methods are more useful for soil invertebrates, plants, and aquatic organisms since other organisms are not easily contained in small plots.

8.7.3 Field Tests

In field tests test chemicals are applied to large areas under natural conditions. The areas are at least several acres and may be either natural or part of some agroecosystem. Because the area is large and in the open, radiolabeled compounds cannot be used and it is not possible to obtain a balance between material applied and material recovered.

The effects are followed over a long period of time, and two types of control may be used: first, a comparison with a similar area that is untreated; and second, a comparison with the same area before treatment. In the first case it is difficult if not impossible to exactly duplicate a large natural area and, in the second, changes can occur that are unrelated to the test material.

In either case, studies of populations are the most important focus of this type of testing, although the disappearance of the test material, its accumulation in various life forms, and the appearance, accumulation, and disappearance of its degradation products are also important. The population of soil organisms, terrestrial organisms, and aquatic organisms as well as plants must all be surveyed and characterized, both qualitatively and quantitatively. Following application of the test material, the populations can be followed through two or more annual cycles to determine both acute and long-term population effects.

8.8 RISK ANALYSIS

The preceding tests for various kinds of toxicity can be used to measure adverse effects of many different chemical compounds in different species, organs, tissues, cells, or even populations, and under many different conditions. This information can be used to predict possible toxicity of related compounds from QSAR or of the same chemical under different conditions (eg, mutagenicity as a predictor of carcinogenicity). It is considerably more difficult to use this information to predict possible risk to other species, such as humans, since little experimental data on this species is available. Some methods are available to predict risk to humans and to provide the risk factor in the risk – benefit assessment that provides the basis for regulatory action, however. The benefit factor is largely economic in nature and the final regulatory action is not, in the narrow sense, a scientific one. It also involves political and legal aspects and, in toto, represents society's evaluation of the amount of risk that can be tolerated in any particular case.

The estimation of risk may be implicit, as in the process by which an acceptable daily intake (ADI) or threshold limit value (TLV) is established, or explicit, as in calculations that lead to a numerical probability of toxic effect for a given dose or a numerical expression of changes in mortality or morbidity rates in exposed populations.

The ADI is calculated by dividing the NOEL by a safety factor. The NOEL is derived from chronic or subchronic studies and is the highest level tested that did not cause any observable effect related to the test chemical — that is, effects observed at higher doses. For all effects other than cancer, the results of a 6-month study are probably adequate. The traditional safety factor is 100, 10 to represent the potential increased sensitivity of humans and 10 to allow for the genetic diversity of the human population. This presents several problems, the most important of which is the fact that the lower the number of animals tested the smaller the probability of detecting an adverse effect at a particular dose. Thus, the NOEL and hence the ADI may be unrealistically high if too few animals are used. The regulation of chemicals such as pesticides, which may appear in many different foodstuffs as well as drinking water, becomes a particularly intractable problem since the ADI must be divided between all of these sources as a maximum permitted residue or tolerance for each one. Because of the many different ethnic groups and diets, meaningful tolerances are difficult to formulate. The safety factor itself lacks any particular scientific rationale, and it should probably be reduced when good epidemiological data are available and increased either when good epidemiological data are not available or when the experimental data are not extensive.

The area of risk assessment for chemical carcinogens is one that has attracted the most attention, but it is still far from resolved. The problems include extrapolation to low doses and extrapolation between species.

Low-dose extrapolation, that is, prediction of the effects of expected environmental levels from results obtained at high levels, is complicated by many factors, but the basic difficulty is that the shape of the dose–response curve is unknown at lower doses. The extremely high doses (maximum tolerated dose) used in carcinogenesis assays are unrealistic in that they may cause metabolic and pharmacokinetic effects not seen at lower doses and thus may not even lie on an upward extrapolation from intermediate doses. They may be valuable for demonstrating the potential of the compound for carcinogenesis but possibly should not be used in extrapolations for the purpose of risk assessment.

In general, models used for low-dose extrapolation fall into the following classes: tolerance distribution; simple linear extrapolation; hit models, such as one-hit and multihit; time-to-tumor models. The tolerance distribution model assumes a lower threshold for each individual below which the individual would not be affected and further assumes that the variation in this threshold can be described by a probability distribution function.

The Mantel-Bryan model is a log-probit extrapolation in which a straight line is extrapolated from the measured values to an acceptable level of risk (eg, 10^{-6}). This model has been subjected to a variety of criticisms, not least of which is that it often does not fit even the observed values, and it has been necessary to propose various corrective factors. Despite the attempted corrections, this type of simple extrapolation is subjected to much criticism, and most risk assessment involves more complex models.

The various hit models assume either a one-hit hypothesis (ie, there is a finite probability of tumor formation if a single target interacts with an effective unit of dose) or a multihit hypothesis, which does not make the single-hit assumption but assumes a more complex set of events prior to tumor formation. This last is probably the most rational but still is problematical.

The most complex of the models based on tumor frequency at different dose levels over the time of the study is the Gamma multihit model of Cornfield and Van Ryzin, which assumes a multihit mechanism and provides a model that can be corrected for spontaneous tumor formation.

Currently, attempts are being made to incorporate time-to-tumor occurrence into predictive models; this shows considerable promise as an improvement in predictability. Even more assurance of accuracy of low-dose predictions should come from the incorporation of pharmacokinetic and metabolic parameters into the model, and much effort is currently being devoted to this end.

The other major problem with risk assessment is extrapolation from one species, the experimental animal in question, to another species, usually humans. Difficulties arise in part from not knowing how a biological function may vary with size. Many physiological functions appear to be related to some exponent of body weight, the exponent varying with the function in question. In toxicity studies, the manner in which the dose is expressed becomes critical, and studies have compared such expressions as milligram per kilogram of body weight per day, milligram per square meter of body surface per day and milligram per kilogram of body weight per lifetime as the basis for extrapolation. The ultimate tests of the utility of such extrapolations to humans are comparisons with actual epidemiological data, and thus it is a difficult question to decide since little data of this type is available. Milligram per kilogram per day and milligram per square meter per day have been said to give more accurate predictions than does milligram per kilogram per lifetime, however; the use of the most sensitive species has been said to require little correction.

8.9 THE FUTURE OF TOXICITY TESTING

Because the public awareness of the potentially harmful effects of chemicals, it is clear that toxicity testing will continue to be an important activity and that it will be required by regulatory agencies before the use of a particular chemical is permitted either in commercial processes or for use by the public. Because of the proliferation of testing procedures, the number of experimental species and other test systems available, as well as the high dose rates usually used, it is clear that eventually some expression of some type of toxicity will be obtained for most exogenous chemicals. Thus, the identification of toxic effects with the intent of banning any chemical causing such effects is no longer a productive mode of attack. The aim of toxicity testing should be to identify those compounds that present an unacceptable potential for risk to humans or the environment and thus ought to be banned, but, at the same time, provide an accurate assessment of the risk to humans and the environment for less toxic compounds so that their use may be regulated.

Subjecting all chemicals to all possible tests is logistically impossible, and the future of toxicity testing must lie in the development of techniques that will narrow the testing process so that highly toxic and relatively nontoxic compounds can be identified early and either banned or permitted unrestricted use without undue waste of time, funds, and human resources. These vital commodities could then be concentrated on compounds whose fate and effects are less predictable. Such progress will come from further development and validation of the newer testing procedures and the development of techniques to select, for any given chemical, the most suitable testing methods. Perhaps of most importance is the development of integrated test sequences that will permit decisions to be made at each step, thereby either abbreviating the sequence or making the next step more effective and efficient. As more data are developed and analyzed, structure activity models should become more predictive. Some current models for predicting the potential for carcinogenesis are accurate in about 90% of cases.

8.10 SUGGESTED FURTHER READING

Balls, M., Riddell, R.J., Worden, A.N. Animals and Alternatives in Toxicity Testing. London: Academic Press, 1983.

Clark, B., Smith, D.A. Pharmacokinetics and toxicity testing, CRC Crit. Rev. Toxicol. 1984; 12:343.

Couch, J.A., Hargis, W.J., Jr. Aquatic animals in toxicity testing, J. Am. College Toxicol. 1984; 3:331.

Dean, J.H., Luster, M.I., Murray, M.J., Laver, L.D. Approaches and methodology for examining the immunological effects of xenobiotics, Immunotoxicology 1983; 7:205.

de Serres, F.J., Ashby, J. (eds.). Evaluation of Short Term Tests for Carcinogens. New York: Elsevier, 1981.

Enslein, K., Craig, P.N. Carcinogenesis: A predictive structure-activity model. J. Toxicol. Environ. Health. 1982; 10:521.

Gillette, J.R., Pohl, L.R. A perspective on covalent-binding and toxicity, J. Toxicol. Environ. Health. 1977; 2:849.

Gorrod, J.W. (ed.). Testing for Toxicity. London: Taylor and Francis, 1981. Relevant chapers include:

Chapter 3. Brown, V.K.H. Acute toxicity testing—A critique.

Chapter 4. Roe, F.J.C. Testing *in vivo* for general chronic toxicity and carcinogenicity.

Chapter 7. Gorrod, J.W. Covalent binding as an indicator of drug toxicity.

Chapter 15. Dewar, A.J. Neurotoxicity testing—With particular reference to biochemical methods.

Chapter 18. Cobb, L.M. Pulmonary toxicity.

Chapter 20. Parish, W.E. Immunological tests to predict toxicological hazards to man.

Chapter 21. Venitt, S. Microbial tests in carcinogenesis studies.

Chapter 22. Styles, J.A. Other short-term tests in carcinogenesis studies.

Gralla, E.J. (ed.). Scientific Consideration in Monitoring and Evaluating Toxicology Research. Washington, D.C.: Hemisphere, 1981.

Hayes, A.W. (ed.). Principles and Methods of Toxicology. New York: Raven Press, 1982. This volume contains the following chapters of particular relevance to this chapter:

Chapter 1. Chan, P.K., O'Hara, G.P., Hayes, A.W. Principles and methods for acute and subchronic toxicity.

Chapter 2. Stevens, K.R., Gallo, M.A. Practical considerations in the conduct of chronic toxicity studies.

Chapter 3. Roberts, J.F., Joiner, J.J., Schueler, R.L. Methods in testing for carcinogenicity.

Chapter 4. Dixon, R.L., Hall, J.L. Reproductive toxicology.

Chapter 5. Manson, J.M., Zenick, H., Costlow, R.D. Teratology test methods for laboratory animals.

Chapter 6. Kennedy, G.L., Jr., Trochimowicz, H.J. Inhalation toxicology.

Chapter 7. Gilman, M.R. Skin and eye testing in animals.

Chapter 8. Brusick, D. Genetic toxicology.

Chapter 10. Edward, A.G. Animal care and maintenance.

Chapter 11. Norton, S. Methods in behavioral toxicology.

Chapter 18. Luster, M.I., Dean, J.H., Moore, J.A. Evaluation of immune functions in toxicology.

Chapter 22. Renwick, A.G. Pharmacokinetics in toxicology.

Chapter 23. Hogan, M.D., Hoel, D.G. Extrapolation to man.

Homburger, F., Hayes, J.A., Pelikan, E.W. (eds.). A Guide to General Toxicology. Basel, New York: Karger, 1983. This volume contains the following chapters of particular relevance to this chapter:

Chapter 4. Wong, S., Natarajan, C. Immunotoxicology.

Chapter 6. Hayes, J.A. Inhalational toxicology.

Chapter 11. Homburger, F. Carcinogenesis—Concepts.

Chapter 15. Rogers, A.E. Factors influencing the results of animal experiments in toxicology.

Chapter 16. Homburger, F. *In vivo* testing in the study of toxicity and safety evaluation.

Chapter 17. Christian, M.S., Voytek, P.E. *In vivo* reproductive and mutagenicity tests.

Chapter 18. Brusick, D.J. Mutagenesis and carcinogenesis in mammalian cells.

Chapter 19. Jagannath, D.R., Brusick, D.J. Mutagens and carcinogens in bacteria.

Jollow, D.J., Roberts, S., Price, V., Longacre, S., Smith, C. Pharmacokinetic consideration in toxicity testing. Drug Metab. Rev. 1982; 13:983.

Loomis, T.A. Essentials of Toxicology. Philadelphia: Lee & Feliger, 1978.

Luotola, M. Use of laboratory model ecosystems for the evaluation of environmental contaminants. In E. Hodgson, (ed.). Reviews in Environmental Toxicology. Amsterdam: Elsevier Biomedical Press, 1985.

McCann, J., Horn, L., Koldor, J. An evaluation of *Salmonella* (Ames) test data in the published literature: Application of statistical procedures and analysis of mutagenic potency. Mutation Res. 1984; 134:1.

Mitchell, C.L., Tilson, H.A. Behavioral toxicology in risk assessment: Problems and research needs. CRC Crit. Rev. Toxicol. 1982; 265–274.

National Toxicology Program. Report of the NTP Ad Hoc Panel on Chemical Carcinogenesis Testing and Evaluation. Washington, D.C.: Department of Health and Human Services, 1984.

Parke, D.V. Significance of the metabolism of xenobiotics for toxicological evaluation. In Bartosek I. et al. (eds.). Animals in Toxicological Research. New York: Raven Press, 1982.

Sperling, F. (ed.). Toxicity: Principles and Practice. Vol. 2. New York: Wiley, 1984. Contains the following chapters of relevance to this chapter:

Chapter 1. Sperling, F. Toxicokinetics: The determinants of toxicity.

Chapter 6. Swanborg, R.H. Immune response in toxicology.

Chapter 9. Kirwin, C.J., Jr. Eye and skin local toxicity testing.

Chapter 10. Sperling, F. Quantitation of toxicity — The dose-response.

WHO-IARC. Monograph Supplement 4 to the Monograph Series on "The Evaluation of the Carcinogenic Risk of Chemicals to Humans." Lyons, France: IARC, 1982.

WHO-GENEVA, Environmental Health Criteria 6. Principles and Methods for Evaluation the Toxicity of Chemicals, Geneva, Switzerland, 1978.

Zbingdon, G., Flury-Roversi, M. Significance of the LD50-Test for the toxicological evaluation of chemical substances. Arch. Toxicol. 1981; 47:77.

chapter nine

THE MEASUREMENT OF TOXICANTS

Ross B. Leidy and Ernest Hodgson

9.1 INTRODUCTION

In the last two to three decades, analytical techniques have improved spectacularly; this is particularly true in the case of toxicants. Although the purpose of toxicant analysis may in experimental work be related to drug toxicity, or in forensic medicine, to determining the cause of poisoning, the needs of the environmental area have provided the biggest impetus to development of analytical methods in toxicology.

The media abound with descriptions of real or potential environmental pollution that may affect the quality of life in a particular region of the world. These news features may list the extent of the pollution, the amounts found, and the length of time that the region will be contaminated. In most cases, these values are accurate to levels that were unattainable 20 years ago, and the primary reason for his improvement is the increased sensitivity of modern analytical instruments. Instrumentation is, however, only one part of the analytical process, which consists of a series of six operations culminating in the determination of the extent and quantity of the toxicant present.

The first step of the analytical process is a definition of the goal, which will differ depending on the circumstances. If, for example, a pollutant has been released into the environment, one must consider, based on the nature of the pollutant, what should be sampled and how the sampling and subsequent analysis should be done. Clearly, in analysis of pesticide metabolism in an experimental setting or in determination of the drugs involved in an accidental overdose, the goals would be quite different. Sampling is the second important step, again varying with the nature of the problem. Isolation, the third step, involves extraction of the compound from the sample. Generally, other interfering materials are released during this step and must be separated (the fourth step) from the toxicant. The separation step precedes the actual identification,

287

which is done by an analytical instrument, and its quantitation. If the reaction used is highly specific, the analysis can be carried out on relatively impure samples. The last step is an evaluation of the data to determine if additional sampling is required, if other samples should be analyzed, and if additional areas should be sampled in the case of environmental pollutants. Within these general categories the particular methods vary considerably depending on the chemical characteristics of the toxicant (Table 9.1).

This chapter is concerned with the sampling, isolation, separation, and measurement of toxicants, including bioassay methods. Bioassay is not strictly the measurement of toxic effects; rather, it is the quantitation of the relative effect of a substance on a test organism as compared with the effect of a standard preparation of a basic toxicant. It is a quantitative measure of the amount present. Although bioassay has many drawbacks, particularly lack of specificity, it provides a rapid analysis of the relative potency of environmental samples.

9.2 CHEMICAL AND PHYSICAL METHODS

9.2.1 Sampling

Even with the most sophisticated analytical equipment available, the resulting data are only as representative as the samples from which the results are derived. This is particularly true in the case of environmental samples. In this case, care must be taken to assure that the sample is representative of the object of study. Often, special attention to sampling procedures is necessary. Sampling accomplishes a number of objectives, depending on the type of area being studied. In environmental areas (eg, wilderness regions, lakes, or rivers) it can provide data not only on the concentration of pollutants but also on the extent of contamination. In urban areas, sampling can provide information on the types of pollutants one is exposed to, either by inhalation or by ingestion over a given period.

In industrial areas, hazardous conditions can be detected and sources of pollution can be identified. Sampling is used in the process of designing pollution controls and can provide a chronicle of the changes in operational conditions as these controls are implemented. Another important application of sampling in industrial areas in the United States is the documentation of compliance with existing Occupational Safety and Health Administration (OSHA) and Environmental Protection Agency (EPA) regulations. The many methods available for sampling the environment can be divided into categories of air, soil, water, and tissue sampling. The fourth category is of particular interest in experimental and forensic studies.

9.2.1.1 Air

Most pollutants entering the atmosphere come from fuel combustion, industrial processes, and solid waste disposal. Additional miscellaneous sources, such as atomic explosions, forest fires, solid dusts, volcanoes, natural gaseous emissions, agricultural burning and pesticide drift, contribute to the level of atmospheric pollution. To affect terrestrial animals and plants, particulate pollutants must be in a size range that allows them to enter the body and remain there; that

TABLE 9.1
Typical Protocols for Analysis of Toxicants

Step	Toxicant		
	Arsenic	TCDD	Furadan
Sampling	Grind solid sample or homogenize tissue to homogeneity; subsample	Grind solid sample or homogenize tissue to homogeneity; subsample	Grind solid sample or homogenize tissue to homogeneity; blend with ethanol and water; subsample
Extraction	Dry ash; redissolve residue; generate arsine and absorb into solution	Extract with ethanol and KOH; remove saponified lipids; column chromatography on H_2SO_4/silica gel followed by basic alumina and then by $AgNO_3$/silica gel followed by basic alumina; reverse-phase HPLC	Extract with petroleum ether; TLC on silica gel G with ethyl ether: xylene
Analysis	Colorimetric analysis using diethyldithio-carbamate and UV/VIS spectrophotometer (Δ A at 535 nm)	GLC-mass spectrometer	GLC

TLC, thin-layer chromatography; HPLC, high-performance liquid chromatography; UV, ultraviolet; VIS, visible; GLC, gas-liquid chromatography.
Source: Everson, R.J., Oehme, F.W. Analytical Toxicology Manual. Manhattan, Kan.: American College of Veterinary Toxicologists, 1981.

is, they must be in an aerosol, defined as an airborne suspension of liquid droplets, or on solid particles small enough to possess a low settling velocity. Suspensions can be classified as liquids—including fogs (small particles) and mists (large particles) produced from atomization, condensation, or entrainment of liquids by gases; and solids—including dusts, fumes, and smokes produced by crushing, metal vaporization, and combustion of organic materials, respectively.

At rest, an adult human inhales 6–8 L of air each minute (1 L = 0.001 m³) and during an 8-hour work day, can inhale from 5 to 20 m³ depending on the level of physical activity. The optimum size range for aerosol particles to get into the lungs and remain there is 0.5–5 μm. Thus, air samplers have been designed to collect the particulate matter in the size range most detrimental to humans.

An air sampler generally consists of an inlet to direct air into a collector, a filter to screen out larger particles that might interfere with an analysis, the collector in which the sample is deposited, a flowmeter and valve to calibrate airflow, and a pump to pull air through the system (Figure 9.1). In recent years, samplers have been miniaturized so that they can be connected to subjects

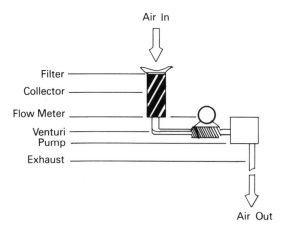

FIGURE 9.1.
Schematic representation of a typical air-sampling device. Source: Leidy, R.B., Detection: Analytical. In Guthrie, F.E., and Perry, J.J. (eds.), Introduction to Environmental Toxicology, New York: Elsevier, 1980.

while they are working, walking, or riding in a given area, thus allowing estimation of individual exposure.

Many air samplers use various types of filters to collect solid particulate matter, such as asbestos, which is collected on glass fiber filters with pores ≤ 20 μm in diameter. Membrane filters with pores $0.01 - 10$ μm in diameter are used to collect dusts and silica. Liquid-containing collectors called impingers are used to trap mineral dusts and pesticides. Mineral dusts are collected in large impingers that have flow rates of $10 - 50$ L of air per minute passing through them, and insecticides can be collected in smaller "midget" impingers that handle flows of $2 - 4.5$ L of air per minute. Depending on the pollutant being sought, the entrapping liquid might be distilled water, alcohol, ethylene glycol, hexylene glycol, or some other solvent. Small glass tubes approximately 7×0.5 cm in diameter containing activated charcoal are used to entrap organic vapors in air. In the last two years, several manufacturers have developed adsorbents to collect specific organic compounds, including industrial organics, pesticides, and formaldehyde. Another type of sampler requires no pump. The compound to be monitored diffuses through a porous membrane and collects on an adsorbent; later, it can be eluted from the adsorbent and analyzed. Polyurethane foam (PUF), which has become a popular trapping medium for pesticides because of the ease of handling and the rapid desorption of compounds from it, is rapidly replacing the use of midget impingers. A large-volume air sampler has been developed by the EPA for detection of chlorinated hydrocarbon insecticides and polychlorinated biphenyls (PCBs): air flows through a polyurethane foam pad at a rate of 225.0 L/min, and the insecticides and PCBs are trapped in the foam. Direct reading instruments are being developed and will be described later.

9.2.1.2 Soil

When environmental pollutants are deposited on land areas, their subsequent behavior is complicated by a series of simultaneous interactions with organic and inorganic components, the existing liquid–gas phases, and the living and nonliving components of the soil. Depending on its chemical and physical structure, the pollutant may remain in one location for long or short periods, be absorbed into plant tissue, or move into the soil by diffusion resulting from random molecular motion. Movement is also affected by mass flow as a result of external forces, such as the pollutant being dissolved or suspended in water or adsorbed onto inorganic and organic soil components. Thus, sampling for pollutants in soils can be simple or very difficult.

To obtain representative samples, the chemical and physical characteristics of the sampling site(s) must be considered, as well as possible reactions of the pollutant with soil components and the degree of variability in the sampling area. With these data, the site(s) can then be divided into homogeneous areas, and the required number of samples can be collected. The number of samples depends on the functions of variance and the degree of accuracy required. Once the correct procedure has been determined, sampling can proceed by random or systematic means.

Many types of soil samplers are available, but various coring devices are preferred because this method of collection allows determination of a pollutant's vertical distribution. These devices can be either steel tubes, which vary from 2.5 to 7.6 cm in diameter and 60–100 cm in length (for hand use), or large boring tubes that are 10×200 cm (operated mechanically). It is possible to sample to uniform depths with such devices. Another type of coring equipment is a wheel to which small tubes are attached so that large numbers of small subsamples can be taken, thus allowing more uniform sampling over a given site. Specialty samplers with large diameters (about 25 cm) incorporate a blade to slice a core of soil after reaching the desired depth.

9.2.1.3 Water

Many factors must be considered to obtain representative samples of water. The most important are the nature of the pollutant and the point at which it entered the aquatic environment. Pollutants may be contributed by agricultural, industrial, municipal, or other sources, such as spills from wrecks or train derailments. The prevailing wind direction and speed, the velocity of stream or river flow, temperature, thermal and salinity stratification, and sediment content are other important factors.

Two questions—where to monitor or sample and what device is best to use to obtain representative samples—are important.

The simplest method of collecting water is the "grab" technique, whereby a container is lowered into the water, rinsed, filled, and capped. A Van Dorn-type sampler is frequently used to obtain water at greater depths.

With the implementation in the United States of the Clean Water Act of 1977, continuous monitoring is required to obtain data for management decisions. A number of continuous monitoring devices are in operation. These consist of a pump (floating, peristaltic, submersible, or tank-mounted) to draw water into collecting devices (generally glass or plastic bottles), metering devices to determine flow rates, and timers to implement periodic sampling. Because large numbers of samples can be generated by such devices, collectors containing membranes with small pores (about 4.5 μm) to entrap metal-containing pollutants, ion-exchange resins, resin-loaded filter paper, or long-chain hydrocarbons (eg, C_{18}) bonded to silica to bind organic pollutants are often used to diminish the number and bulk of the samples by allowing several liters of water to pass through and leave only the pollutants entrapped in a small cylinder or container.

Once samples have been collected, they should be frozen immediately in solid CO_2 (dry ice) and returned to the laboratory. If they are not analyzed at that time, they should be stored frozen at temperatures of -20 °C or lower.

9.2.1.4 Tissues

9.2.1.4a Environmental Studies

When environmental areas are suspected of being contaminated, surveys of plants and animals are conducted. Many of the surveys, conducted during hunting and fishing seasons, determine the number of animals killed, and organs and other tissues are removed for analysis for suspected contaminants by federal and state laboratories. Sampling is conducted randomly throughout an area; the analysis can help determine the concentration, extent of contamination within a given species, and areas of contamination.

Many environmental pollutants are known to concentrate in bone, certain organs, or specific tissues (eg, adipose). These organs are removed from recently killed animals for analysis. In many instances, the organs are not pooled with others from the same species but are analyzed separately as single subsamples.

When plant material is gathered for analysis, it is either divided into roots, stems, leaves, and flowers and/or fruit, or the whole plant is analyzed as a single entity. Pooling of samples from a site can also provide a single sample for analysis. The choice depends on the characteristics of the suspected contaminant.

9.2.1.4b Experimental Studies

Experimental studies, particularly those involving the metabolism or mode of action of toxic compounds in animals (or, less often, plants) may be conducted either in vivo or in vitro. Because individual organisms or enzyme preparations are treated with known compounds, the question of random sampling techniques does not arise as it does with environmental samples. Enough replication is needed for statistical verification of significance, and it should always be borne in mind that repeated determinations carried out on aliquots of the same preparation do not represent replication of the experiment; at best, they test the reproducibility of the analytical method.

In environmental studies, the analyst is concerned with stable compounds or stable end-products; in metabolic studies, the question of reactive (therefore unstable) products and intermediates is of critical concern. Thus, the reaction must be stopped, and the sample must be processed using techniques that minimize degradation. This is facilitated by the fact that the substrate is known, and the range of possible products can be the subject of much informed hypothesis.

The initial sampling step is to stop the reaction, usually by a protein precipitant. Although traditional compounds such as trichloroacetic acid are effective protein precipitants, they are usually undesirable. Water-miscible organic solvents such as ethanol or acetone are milder, whereas a mixture of a miscible and an immiscible solvent (chloroform/methanol, for example) not only denatures the protein but effects a preliminary separation into water-soluble and organosoluble products. Rapid freezing is a mild method of stopping reactions, but low temperature during the subsequent handling is necessary.

In toxicokinetic studies involving sequential killing and tissue examination, it is critical to obtain uncontaminated organ samples. Apart from contamination by blood, this can be avoided by careful dissection and rinsing of the organs in ice-cold buffer, saline, or other appropriate solution. Blood samples themselves are obtained by cardiac puncture, and blood contamination of organ samples is minimized by careful bleeding of the animal at the time of killing or, if necessary, by perfusion of the organ in question.

9.2.1.4c Forensic Studies

Because forensic toxicology deals primarily with sudden or unexplained death, the range of potential toxicants is extremely large. The analyst does not usually begin examination of the samples, however, until all preliminary studies are complete, including necropsy and microscopic examination of all tissues. Thus, the analyst is usually able to begin with some working hypothesis as to the possible range of toxicants involved.

Because further sampling usually involves exhumation and is therefore unlikely or, in the case of cremation, impossible, adequate sampling and sample preservation is essential. For example, various body fluids must be collected in a proper way: blood by cardiac puncture, never from the body cavity; urine from the urinary bladder; bile collected intact as part of the ligated gall bladder; etc. Adequate sample size is important. Blood can be analyzed for carbon monoxide, ethanol and other alcohols, barbiturates, tranquilizers, and other drugs; at least 100 mL should be collected. Urine is useful for analysis of both endogenous and exogenous chemicals and the entire content of the bladder is retained. Liver frequently contains high levels of toxicants and/or their metabolites, and it and the kidney are the most important solid tissues for forensic analysis; 100 – 200 g of the former and the equivalent of one kidney are usually retained.

An unusual requirement with important legal ramifications is that of possession. An unbroken chain of identifiable possession must be maintained. All transfers are marked on the samples as to time and date, and all transfers must be signed by both parties. The security of samples during time of possession must be verifiable as a matter of law.

9.2.2 Extraction

In most cases, the analysis of a pollutant or other toxicant depends on its physical removal from the sample medium. This process is called extraction and involves bringing a suitable solvent into intimate content with the sample, generally in a ratio of 5 – 25 vol of solvent to 1 vol of sample. One or more of four different procedures can be used, depending on the chemical and physical characteristics of the toxicant and the sample matrix. Other extraction methods such as boiling, grinding, or distilling the sample with appropriate solvents are used less frequently.

9.2.2.1 Blending

The use of an electric or air-driven blender is currently the most common method of extraction of biological materials. The weighed sample is placed in a container, solvent is added, and the tissue is homogenized by motor-driven blades. Blending for 5 – 15 minutes followed by a repeat blending will extract most environmental toxicants. A homogenate in an organic solvent can be filtered through anhydrous sodium sulfate to remove water that might cause problems in the quantitation phase of the analysis. The use of sonication is a popular method for extracting tissue samples, particularly when the binding of toxicants to subcellular fractions is of interest. Sonicator probes rupture cells rapidly, thus allowing the solvent to come into intimate contact with all cell components. Differential centrifugation can then be used to isolate fractions of interest.

9.2.2.2 Shaking

Pollutants are generally extracted from water samples, and in some cases soil samples, by shaking with an appropriate solvent or solvent combination. Mechanical shakers have been developed to handle several water or soil samples at once. These devices allow the analyst to conduct long-term extractions (eg, 24 hours) if required. Two or more shakings normally are required for complete removal (ie, > 98%) of the toxicant from the sample matrix.

9.2.2.3 Washing

With some environmental samples such as plants or fruits, a simple surface washing with water and a detergent or with a solvent is sufficient to determine surface contamination.

9.2.2.4 Continuous Extraction

The procedure is performed on solid samples (eg, soil) and involves the use of an organic solvent or combination of solvents. The sample is weighed into a cup (thimble) of specialized porous material such as cellulose or fiberglass and Soxhlet extractor is used to remove the toxicant from the sample matrix. This consists of a boiling flask, in which the solvent is placed, an extractor, which holds the thimble, and a water-jacketed condensor. When heated to boiling, the solvent vaporizes, is condensed, and fills the extractor, thus bathing the sample and extracting the toxicant. A siphoning action drains the solvent back into the boiling flask, and the cycle begins again. Depending on the nature of the toxicant and sample matrix, the extraction can be completed in as little as 2 hours but may take as long as 3 – 4 days.

9.2.3 Separation and Identification

During extraction processes, many undesirable components are also released from the sample matrix; these must be removed to obtain quantitative results from certain instruments. These components include plant and animal pigments, lipids, organic material from soil and water, and inorganic compounds. If not removed, the impurities decrease the sensitivity of the detectors and columns in the analytical instrument, mask peaks, or produce extraneous peaks on chromatograms. Although some instruments developed in recent years automatically remove these substances and concentrate to small volumes for quantitative analysis, they are expensive; most laboratories rely on other methods. These include adsorption chromatography, thin-layer chromatography (TLC), and solvent partitioning. Before the separation step is conducted, the solvent containing the extracted toxicant must be concentrated to a small volume (usually < 5 mL). This is accomplished by removal of the solvent by distillation, evaporation under a stream of air or an inert gas such as nitrogen, or evaporation under reduced pressure. Once the working volume is reached, extracts can be further purified by one or more procedures.

Once the toxicant has been extracted and separated from extraneous materials, the actual identification procedure can begin, although it should be remembered that the purification procedures are themselves often used in identification, eg, peak position in gas–liquid chromatography (GLC) and high-performance liquid chromatography (HPLC). Thus no definite line can be drawn between the two types of procedures. Recent advances in circuit miniaturization and column technology, the development of microprocessors, and new concepts in instrument design have allowed sensitive measurement at the parts per billion and parts per trillion levels for many toxicants. This increased sensitivity has focused public attention on the extent of environmental pollution, because many toxic materials present in minute quantities could not be detected until technological advances reached the present state of the art. At present, most environmental pollutants are identified and quantified by chromatography, spectroscopy, and bioassays.

9.2.3.1 Solvent Partitioning

Many organic toxicants will distribute between two immiscible solvents (eg, chloroform and water or hexane and acetonitrile). When shaken in a separatory funnel and then allowed to equilibrate into the two original solvent layers, some of the toxicant will have transferred from the original extracting solvent into the other layer. With repeated additions (eg, 4–5 vol), mixing, and removal, most or all of the compound of interest will have been transferred, leaving many interfering compounds in the original solvent. Regardless of the separation method or combination of methods used, the toxicant will be in a large volume of solvent in relation to its amount; however, the volume of solvent can be reduced by evaporation.

9.2.3.2 Chromatography

All chromatographic processes such as TLC, GLC, or HPLC use an immobile and a mobile phase to effect a separation of components. In TLC, the immobile phase is a thin layer of adsorbent placed on glass, resistant plastic, or fiberglass, and the mobile phase is the solvent. The mobile phase can be a liquid or gas, whereas the immobile phase can be a liquid or solid. Chromatographic separations are based on the interactions of these phases or surfaces. All chromatographic procedures use the differential distribution or partitioning of one or more components between the phases, based on the absorption, adsorption, ion-exchange, or size exclusion properties of one of the phases.

9.2.3.2a Paper

Although the introduction of paper chromatography to common laboratory use about 30 years ago revolutionized experimental biochemistry and toxicology, it has been largely superseded by TLC—even in laboratories that lack the expensive instruments necessary for GLC or HPLC—because of the speed and greater revolving power of TLC. The stationary phase is represented by the aqueous constituent of the solvent system, which is adsorbed onto the paper; the moving phase is the organic constituents. Separation is effected by partition between the two phases as the solvent system moves over the paper. Although many variations exist, including reverse-phase paper chromatography in which the paper is treated with a hydrophobic material, ion-exchange cellulose paper, etc., all have been superseded by equivalent systems involving thin layers.

9.2.3.2b Thin-Layer Chromatography

Many toxicants can be separated from interfering substances with TLC. In this form of chromatography, the adsorbent is spread as a thin layer (250–2,000 μm) on a glass plate, resistant plastic, or fiberglass backings. When the extract is placed near the bottom of the plate and the plate is placed in a tank containing a solvent system, the solvent migrates up the plate and the toxicant and other constituent move with the solvent; differential rates of movement result in separation. The compounds can be scraped from the plate and eluted from the adsorbent with suitable solvents. Recent developments in TLC adsorbents allow toxicants and other materials to be quantitated at the nanogram (10^{-9} g) and picogram (10^{-12} g) levels.

9.2.3.2c Column: Adsorption, Hydrophobic, Ion Exchange

Adsorption-column chromatography involves the use of glass columns with Teflon stopcocks to control flow rate. The adsorbent can be activated charcoal, aluminum oxide, Florisil, silica, silicic acid, or mixed adsorbents. The characteristics of the toxicant determine the choice of adsorbent. Once the concentrated extract is placed on the column, the toxicant can be removed selectively by passing one or more solvents through the column while the coextracted materials remain. In some instances, selected solvents are used to remove contaminating material first; the toxicant is then eluted by another solvent system. In the most common sequence, the column is packed in an organic solvent of low polarity; the sample is added in the same solvent, and the column is then developed with a sequence of solvents or solvent mixtures of increasing polarity. Such a sequence might include (in order of increasing polarity) hexane, benzene, chloroform, acetone, and methanol. Once removed, the eluate containing the toxicant is reduced to a small volume for quantitation. A number of miniaturized columns have been introduced over the last 5 years. Most contain 2–4 g of the adsorbent in a plastic tube with fritted ends. The columns can be attached to standard Luer Lock syringes. Other companies have designed vacuum boxes that hold the collecting device. The column is placed on the apparatus, vacuum is applied, and the solvent is "pulled" through the column. Advantages of these systems include preweighed amounts of adsorbent for uniformity, easy disposal of the coextractives remaining in the cartridge, no breakage, and decreased cost of the analysis because less solvent and adsorbent are used.

Other forms of column chromatography may be used. They include ion-exchange chromatography, permeation chromatography, and affinity chromatography.

Ion-exchange chromatography depends on the attraction between charged molecules and opposite charges on the ion exchanger, usually a resin. Compounds so bound are eluted by changes in pH and, since the net charge depends on the relationship between the pH of the solution and the isoelectric point of the compounds, compounds of different isoelectric point can be sequentially eluted. Both ionic and anionic exchangers are available.

Permeation chromatography utilizes the molecular sieve properties of porous materials. Molecules large enough to be excluded from the pores of the porous material will move through the column faster than those not excluded and thus can be separated from them. Cross-linked dextrans such as Sephadex or agarose (Sepharose) are commonly used materials.

Affinity chromatography is a potent tool for biologically active macromolecules but is seldom used for purifying small molecules, such as most toxicants. It depends on the affinity of an enzyme for a substrate (or substrate analog) that has been incorporated into a column matrix or the affinity of a receptor for a ligand.

9.2.3.2d Gas-Liquid Chromatography (GLC)

Gas-liquid chromatography has become the method most commonly used for the separation and quantitation of organic toxicants. It consists of an injector port, oven, detector, amplifier (electrometer), and supporting electronics (Figure 9.2). Contained within the oven is a column of glass, nickel, stainless steel, or perhaps a polymer, filled or coated with the immobile phase. The immobile or stationary phase is a liquid coated on an inert support material such as diatomaceous earth. The mobile phase is an inert gas (called a carrier gas), such as helium or nitrogen, which passes through the column.

When a sample is injected into or onto the column, the injector port is at a temperature sufficient to vaporize the sample components. Based on the solubility and volatility of these components with respect to the stationary phase, the components separate and are swept through the column by the carrier gas to a detector, which responds to the concentration of each component. The detector may not respond to all components. The electronic signal produced as the component passes through the detector is amplified by the electrometer, and the resulting signal is sent to a recorder, computer, or electronic data-collecting device for quantitation.

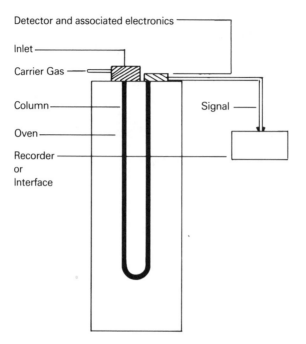

FIGURE 9.2.
Schematic representation of a typical gas–liquid chromatograph. Source: Leidy, R.B., Detection: Analytical. In Guthrie, F.E., and Perry, J.J. (eds.), Introduction to Environmental Toxicology, New York: Elsevier, 1980.

COLUMN TECHNOLOGY.   Increased sensitivity has resulted from advances in solid-state electronics, column, and detector technology. In the field of column technology, the capillary column has revolutionized toxicant detection in complex samples. Capillary columns differ from conventionally packed ones in four ways: (1) there is an open unrestricted path through the column rather than the obstructed path in conventional columns that are filled with material; (2) the inner tubing has a diameter of approximately 0.2 mm, as compared with 2–6.3 mm in conventional columns; (3) the length varies from 15 to 100 m as opposed to 0.6–6.7 m in packed columns; and (4) the carrier gas flow rates are quite low (eg, 1–2 mL/min) as compared with 50–100 mL/min through packed columns.

Two types of capillary columns are receiving widespread use: the support-coated, open tubular (SCOT) column and the wall-coated, open tubular (WCOT) column. The SCOT column has a very fine layer of diatomaceous earth coated with liquid phase which is deposited on the inside wall. The WCOT column is pretreated and then coated with a thin film of liquid phase. Of the two columns, the SCOT is claimed to be more universally applicable because of large sample capacity, simplicity in connecting it to the chromatograph, and lower cost. For difficult separations or highly complex mixtures, the WCOT is the more efficient type. Many older chromatographs are not designed to accomodate capillary columns, and because of these design restrictions, some manufacturers have introduced the wide-bore capillary column along with the fittings and valving required to adapt the columns to older instruments. With inner diameters of 0.55 mm, flow rates of 25–30 mL/min of carrier gas can be used to affect separations of components approaching that of the narrow-bore columns. Water samples chromatographed on capillary columns routinely separate 400–500 compounds, as compared with 90–120 resolved compounds from conventional compounds.

DETECTOR TECHNOLOGY.   The second advance in GLC is detector technology. Five detectors are used widely in toxicant detection: the flame ionization (FID), flame photometric (FPD), electron capture (ECD), alkali flame, and conductivity detectors (Figure 9.3). New detectors are being introduced that could have an impact on toxicant analysis, however, including the Hall conductivity detector, the nitrogen-phosphorus detector, and the photoionization detector.

The FID operates on the principle of ion formation from compounds being burned in a hydrogen flame as they elute from a column. The concentrations of ions formed are several orders of magnitude greater than those formed in the uncontaminated flame. The ions cause a current to flow between two electrodes held at a constant potential, thus sending a signal to the electrometer.

The FPD is a specific detector in that it detects either phosphorus or sulfur-containing compounds. When atoms of a given element are burned in a hydrogen-rich flame, the excitation energy supplied to these atoms produces a unique emission spectrum. The intensity of the wavelengths of light emitted by these atoms is directly proportional to the number of atoms excited. Larger concentrations cause a greater number of atoms to reach the excitation energy level, thus increasing the intensity of the emission spectrum. The change in intensity is detected by a photomultiplier, amplified by the electrometer, and recorded. Filters that allow only the emission wavelength of phosphorus (526 nm) or sulfur (394 nm) are inserted between the flame and the photomultiplier to give this detector its specificity.

The ECD is used to detect halogen-containing compounds, although it will produce a response to any electronegative compound. When a negative DC voltage is applied to a radioactive source (eg, ^{63}Ni or ^{3}H), low-energy β particles are emitted, producing secondary electrons by ionizing the carrier gas as it passes through the detector. The secondary electron stream flows from the source (cathode) to a collector (anode), where the amount of current generated (called a standing current) is amplified and recorded. As electronegative compounds pass from the column into the detector, electrons are removed or "captured," and the standing current is reduced. The reduction is related to both the concentration and electronegativity of the compound passing through, and this produces a response that is recorded. The sensitivity of the ECD is greater than that of any of the other detectors currently available.

Early electrolytic conductivity detectors operated on the principle of component combustion, which produced simple molecular species that readily ionized, thus altering the conductivity of deionized water. The changes were monitored by a DC bridge circuit and recorded. By varying the conditions the detector could be made selective for different types of compounds (eg, chlorine-containing or nitrogen-containing).

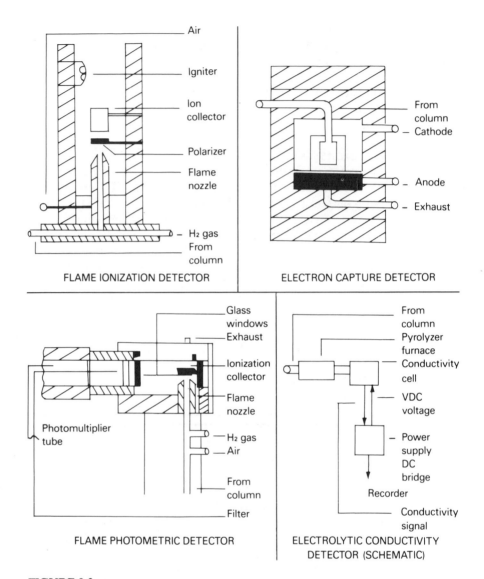

FIGURE 9.3.
Schematic representations of four frequently used gas chromatography detectors.
Source: Leidy, R.B., Detection: Analytical. In Guthrie, F.E., and Perry, J.J. (eds.),
Introduction to Environmental Toxicology, New York: Elsevier, 1980.

The alkali flame detector can also be made selective. Enhanced response to
compounds containing arsenic, boron, halogen, nitrogen, and phosphorus results when the collector (cathode) of an FID is coated with different alkali metal
salts such as KBr, KCl, Na_2SO_4, and Rb_2SO_4. As with conductivity detectors,
by varying gas flow rates, type of salt, and electrode configuration, enhanced
responses are obtained.

New detectors are also being used in the field of toxicant analysis. The Hall
electrolytic conductivity detector uses advanced designs in the conductivity
cell, furnace, and an AC conductivity bridge to detect chlorine, nitrogen, and

sulfur-containing compounds at sensitivities of 0.01 ng. It operates on the conductivity principle described previously. A nitrogen-phosphorus alkali detector was introduced recently. In this detector, the alkali salts are embedded in a silica gel matrix and are heated electrically. The detector allows routine use of chlorinated solvents and derivatizing reagents to prevent contamination of the salts. It will also reduce a response to phosphorus by 30% while maintaining the normal response to nitrogen for confirmation purposes. Another new detector, the photoionization detector, uses an ultraviolet (UV) light source to ionize molecules by absorption of a photon of UV light. The ion formed has an energy greater than the ionization potential of the parent compound, and the formed ions are collected by an electrode. The current, which is proportional concentration, is amplified and recorded. The detector can measure a number of organic and inorganic compounds in air, biological fluids, and water.

9.2.3.2e High-Performance Liquid Chromatography (HPLC)

Although it is a relatively new method in the field of analytical chemistry, HPLC has become very popular for the following reasons: it can be run at ambient temperatures; it is nondestructive to the compounds of interest, which can be collected intact; in many instances, derivatization is not necessary for response; and columns can be loaded with large quantities of the material for detection of low levels.

The instrument consists of a solvent reservoir, gradient-forming device, high-pressure pumping device, injector column, and detector. The principle of operation is very similar to that of GLC except that the mobile phase is a liquid instead of a gas. The composition of the mobile phase and its flow rate effect separations. The columns being developed for HPLC are too numerous to discuss in detail. Most use finely divided packing ($3 – 10 \ \mu m$ in diameter), some have bonded phases, and others are alumina or silica. The columns normally are 15–20 cm in length, with small diameters (approximately 4.6-mm inner diameter). A high-pressure pump is required to force the solvent through this type of column. The major detectors presently used for HPLC are UV fluorescent spectrophotometers or differential refractometers, although others are being developed.

9.2.3.3 Spectroscopy

To discuss spectroscopy, one must review radiation briefly. In certain experiments involving radiation, observed results cannot be explained on the basis of the wave theory of radiation. One must assume that radiation comes in discrete units, called quanta. Each quantum of energy has a definite frequency v, and the quantum energy can be calculated by the equation $E = hv$, where h is Planck's constant (6.6×10^{-27} erg-sec). Matter absorbs radiation one quantum at a time, and the energy of radiation absorbed becomes greater as either the frequency of radiation increases or the wavelength decreases. Therefore, radiation of shorter wavelength causes more drastic changes in a molecule than does that of longer wavelength.

Spectroscopy is concerned with the changes in atoms and molecules when electromagnetic radiation is absorbed or emitted. Instruments have been designed to detect these changes, and these instruments are important to the field of toxicant analysis. Discussions of atomic absorption (AA) spectroscopy, mass

TABLE 9.2
Characteristics of Spectroscopic Techniques

Type	Principle	Uses
Visible and UV spectrometry	Energy transitions of bonding and nonbonding outer electrons of molecules, usually delocalized electrons	Routine qualitative and quantitative biochemical analysis including many colorimetric assays. Enzyme assays, kinetic studies, and difference spectra
Spectrofluorimetry	Absorbed radiation emitted at longer wavelengths	Routine quantitative analysis, enzyme analysis and kinetics. More sensitive at lower concentrations than visible and UV absorption
Infrared and Raman spectroscopy	Atomic vibrations involving a change in dipole moment and a change in polarizability, respectively	Qualitative analysis and fingerprinting of purified molecules of intermediate size
Flame spectrophotometry (emission and absorption)	Energy transitions of outer electrons of atoms after volatilization in a flame	Qualitative and quantitative analysis of metals; emission techniques; routine determination of alkali metals; Absorption technique extends range of metals that may be determined and the sensitivity
Electron spin resonance spectrometry	Detection of magnetic moment associated with unpaired electrons	Research on metalloproteins, particularly enzymes and changes in the environment of free radicals introduced into biological assemblies, eg, membranes
Nuclear magnetic resonance spectrometry	Detection of magnetic moment associated with an odd number of protons in an atomic nucleus	Determination of structure of organic molecules of mol wt $< 20,000$ daltons
Mass spectrometry	Determination of the abundance of positively ionized molecules and fragments	Qualitative analysis of small quantities of material (10^{-6}–10^{-9} g), particularly in conjunction with gas liquid chromatography

Source: Modified from Williams, B.W., Wilson, K., Principles and Techniques of Practical Biochemistry. London: Edward Arnold, 1975.

spectroscopy (MS), infrared (IR), and UV spectroscopy follow. A summary of spectroscopic techniques is given in Table 9.2.

9.2.3.3a AA Spectroscopy

One of the more sensitive instruments used to detect metal-containing toxicants is the AA spectrophotometer. Samples are vaporized either by aspiration into an acetylene flame or by carbon rod atomization in a graphite cup or tube (flameless AA). The atomic vapor formed contains free atoms of an element in their ground state and, when illuminated by a light source that radiates light of a frequency characteristics of that element, the atom absorbs a photon of wavelength corresponding to its AA spectrum, thus exciting it. The amount of absorption is a function of concentration. The flameless instruments are much more sensitive than conventional flame AA. For example, arsenic can be detected at levels of 0.1 ng/mL and selenium at 0.2 mg/mL, which represent sensitivity three orders of magnitude greater than that of conventional flame AA.

9.2.3.3b   Mass Spectroscopy (MS)

The mass spectrometer is an outstanding instrument for the identification of compounds. In toxicant analysis, MS is used widely as a highly sensitive detection method for GLC and is increasingly used with HPLC since these instruments can be interfaced to the mass spectrometer. GLC or HPLC is used to separate individual components as previously described. A portion of the column effluent passes into the mass spectrometer, where it is bombarded by an electron beam. Electrons or negative groups are removed by this process, and the ions produced are accelerated. After acceleration, they pass through a magnetic field, where the ion species are separated by the different curvatures of their paths under gravity. Normally, only single positive ions are detected. The resulting pattern is characteristic of the molecule under study. By interfacing the detector with a computer system, data reduction, analysis, and quantitation are performed automatically. Large libraries of mass spectra have been developed for computing systems and, with technological advances, substances in femtogram (10^{-15} g) quantities are detected and quantitated. One disadvantage of MS is its high cost ($250,000 – 750,000 per instrument), and many laboratories cannot afford the capital outlay required. In the last 2 years, table-top MS detectors have been introduced that can be adapted to almost any GLC. The cost of these instruments is about one-tenth that of the conventional ones, and they are equipped with computer-driven libraries.

9.2.3.3c   IR Spectrophotometry

Within molecules, atoms are in constant motion, and associated with these motions are molecular energy levels that correspond to the energies of quanta of IR radiation. These motions can be resolved into rotation of the whole molecule in space and into motions corresponding to the vibration of atoms with respect to one another by bending or stretching of covalent bonds. The vibrational motions are very useful in identifying complex molecules, because functional groups (eg, OH, C, O, and S-H) within the molecule have characteristic absorption bands. The principle functional groups can be determined and used to identify compounds in cases in which chemical evidence permits relatively few possible structures. Standard IR spectrophotometers cover the spectral range from 2.5 to 15.4 μm (wave number equivalent to $4,000 – 650$ cm^{-1}) and use a source of radiation that passes through the sample and reference cells into a monochromator (a device used to isolate spectral regions). The radiation is then collected, amplified, and recorded. Current instruments use microprocessors, allowing a number of refinements that have increased the versatility of IR instruments so that more precise qualitative and quantitative data can be obtained.

9.2.3.3d Ultraviolet/Visible Spectrophotometry

Transitions occurring between electronic levels of molecules produce absorptions and emissions in the visible (VIS) and UV portions of the electromagnetic spectrum. Many inorganic and organic molecules show maximum absorption at specific wavelengths in the UV/VIS range, and these can be used to identify and quantitate compounds. Instruments designed to measure absorbance in the UV/VIS portions of the spectrum (200–800 nm) have been used in many disciplines for years. Today's instruments are being designed to be used for specific purposes, such as detectors in HPLC. Basic spectrophotometers have the same components as the IR instruments described previously, including a source (usually a tungsten lamp for VIS measurements or a hydrogen discharge lamp for UV), sample chamber, monochromator, and detector.

9.2.3.3e Nuclear Magnetic Resonance (NMR)

Nuclear magnetic resonance detects atoms which have nuclei that possess a magnetic moment. These are usually atoms containing nuclei with an odd number of protons (charges). Such nuclei can exist in two states, a low energy state with the nuclear spin aligned parallel to the magnetic field and a high energy state with the spin perpendicular to the field. Basically, the instrument measures the absorption or radiowave necessary to change the nuclei from a low to a high energy state as the magnetic field is varied. It is most commonly used for hydrogen atoms, although ^{13}C and ^{31}P are also suitable. Because the field seen by a proton varies with its molecular environment, such molecular arrangements as CH_3, CH_2, CH, etc., all give different signs, providing much information about the structure of the molecule in question.

9.2.3.3f Other Analytical Methods

As previously mentioned, the above instruments are the primary ones used in toxicant analysis, but an enormous number of analytical techniques are used in the field. Many of the instruments are expensive (eg, Raman spectrometer and x-ray emission spectrometer), and few laboratories possess them. Many other instruments are available, however, such as the specific-ion electrode, which is both sensitive and portable. Specific-ion electrodes have many other advantages in that sample color, suspended matter, turbidity, and viscosity do not interfere with analysis; therefore, many of the sample preparations steps are not required. Some of the species that can be detected at parts-per-billion levels are ammonia, carbon dioxide, chloride, cyanide, fluoride, lead, potassium, sulfide, and urea. Analytical pH meters or meters designed specifically for this application are used to calculate concentrations.

Finally, an increasing number of portable, direct reading instruments are now available to detect and quantitate environmental pollutants. Most of these measure airborne particulates and dissolved molecules and operate on such diverse principles as aerosol photometry, chemiluminescence, combustion, and polarography. Striking advances are being made in this area, and these instruments can be interfaced to remote samplers and automatic data collection systems.

9.2.4 Data Handling

Automatic data handling systems are used widely with current instruments. Many of the more sophisticated systems such as GC/MS are connected directly to computers to facilitate rapid identification and quantitation. Integrating calculators are used to handle data from GLCs, and, as mentioned previously, microprocessor-equipped IR and UV spectrophotometers simplify data manipulation.

Many data are calculated by hand, by measuring either peak heights or areas; by comparing these with known standards, one can quantitate amounts. Although many data are based on either external or internal standards, the calculated values are only as good as the efficiency of the analytical method. That is, does the method used in extracting and analyzing give a true concentration? This can be determined to a great extent by adding known amounts of the material being analyzed to a sample matrix known to be free of the toxicant. Analyzing these fortified or "spiked" samples along with the unknown will allow the analyst to determine the efficiency of the analytical method. Adding the same amount of material to solvent and analyzing it without performing the extraction and cleanup allows a further check on efficiency. Generally, at least an 80% recovery is considered necessary for an analytical method to be adequate, although some analytical methods effect only a 50–60% recovery. Recovery samples, in addition to indicating efficiency, can tell an analyst how well the instruments are functioning. Thus, one can correct data from a particular set of samples to reflect daily variation.

9.3 BIOASSAY

The term bioassay is used in two distinct ways. First, the narrow definition is the use of a living organism in an assay designed to measure the amount of a toxicant present in a sample or the toxicity of a sample. This is done by comparing the toxic effect of the sample with the toxic effect of a graded series of known amounts of a standard toxicant, ie, a standard curve. The second and less appropriate way is to use the word bioassay to include the use of animals to investigate the toxic effect of a toxicant. This latter is considered to be toxicity testing and is covered, in most of its many forms, in Chapter 8.

The bioassay technique has both advantages and disadvantages. It is the most nonspecific assay used for toxic chemicals since the endpoint most often used, the death of the organism, is common to many toxicants. On the other hand, it is rapid, inexpensive, and useful for obtaining an early indication of the equivalent toxicity of environmental samples. The effect of the environment on the toxicant can also be quickly ascertained.

The organisms most commonly used are aquatic and include plants as well as vertebrate and invertebrate animals. Some examples follow, and a list of species commonly used is shown in Table 9.3.

DAPHNIA.   Several tests using the water flea *Daphnia* are routinely conducted. They include screening tests to obtain an index of the toxicity of pure or mixed

TABLE 9.3
Some Organisms Commonly in Bioassay Procedures

Vertebrates
Fathead minnow, *Pimephales promelas*
Brook trout, *Solvelinus fontinalis*
Sheepshead minnow, *Cyprinodon variegatus*

Invertebrates
Water fleas, *Daphnia sp.*
Grass shrimp, *Palaemonetes sp.*
Shrimp, *Penaeus sp.*

Algae
Green algae (Chlorophytes): *Selenastrum capricornutum, Chlorella sp.*
Blue-green algae (Cyanophytes), *Anabaena flos-aquae*
Red algae (Rhodophyta), *Porphyridium cruentum*

compounds in water or waste treatment processes or to determine which of several processes may contribute to the eventual toxicity of plant effluents. A more standardized test is used for compliance with the National Pollution Discharge Elimination System, for which an index of the toxicity of effluents is required. The endpoint of the tests is acute lethality over a 24 to 48-hour period. The *Daphnia* used are cultured and the culture conditions must be carefully controlled to assure reproducibility. Factors of importance are species selection (eg, *D magna* or *D pulex*), age, nutrition, osmotic and ionic balance of the medium, light, and temperature. A variety of chronic and multigeneration tests can also be carried out using *Daphnia.*

Grass shrimp (*Palaemonetes* sp.) have been used in a variety of bioassays. They are used to identify toxic effluents and estimate pure compounds and to measure the toxic potential of dissolved pesticides, chlorine, metals, and industrial wastes. Several species have been used, but *P pugio* is used most commonly. Care must be taken with shipping and acclimatization to the medium. Mortality is usually the endpoint used with groups of 10–20 shrimp being exposed to each of five or six concentrations of the test compound. A positive control is also conducted using a compound of known toxicity.

ALGAE. Algal cultures are exposed to a range of concentrations of the test chemical or effluent and their growth rates are determined over a 4 to 5-day period. Physical conditions and the composition of the medium must be closely controlled and some convenient method must be used to determine growth rate. Because growth rate is quite variable, not only a number of concentrations are used, but also enough replicates to permit statistical analysis. Negative controls, without the test compound, and positive controls, with a compound of known toxicity to the species in question, are routinely included. Growth can be determined in one of many ways, including counting the cells manually under the light microscope, counting the cells in a cell counter, measuring chlorophyll fluorometrically, measuring ATP or measuring the assimilation of a suitable ^{14}C-labeled precursor.

FISH. Fish are also used as bioassay organisms. Although these bioassays require more time and laboratory space than the above, they have the advantage of using a vertebrate organism, presumably closer to mammals in activation and detoxication pathways as well as in mode of toxic action. The most useful species among freshwater species is the fat-head minnow, *Pimephales promelas,* and among saltwater species is the sheepshead minnow, *Cyprinodon variegatus.*

9.4 SUGGESTED FURTHER READING

American Public Health Association, American Water Works Association, and Water Pollution Control Federation. Standard Methods for the Examination of Water and Wastewater. 14th ed. New York: American Public Health Association, 1976.

Buikema, A.L., Cairns, J. (eds.). Aquatic Invertebate Bioassays. ASTM, Special Technical Publication No. 715. Philadelphia: ASTM, 1980.

Cairns, J., Dickson, K.L. Biological Methods for the Assessment of Water Quality. ASTM Special Technical Publication 528. Philadelphia: American Society for Testing and Materials, 1973.

Everson, R.J. Oehme, F.W. Analytical Toxicology Manual. Manhattan, Kan.: American College of Veterinary Toxicologists, 1981.

Frei, R.W., Hutzinger, O. (eds.). Analytical Aspects of Mercury and Other Heavy Metals in the Environment. New York: Gordon & Breach, 1975.

Glass, G.E. Bioassay Techniques and Environmental Chemistry. Ann Arbor, Mich.: Ann Arbor Science, 1973.

Keith, L.H. Identification and Analysis of Organic Pollutants in Water. Ann Arbor, Mich.: Ann Arbor Science, 1976.

National Academy of Sciences. Decision Making for Regulatory Chemicals in the Environment. Washington, D.C., National Academy of Sciences, 1975.

Pickering, W.F. Pollution Evaluation: The Quantitative Aspects. New York: Dekker, 1977.

Rand, G.M., Petrocelli, S.N. Fundamentals of Aquatic Toxicology. Washington, D.C.: Hemisphere, 1985.

Thoma, J.J., Bond, P.B., Sunshine, I. (eds.). Guideline for Analytical Toxicology Programs. Vols. 1 and 2. Cleveland: CRC Press, 1977.

Zweig, G. (ed.). Analytical Methods for Pesticides and Plant Growth Regulators. New York: Academic Press. (This is a multivolume series appearing since 1973 that contains analytical methods for the analysis of food and food additives, fungicides, herbicides, nematocides, pheromones, rodenticides, and soil fumigants.)

chapter ten

PREVENTION OF TOXICITY

Ernest Hodgson

10.1 INTRODUCTION

Laws and regulations provide the framework for organized efforts to prevent toxicity, and sanctions are necessary to prevent those without social conscience from deliberately exposing their fellows to risks from toxic chemicals. This is not enough, however, since without a population educated to toxic hazards and their prevention, the laws could never be properly administered. Moreover, in many circumstances, and particularly in the home, wisdom dictates courses of action not necessarily prescribed by law. The key to toxicity prevention lies in information and education, with legislation, regulation, and penalties as final safeguards. In all probability, the better the general population is educated and informed, the less likely are laws to be necessary.

10.2 LEGISLATION AND REGULATION

In the best sense, legislation provides an enabling act describing the areas to be covered under the particular law and the general way they are to be regulated, and designating an executive agency to write and enforce specific regulations within the intent of the legislative body. For example, the Toxic Substances Control Act was passed by Congress to regulate the introduction of chemicals into commerce, to determine their hazards to the human population and the environment, and to regulate or ban those deemed hazardous. The task of writing and enforcing specific regulations was assigned to the Environmental Protection Agency (EPA).

Legislative attempts to write specific regulations into laws usually fail. The resultant laws lack flexibility and, since they are written by lawyers rather than toxicologists, seldom address the problem in an appropriate manner.

It should be borne in mind that legislation is a synthesis of science, politics, and public and private pressure. It represents a society's best estimate, at that moment, of the risks it is prepared to take and those it wishes to avoid, as well as the price it is prepared to pay. Such decisions properly include more than science. The task of the toxicologist is to see that the science that is included is accurate and is logically interpreted.

This section (10.2) is based primarily on regulations in the United States, not because these are the best but because in toto they are the most comprehensive. In many respects, they are a complex mixture of overlapping laws and jurisdictions, providing unnecessary work for the legal profession. At the same time, few if any toxic hazards in the home, workplace, or environment are not addressed.

10.2.1 Federal Government: United States

The following is a summary of the most important federal statutes concerned in whole or in part with the regulation of toxic substances.

CLEAN AIR ACT. The Clean Air Act is administered by the EPA. Although the principal enforcement provisions are the responsibility of local governments, overall administrative responsibility rests with the EPA. This act requires criteria documents for air pollutants and sets both national air quality standards and standards for sources that create air pollutants, such as motor vehicles, power plants, etc. Important actions taken under this law include standards for a phased-out elimination of lead in gasoline and the setting of sulfuric acid air emission guidelines for existing industrial plants.

CLEAN WATER ACT. (Amends *Federal Water Pollution Control Act*) Also administered by the EPA, the Clean Water Act provides for funding of municipal sewage treatment plants but, with respect to toxicity prevention, it is more important that it regulates emissions from municipal and industrial sources. Some of the more important actions taken under this statute include setting standards for emissions of inorganics from smelter operations and publishing priority lists of toxic pollutants. This act allows the federal government to recover clean-up and other costs as damages from the polluting agency, company, or individual.

CONSUMER PRODUCTS SAFETY ACT (AND CONSUMER PRODUCTS SAFETY COMMISSION IMPROVEMENTS ACT). Administered by a Consumer Products Safety Commission, the Consumer Products Safety Act is designed to protect the public against risk of injury from consumer products and to set safety standards for such products.

CONTROLLED SUBSTANCES ACT. The Controlled Substances Act not only strengthens law enforcement in the field of drug abuse but also provides for research into the prevention and treatment of drug abuse.

FEDERAL FOOD, DRUG AND COSMETIC ACT. The Federal Food, Drug and Cosmetic Act is administered by the Food and Drug Administration (FDA). It establishes limits for food additives and cosmetic components, sets criteria for drug safety for both human and animal use and requires the manufacturer to prove both safety and efficacy. The FDA is authorized to define the required toxicity testing for each product. This act contains the Delaney clause, which states that food additives that cause cancer in humans or animals at any level shall not be considered safe and are, therefore, prohibited from such use. This law also empowers the FDA to establish and modify the generally recognized as safe list (GRAS) and to establish good laboratory practice (GLP) rules.

FEDERAL INSECTICIDE, FUNGICIDE AND RODENTICIDE ACT (FIFRA). Administered by the EPA, this act regulates all pesticides (and other agricultural chemicals, such as plant growth regulators) used in the United States. It includes registration requirements, with appropriate chemical and toxicological tests prescribed by the agency. This act also permits the agency to specify labels, to restrict application to certified applicators and to deny, rescind, or modify registration. Under this act, the EPA also establishes tolerances for residues on raw agricultural products.

OCCUPATIONAL SAFETY AND HEALTH ACT. Administered by the Occupational Safety and Health Administration (OSHA), the Occupation Safety and Health Act concerns health and safety in the workplace. OSHA sets standards for worker exposure to specific chemicals, for air concentration values, and for monitoring procedures. Construction and environmental controls also come under this act. It also provides for research, information, education, and training in occupational safety and health. By establishing NIOSH (National Institute for Occupational Safety and Health) the act provided for appropriate studies to be conducted so that regulatory decisions could be based on the best available information.

NATIONAL ENVIRONMENTAL POLICY ACT. The National Environmental Policy Act is an umbrella act covering all US government agencies, requiring them to prepare environmental impact statements for all federal actions affecting the quality of the human environment. Environmental impact statements must include not only an assessment of the effect of the proposed action on the environment but also alternatives to the proposed action, the relationship between local short-term use and enhancements of long-term productivity, and a statement of irreversible commitment of resources.

This act also created the Council on Environmental Quality, which acts in an advisory capacity to the president on matters affecting or promoting environmental quality.

RESOURCE CONSERVATION AND RECOVERY ACT. Also administered by the EPA, the Resource Conservation and Recovery Act is the most important act governing the disposal of hazardous wastes; it promulgates standards for identification of hazardous wastes, their transportation, and their disposal. Included in the latter are siting and construction criteria for landfills and other disposal facilities as well as the regulation of owners and operators of such facilities.

TOXIC SUBSTANCES CONTROL ACT. Administered by the EPA, the Toxic Substances Control Act is mammoth, covering almost all chemicals manufactured in the United States for industrial and other purposes, excluding certain compounds covered under other laws such as FIFRA. EPA may control or stop production of compounds deemed hazardous. Producers must give notice of intent to manufacture new chemicals or significantly increase production of existing chemicals. They may be required to conduct toxicity and other tests.

This law is as yet incompletely applied due to the enormous number of existing chemicals that must be evaluated. Once fully applied, it will be the most important statute affecting toxicology.

OTHER STATUTES WITH RELEVANCE TO THE PREVENTION OF TOXICITY. It should be noted that some of these statutes have been superseded by others, either in whole or in part.

Air Pollution Control Act, Air Quality Act

Comprehensive Employment and Training Act

Dangerous Cargo Act

Federal Coal Mine Health and Safety Act, Federal Coal Mine Safety and Health Amendment Act

Federal Caustic Poison Act

Federal Railroad Safety Authorization Act

Hazardous Materials Transport Act

Lead-Based Paint Poison Prevention Act

Marine Protection Research and Sanctuaries Act

Poison Prevention Packaging Act

Ports and Waterways Safety Act

10.2.2 State Governments

States are free to adopt legislation with toxicological significance although their jurisdiction does not extend beyond their geographic boundaries. In other cases, enforcement by the states of federal statutes is permitted under certain circumstances. For example, if regulations promulgated by the states for hazardous waste disposal are neither less comprehensive nor less rigorous than the federal statute, enforcement is delegated to the states. Similarly, certain aspects of FIFRA are enforced by individual states.

In some cases (California is notable in this respect), states have passed laws considerably more comprehensive and more rigorous than the corresponding federal statute.

10.2.3 Legislation and Regulation in Other Countries

It would serve little purpose to enumerate all the laws affecting toxicology, toxicity testing, and the prevention of toxicity that have been promulgated in all countries that have such laws. Legislation in this area has been adopted in most countries of western Europe and in Japan, however. Although the laws in use in the United States are a complex mixture of overlapping statutes and enforcement agencies, they are probably the most comprehensive set of such laws in existence. Most other industrialized countries have some legislation in the same areas, although the emphasis varies widely from one country to another. Many undeveloped countries, due to the lack of both trained manpower and financial resources, are unable to write and enforce their own code of regulations and instead adopt the regulatory decisions of either the United States or some other industrialized nation. For example, they will permit the use, in their own territory, of pesticides registered under FIFRA by the US EPA, but will prohibit the use of pesticides not so registered.

10.3 PREVENTION IN DIFFERENT ENVIRONMENTS

Humans spend their time in many environments. Homes vary with climate, family income, and personal choice. The workplace varies from pristine mountains to industrial jungles, whereas the outdoor environment from which recreation, food, and water are derived varies through the same extremes. Each of these environments has its own specific complex of hazards and thus requires its own set of rules and recommendations if these hazards are to be avoided.

10.3.1 Home

Approximately 50% of all accidental poisoning fatalities in the United States involve preschool children; thus, prevention of toxicity is particularly important in homes with young children.

Prescription drugs should always be kept in the original container (in the United States, these are now required to have safety closures). They should only be taken by the persons for whom they were prescribed, and excess drugs should be safely discarded when the illness is resolved. When children are present, prescription drugs should be kept in a locked cabinet, since few cabinets are inaccessible to a determined child. Although nonprescribed drugs are usually less hazardous, they are frequently flavored in an attractive way. Thus, it is prudent to follow the same rules as for prescription drugs.

Household chemicals such as lye, polishes, and kerosene should be kept in locked storage if possible but, if not, in as secure a place as possible, out of the reach of children. Such chemicals should never be stored in anything but the original containers—certainly beverage bottles, kitchen containers, etc., should never be used. Unnecessary materials should be safely disposed of in appropriate disposal sites.

Certain household operations such as interior painting, etc., should be done only with adequate ventilation. Insecticide treatment should be done precisely in accordance with instructions on the label.

Increasing fuel costs have caused several changes in life style, and some of these changes carry potential toxic hazards. They include more burning of wood and coal and the construction of heavily insulated houses with a concomitant reduction in ventilation. In the latter circumstances, improperly burning furnaces can generate high levels of CO and aromatic hydrocarbons, whereas even those burning properly may still generate oxides of nitrogen (NOx) at levels high enough to cause respiratory tract irritation in sensitive individuals. These effects can be avoided by ensuring that all heating equipment (furnaces, wood stoves, heaters, etc.) are properly maintained and regularly checked. In addition, some ventilation should always be provided. Less ventilation is needed when the temperature is either excessively high or excessively low and more is needed when the temperature is in the midrange, but under no circumstances should the homeowner strive for a completely sealed house.

10.3.2 Workplace

Exposure levels of hazardous chemicals in the air of work environments are mandated by OSHA as exposure limit values. The studies necessary to establish these limits are carried out by NIOSH. The more complete list of the better-known threshold limit values (TLVs) is established by the American Conference of Governmental Industrial Hygienists, however. Although TLVs are not binding in law, they are an excellent guide to the employer. In fact, they are often adopted by OSHA as exposure limit values. The concentrations thus expressed are the weighted average concentration normally considered safe for an exposure of 8 h/day, 5 days/week. Absolute upper limits (excursion values) may also be included. Some exposure limits are shown in Table 10.1.

Concentrations at or lower than those normal or working exposures are usually maintained by environmental engineering controls. Operations that generate large amounts of dusts or vapors are conducted in enclosed spaces that are separately vented or under hoods. Other spaces are adequately ventilated, and temperature and humidity controls are installed where necessary.

Other precautions must be taken to prevent accidental or occasional increases in concentrations. Materials should be transported in "safe" containers,

TABLE 10.1
Some Selected Threshold Limit Values (1982)

Chemical	TLV–TWA[a] (mg/m³)	TLV-STEL[b] (mg/m³)	TLV–C[c] (mg/m³)
Acetaldehyde	180	270	—
Boron trifluoride	—	—	3
Carbaryl	5	10	—
O-Dichlorobenzene	—	—	300
p-Dichlorobenzene	450	675	—
N-Ethylmorpholine	40	95	—
Phosgene	0.4	—	—
Trichloroethylene	270	805	—

[a] TLV–TWA, threshold limit value: time-weighted average concentration for a normal 8-hour work day and 40-hour work week to which nearly all workers may be repeatedly exposed without adverse effect.

[b] TLV–STEL, threshold limit value: short-term exposure limit concentration. This time-weighted 15-minute average exposure should not be exceeded at any time during a work day even if the TLV–TWA is within limits. Intended as supplement to TLV–TWA.

[c] TLV–C, threshold limit value–ceiling, a concentration that should not be exceeded at any time.

spilled material rapidly removed, and floor and wall materials selected to prevent contamination and allow easy cleaning.

Other methods for the prevention of toxicity in the workplace include the use of personal safety equipment — protective clothing, gloves, and goggles are the most important. In particularly hazardous operations, closed-circuit air masks, gas masks, etc., may also be necessary.

Preemployment instruction and preemployment physical examinations are of critical importance in most work situations involving hazardous chemicals. The former should make clear the hazards involved, the need to avoid exposure under normal working conditions, and the mechanisms by which exposure is limited. Furthermore, employees should understand how and when to contain spills and how and when to evacuate the area around the spill. Location and use of emergency equipment, showers, eye washes, etc., should also be given, and the most important procedures should be posted in the work area.

10.3.3 Pollution of Air, Water, and Land

The toxicological significance of pollution of the environment may be work related, as in the case of agricultural workers, or related to the outside environment encountered in daily life.

In the case of agricultural workers, numerous precautions are necessary for the prevention of toxicity. For example:

1. Pesticides and other agricultural chemicals should be kept only in the original container, carrying the label prescribed by EPA under FIFRA.
2. Empty containers and excess chemicals should be properly disposed of in safe hazardous waste disposal sites, incinerated when possible or, in some cases, decontaminated.
3. Workers should not reenter treated areas until the safe reentry period has elapsed.
4. Certain workers such as applicators, those preparing tank mixes, etc., should wear appropriate protective clothing, gloves, face masks, etc. The development of closed systems for mixing pesticides should help protect mixers and loaders of pesticides from exposure.
5. Spraying operations should be carried out in such a way as to minimize drift, contamination of water, etc.

Pesticides have caused a number of fatalities in the past. The current practice of restricting the most hazardous chemicals for use only by certified operators should greatly minimize pesticide poisoning.

Individuals can do little to protect themselves from poisoning by chemicals that pollute the air and water except to insist that discharge of toxicants into the environment be minimized. The exposure levels are low as compared with those in acute toxicity cases, and the effects may be indirect, as in the increase in preexisting respiratory irritation during smog. Thus, only at the epidemiological level can the effects be seen. Because many persons are not affected or may not be affected for years, it is often argued that environmental contamination is not very important. A small percentage increase may represent a large number of people when the whole population is considered, however. Furthermore, chronic toxicity is not often reversible. Because in most industrialized countries laws already exist to control emission problems, if such problems exist they are usually problems of enforcement.

One of the most critical areas for the prevention of toxicity caused by environmental contamination is that of disposal of hazardous wastes. It is now apparent that past practices in many industrialized countries have created large numbers of waste sites in which the waste is often unidentified, improperly stored, and leaching into the environment. The task of rectifying these past errors is an enormous one just now being addressed.

The ideal situation for current and future practices is to reduce chemical waste to an irreducible minimum and then to place the remainder in secure storage. Waste reduction can be accomplished in many ways.

1. Refine plant processes so that less waste is produced.
2. Recycle waste into useful products.
3. Concentrate wastes.
4. Incinerate. The technology is available to incinerate essentially all waste to inorganic slag.

Safe storage for the remaining waste may be in dump sites or in above-ground storage. In either case, such storage should ideally be properly sited, constructed, maintained, and monitored.

Because of the nature of commerce, probably none of these measures will be successful unless the laws, penalties, and incentives are manipulated in such a way as to make safe disposal more attractive economically than unsafe disposal.

10.4 EDUCATION

Because chemicals, many of them hazardous, are an inevitable part of life in industrialized countries, education is probably the most important method for the prevention of toxicity. Unfortunately, it is also one of the most neglected. In a typical public debate concerning a possible chemical hazard, the principle protagonists tend to fall into two extreme groups. The "everything is ok" protagonists and the "ban it completely" protagonists. The media seldom seem to educate the public, usually serving only to add fuel to the flames.

The educational role of the toxicologist should be the voice of reason, presenting a balanced view of risks and benefits, and outlining alternatives whenever possible. The simple lesson that science deals not in certainty, but rather degrees of certitude, must be learned by all involved.

In terms of ongoing educational programs, there should be opportunities at all levels: elementary schools, high schools, university, adult education, and media education. Several approaches can be used to educate the general public, in ideal situations:

Elementary schools—teach the rudiments of first aid and environmental concerns—proper disposal, etc.

High school—teach concepts of toxicology (dose response, etc.) and environmental toxicology (bioaccumulation, etc.). These concepts can be introduced into general science courses.

University—in addition to toxicology degrees, in general courses for nontoxicology and/or nonscience majors stress a balanced approach, with both responsible use and toxicity prevention as desirable endpoints.

Media—encourage a balanced approach to toxicity problems. Toxicologists should be available to media representatives and, where appropriate, should be involved directly.

10.5 SUGGESTED FURTHER READING

American Conference of Governmental Industrial Hygienists. TLVs—Threshold Limit Values for Chemical Substances and Physical Agents in the Work Environment with Intended Changes. Cincinnati (published annually).

American Conference of Governmental Industrial Hygienists. Documentation of the Threshold Limit Values for Substances in Workroom Air. Cincinnati (published annually).

Arena, J.M. Poisoning: Toxicology, Symptoms and Treatments. 4th ed. Springfield, Ill.: Charles C Thomas, 1979.

Dreisbach, R.H. Handbook of Poisoning: Prevention, Diagnosis and Treatment. 11th ed. Los Altos, Calif.: Lange Medical, 1983.

Environmental Regulation: An International View. A series of papers on: I. Britain—T.W. Hall; II. European Economic Community—S.P. Johnson; III. The United States—J.B. Ritch, Jr.; IV. An Industry View—R.C. Tineknell. Chem. Soc. Rev. 1976; 5:431–471.

Sandmeyer, E.E. Regulatory Toxicology. Chapter 20. In A Guide to General Toxicology. Homberger, F., Hayes, J.A., Pelikan, E.W. (eds.). Basel: Karger, 1983.

chapter eleven

DIAGNOSIS AND TREATMENT OF TOXICITY

Ernest Hodgson

11.1 INTRODUCTION

It should be made clear at the outset that this chapter is not a manual on how to treat the poisoned individual. It is a brief summary without the necessary details even for adequate first aid and designed only to introduce the student to the most important principles involved. Except for first aid, treatment of poisoning is the province of the medical practitioner, and even first aid is best rendered by those with specific training in the area, or at the very least those who have carefully reviewed such manuals as those written by Dreisbach or Arena (see Section 11.6). After removing the victim from contact with the suspected poison, the most useful action to be taken by someone without appropriate training is to call the nearest source of emergency medical care, Emergency Rescue Squad, the local police, or the nearest hospital emergency room. Poison Control Centers are available as sources of information. They are invaluable as a backup for physician and emergency medical personnel.

Most of the material in this chapter is related to acute toxicity. Chronic toxicity rarely constitutes an immediately life-threatening crisis and is, in any case, less responsive to therapy.

11.2 DIAGNOSIS

11.2.1 Introduction

Following appropriate first aid (see Section 11.3.1), the removal of the poisoning victim from contact with the poison, and steps to prevent further absorption of the poison, the physician is required to make a diagnosis so that the treatment most appropriate to the specific compound can be initiated. Because the poisoning victim is frequently a child or, if an adult, may be comatose, it is often

319

necessary to rely on parents, friends, eye-witnesses or an examination of the scene (containers, etc.) for useful background details.

Relative to the toxicant involved, patients will fall into three classes. In the first class are those patients who have absorbed a known poison. The physician must initiate appropriate emergency treatment and estimate the quantity absorbed in order to approach further therapy with greater confidence. A maximum estimate can sometimes be determined from the amount missing from the container. Although fatal doses determined on experimental animals may not be similar to those for humans, they do give a rough idea of relative toxicity.

In the second class of poisoning, patients are known to be poisoned but the actual toxicant is unknown, usually because the poison is a complex mixture. The physician's task is to attempt to identify the toxicant, a task made difficult by the numerous trade names and proprietary mixtures. Some lists and reference sources are available, however (Table 11.1). In addition, the nearest poison control center is a source of information, as is the manufacturer. It is important that the first person on the scene or anyone rendering first aid to a poisoning victim sends the container, if available, with the patient when the patient is moved to the hospital or emergency center. Naturally, it should be resealed and properly packed to ensure that it does not cause further problems. Similarly, if the victim vomits, the vomitus should be collected and placed in a jar, and should accompany the patient. If the toxicant can be identified, appropriate therapy can be initiated; otherwise, the physician must rely on nonspecific life-support measures while the vomitus, urine, feces, or blood is analyzed.

In the third class are those patients in whom the physician must carry out the differential diagnosis of a disease that may or may not be the result of poisoning. This consists of a complete case history, a complete physical examination, and appropriate laboratory tests.

11.2.2 Case History

The case history may be obtained from the victim or from parents, friends, neighbors, or eye-witnesses. The various individuals should be questioned separately to avoid overlooking important items. It is important to consider the occupation of the patient and whether the patient was at his normal job at the time of the poisoning.

There are many known occupational hazards, including the following types of poisoning:

CO poisoning may occur among blacksmiths, furnace or foundry workers, brick or cement makers, chimney cleaners, service-station attendants, parking attendants, garage workers, miners, refinery workers, plumbers, police officers, and sewer workers.

Poisoning by chlorinated hydrocarbons, particularly solvents, occurs among rubber cement and plastic cement workers or users, leather workers, dry cleaners, painters, furniture finishers, cloth finishers, paint removers, and rubber workers.

Lead poisoning occurs among welders, steamfitters, plumbers, painters, ceramic workers, battery makers, miners, pottery makers, electroplaters, printers, service-station attendants, and junk-metal refiners.

TABLE 11.1
Some Sources of Information on the Identity of Toxic Chemicals

A. Published works
1. *General*
Likes, K.E. (ed.). Toxifile. Chicago: Chicago Micro Corporation (microfiche).
Rumack, B.H. (ed.). Poisindex. Denver: National Center for Poison Information (microfiche).
———. The Merck Index. Rahway, N.J.: Merck and Co. 10th Ed., 1983.
Wexler, P. Information Resources in Toxicology. New York: Elsevier. Important guide to directories, reference works, data bases, organizations, etc.

2. *Commercial and Industrial Chemicals*
———. Trade Names Index. American Conference of Governmental Industrial Hygienists. Cincinnati. 1965 with annual supplements.
Gosselin, R.E., et al. Clinical Toxicology of Commercial Products. Baltimore: Williams & Wilkins. 4th Ed., 1976.

3. *Prescription Drugs*
Wilson, C.O., Jones, T.E. American Drug Index. Philadelphia: Lippincott. Published annually.
———. Physicians Desk Reference. Oradell, N.J.: Medical Economics. 40th Ed., 1986.
———. Hospital Formulary. Washington, D.C.: American Society of Hospital Pharmacists, Published annually.

4. *Non-Prescription Drugs*
Griffenhagen, G.G. (ed.). Handbook of Non-Prescription Drugs. American Pharmaceutical Association. Washington, D.C. Published annually.

5. *Drugs of Abuse*
Lowry, W.T., Gamiott, J.C. Forensic Toxicology: Controlled Substances and Dangerous Drugs. NY: Plenum Press, 1979.

6. *Pesticides*
Caswell, R.L. (ed.). Pesticide Handbook. College Park, Md.: Entomological Society of America. Published annually.
Farm Chemicals Handbook. Willoughby, Ohio: Meister. Published annually.

B. Computer data bases
1. Toxicology Data Base, Toxicology Information Science. National Library of Medicine. 8600 Rockville Pike, Bethesda, MD 20014.

2. TOXLINE. Toxicology Information Science. National Library of Medicine. 8600 Rockville Pike, Bethesda, MD 20014.

C. Telephone sources
1. Poison Control Center—See Directory of Poison Control Centers. Bulletin of National Clearinghouse for Poison Control Centers 1980:24(8). Also Wexler (Section A.1. this table).

2. Chemical manufacturers.

Methanol poisoning occurs among bookbinders, bronzers, rubber and plastic cement users, dry cleaners, leather workers, printers, painters, and woodworkers.

Many other types of poisoning are characteristic of particular tasks; the above are illustrative examples.

If the poisoning incident occurred in the home, the patient, the patient's home, and the immediate surroundings must be searched for poison containers. It is also important to check for possible ingestion of food, drink, and medicines; contact with insecticides or other agricultural chemicals; exposure to fumes; smoke or gases; or skin contact with liquids such as insecticides or cleaning solvents.

11.2.3 Systemic Examination

The systemic examination covers various general aspects of function as well as observations that bear on particular organ systems. Although such examinations are useful and should always be performed, it should also be borne in mind that individual variation in humans is so great that in any particular case typical symptoms may not be present.

Blood pressure and pulse rate are often important general indicators. For example, blood pressure may be high in nicotine poisoning or low in poisoning by nitrites, arsenic, or fluorides. Similarly, a fast pulse may indicate poisoning by atropine, and a slow or irregular pulse may indicate poisoning by nitrites. Weight loss, lethargy, and weakness are often symptoms of chronic poisoning by such toxicants as lead and mercury, whereas an elevated body temperature is typical of poisoning with nitrophenols.

The skin is among the first tissues examined in a systemic examination. For example, cyanosis (a bluish color, especially of the lips) may indicate hypoxia or methemoglobinemia caused by nitrites, aniline, etc., whereas redness or flushing may indicate poisoning by CO or cyanide. Jaundice, a yellow color visible in the skin and the eyes, may be due to quite different forms of poisoning—for example, liver injury, caused by compounds such as carbon tetrachloride, and hemolysis, caused by compounds such as aniline or arsine. Overt damage to the skin, such as burns or corrosion, may be caused by acids, alkalis, or strong oxidizing agents such as permanganate or dichromate.

Effects on the central nervous system (CNS) may be indicated by a variety of physical, behavioral, or psychological symptoms. Muscular twitching and convulsions may be caused by a number of different insecticides, by nicotine, by amphetamines, or by many other toxicants. Headaches may be caused by poisoning with organophosphate insecticides, CO, etc. Depression, drowsiness, and coma often follow barbiturate overdose or poisoning by ethanol, various industrial solvents, and many other chemicals. Delirium or hallucinations may follow ingestion of excessive alcohol, amphetamines, cocaine, or other chemicals. Metals such as thallium, lead, or mercury, as well as drugs such as antihistamines and barbiturates, may cause confusion or similar mental changes.

Examination of the head, including the eyes, ears, nose, and mouth may provide valuable clues as to the nature of the toxicant involved in poisoning cases, with the eyes being perhaps the most valuable diagnostic indicator. For example, blurred vision may result from poisoning with such chemicals as atropine, phosphate ester insecticides, cocaine, or methanol, whereas double vision can result from alcohol, barbiturates, nicotine, or phosphate ester insecticides. Dilated pupils can be caused by atropine and related drugs, cocaine, nicotine, solvents, and depressants. Contracted pupils can be due to morphine and related drugs, physostigmine and related drugs, or phosphate ester insecticides.

Indicators of toxicity problems related to the ears include tinnitus, deafness, or disturbances of equilibrium, any of which may be caused by compounds such as quinine or salicylates.

Examples of diagnostic features associated with the mouth include loosening of teeth and painful teeth due to heavy metal poisoning, dry mouth associated with atropine and related drugs, and excessive salivation due to poisoning by phosphate ester insecticides and heavy metals.

Symptoms related to the cardiorespiratory system are respiratory difficulty, including dyspnea or exertion, chest pain, and decreased vital capacity caused by a wide variety of toxicants, including salicylates, cyanide, CO, atropine, strychnine, and ethanol. Rapid respiration may be due to cyanide, atropine, cocaine, carbon monoxide, salicylates, alcohol, or amphetamine. Slow respiration, on the other hand, may be due to such chemicals as barbiturates, morphine or antihistamines but, paradoxically, may also be caused by cyanide, CO, etc.

Although symptoms related to the GI system may be valuable in diagnosis, some, such as vomiting, diarrhea, and abdominal pain, may be caused by almost any poison. A less common symptom, blood in the stool, may be caused by coumarin anticoagulants, thallium, iron, salicylates, and a number of corrosive materials.

Dysfunctions of the urinary system include anuria, the inability to excrete urine, which may result from poisoning with mercurials, carbon tetrachloride, formaldehyde, turpentine, oxalic acid, chlordane, castor beans, and many other compounds; proteinuria, the appearance of protein in the urine, may result from arsenic, mercury, or phosphorus poisoning, for example. Hematuria, hemoglobinuria, or myoglobinuria, the appearance of blood, hemoglobin or myoglobin, respectively, in the urine, may also be indicative of particular poisons and, in some of these cases, the color of the urine may also be a useful indicator.

Effects on the neuromuscular system may often be difficult to distinguish from effects on the CNS, particularly muscular weakness or paralysis, which may be due to lead, arsenic, organic mercurials, thallium, triorthocresyl phosphate, carbon disulfide, and other compounds. Tremors, muscle stiffness, and muscle cramps may also be useful diagnostic indicators.

The laboratory examination is a critical part of the diagnostic process and deals primarily with the blood or other body fluids. A brief summary of the appropriate tests is shown in Table 11.2.

11.3 NONSPECIFIC THERAPY

Nonspecific therapy may be defined as therapy designed to maintain vital signs, decrease uptake, and increase elimination of the toxicant but which, at the same time, is not related directly to the specific mode of action of the toxicant.

11.3.1 First Aid and Emergency Management

Untrained people should rarely find it necessary to render first aid, but should never do so if the victim is either unconscious or is having convulsions. In any case of poisoning or suspected poisoning professional help — the nearest Poison

TABLE 11.2
Summary of Laboratory Tests Performed During Systemic Examination of Poison Victims

Test Type	Symptom	Example of Possible Cause
A. Blood, gross and microscopic appearance	Leukopenia, agranulocytosis	Aminopyrine, phenylbutazone
	Anemia	Lead, naphthalene, chlorates, solanine, and other plant poisons
	Cherry-red color	CO, cyanide
	Chocolate color (methemoglobin)	Nitrates, nitrites, aniline, dyes, chlorates
B. Blood, serum, or plasma chemistry	Glucose (whole blood)	Increased after thiazide diuretics or adrenal glucocorticoids; decreased after salicylates, lead or ethanol
	Uric acid (serum)	Increased after thiazide diuretics or ethanol
	Potassium (serum or plasma)	Increased after thiazide diuretics or ethanol
	Bromide	Serum chloride is spuriously increased in bromism because the standard tests (eg, AutoAnalyzer) measure total halides

C. Special chemical examinations useful in diagnosis of poisoning: Analysis of lead or other heavy metals, insecticides, cholinesterase, barbiturates, alkaloids, etc., may be necessary in the diagnosis of poisoning.

Source: Dreisbach, R.H. Handbook of Poisoning. 11th ed. Los Altos, Calif.: Lange Medical, 1983.

Control Center, hospital emergency room, or Emergency Rescue Squad — should be contacted immediately. With conscious patients, vomiting will then probably be induced, preferably with syrup of ipecac. This is never done, however, in cases of ingestion of acids, bases, or any petroleum product. In cases of inhaled toxicants, the victim is moved to fresh air. In cases of poisoning by dermal contamination, the skin is drenched with water; the clothing is removed from the affected area, after which the affected area is washed with soap and water. With eye contamination, the eye is washed with a gentle stream of water at fountain or under a faucet.

In any poisoning case in which the patient's breathing is depressed, artificial respiration is given, preferably by direct inflation. If available, oxygen may be given. Chemical antidotes should not be given. In the case of an overdose of an injected drug, either prescription or drug of abuse, a tourniquet may be applied at the proximal side of the injection site.

In all poisoning cases, the patient should be kept warm, and either a physician should be brought to the site or transport of the patient to a treatment facility should be arranged. Because identification of the poison may be critical, anyone rendering first aid should be sure that the poison (in a properly sealed container) or vomited material, is sent to the treatment facility with the patient. Any information as to what the victim was doing at the time of the poisoning, which chemicals are in use at the site, the physical characteristics and trade names of bulk chemicals at the site, etc., should all be communicated to the treating physician.

11.3.2 Life Support

Further emergency treatment that may be carried out at the treatment center includes:

MAINTENANCE OF RESPIRATION AND CIRCULATION.   Maintenance of respiration involves maintaining an adequate airway, if necessary by catheter, tracheostomy, or cricothyroid puncture, and also maintaining adequate pulmonary ventilation. This last may be by direct, mouth-to-mouth inflation or by a portable resuscitator. Oxygen can be administered if available.

Circulatory failure is usually the result of shock; in this case, emergency therapy appropriate to shock is initiated immediately. The patient is placed in a supine position with lower limbs elevated, body warmth is maintained by blankets, an adequate airway is assured, and adequate circulating blood volume is restored and maintained. If the fall in blood pressure is severe, appropriate drug therapy is initiated along with plasma transfusion.

EMESIS.   Emesis is best accomplished with syrup of ipecac but never after poisoning with corrosives (acids or bases) or petroleum derivatives. In the former case, the esophagus is subjected to further corrosive attack; in the latter, the risk of aspirating stomach contents is unacceptably high.

GASTRIC LAVAGE.   In gastric lavage, special precautions are taken in the case of corrosives since the lavage tube may damage the esophagus or, in the case of petroleum derivatives, when the trachea should be intubated with a tube with an inflatable cuff. In convulsing patients, the convulsions should first be controlled. Materials used for gastric lavage include milk (for corrosives or to retard uptake), lemon juice (for alkali poisoning), activated charcoal suspension, saline, sodium bicarbonate, or milk of magnesia. Sodium bicarbonate is never given in the case of poisoning by acids, since the carbon dioxide generated may damage the stomach.

GASTROTOMY.   Gastrotomy may be necessary if large quantities of solid matter (eg, tablets, capsules, etc.) are present that cannot be removed by lavage.

CATHARSIS OR INTESTINAL LAVAGE.   Catharsis or intestinal lavage is not used in poisoning with corrosives, if electrolyte balance is disturbed, or if there is renal impairment.

11.3.3 Nonspecific Maintenance Therapy

Nonspecific maintenance therapy is largely a continuation of the procedures outlined above and is designed to maintain vital signs on a long-term basis. One should bear in mind that during this phase of the treatment good nutrition is important. This can be done intravenously (IV) or by stomach tube if necessary, but per os is preferable. In general, energy metabolism is most important, and excess fat and protein is avoided to reduce stress on the liver and kidneys. Pain can also contribute to functional difficulties, particularly in the case of shock. The treating physician may elect to relieve pain with meperidine (Demerol), since morphine is often counterindicated. This is particularly true in the case of CNS depression, respiratory difficulties, or liver involvement.

MAINTENANCE OF WATER AND ELECTROLYTE BALANCE.   The means by which water and electrolytes are replaced are usually not critical in the absence of kidney impairment; however, they may become critical if renal function is impaired. Electrolytes and/or water are lost in urine, feces, expired air, sweat, and vomiting, and must be replaced either orally or IV. Simple calculations that indicate the necessary amount can be made based on body weight and serum ion analysis. Glucose may also be given to provide an energy source.

Acidosis may be due to the generation of an acidic metabolite such as formic acid from methanol, by loss of base, or by CO_2 retention. These problems are usually addressed by maintaining an adequate airway and giving artificial respiratory to prevent CO_2 retention or by giving sodium bicarbonate either IV or orally.

MAINTENANCE OF NORMAL BODY TEMPERATURE.   Neither hyperthermia nor hypothermia is desirable in the poisoned patient. The former increases metabolic rate and hence the O_2 requirement as well as the requirements for food and water. The latter, while reducing the metabolic rate, also reduces the rate of detoxication and the elimination of both the toxicant and its metabolites.

Because of the additional involvement of the detoxication system which would be entailed, chemical intervention in the case of hyperthermia is not recommended. The use of wet towels, cooling blankets, and air circulation is more appropriate. Similarly, in the case of hypothermia, total or partial immersion in warm water is recommended. Local heating is not appropriate because of the effect on skin capillaries.

CNS INVOLVEMENT.   Toxic chemicals can cause convulsions by a number of mechanisms such as stimulation of peripheral receptors that affect the CNS by causing O_2 lack (hypoxia) or by inducing hypoglycemia. Because convulsions can be life-threatening, due to effects such as respiratory failure caused by spasms of the respiratory muscles or to postconvulsion depression, the treating physician will usually take emergency measures. Such measures may include artificial respiration in the postconvulsion period and restraint to prevent injury. The patient is kept in quiet surroundings and neither emesis nor gastric lavage is attempted unless failure to do so might cause death. Anticonvulsant drugs can be used but none which might cause either coma or respiratory depression. Fluid balance is maintained, an adequate airway is assured, and glucose is given to treat hypoglycemia.

Coma caused by poisons generally results from effects on brain cell function. Emergency measures include maintaining an adequate airway, aspirating mucus from the nose and mouth, giving artificial respiration, treating for shock, and giving gastric lavage with activated charcoal. These treatments are continued; attention is given to fluid balance, renal function and, eventually, if the coma persists, to tube feeding and to dialysis to eliminate the toxicant.

Hyperactivity and delirium occur with certain toxicants. Treatment is in part psychological and is designed to reduce tension. Hydrotherapy may be used for the same reason and, if absolutely necessary, drugs such as paraldehyde or scopolamine may be administered.

Hypoglycemic convulsions and coma are treated by administration of glucose, using the most appropriate route.

RESPIRATORY INVOLVEMENT.   Many poisons affect respiration, either directly or indirectly. The effects include hypoxia, respiratory depression, and pulmonary edema. Several principles are involved in all respiratory problems, including maintaining an adequate airway, adequate pulmonary ventilation, and an adequate O_2 supply. Adequate airway is maintained either by the oropharyngeal method, using a metal or plastic airway or the tracheal method using a catheter, tracheostomy, or cricopharyngeal puncture (an opening in the cricopharyngeal cartilage), a procedure that can be done by a physician when other methods are not immediately possible. Adequate pulmonary ventilation can be assured by artificial respiration or a respirator while O_2 can be administered directly. Pulmonary edema is first treated with morphine sulfate, oxygen, and aminophylline. Subsequently, diuretics and corticoid anti-inflammatory agents may be prescribed.

CIRCULATORY SYSTEM INVOLVEMENT.   The treatment of one of the most common involvements, shock, has been mentioned. Congestive heart failure may result from poisons that cause myocardial damage. This is treated with rest, sodium restriction and, in serious cases, digitalis. Cardiac arrest may result from asphyxiation, CO, etc. Emergency treatment consists of chest massage and artificial respiration. Subsequently, 0.9% saline is given IV, and epinephrine is injected and/or defibrillation is attempted. In short, all of the techniques available to the physician for the treatment of cardiac arrest, whatever the cause, may be attempted.

URINARY TRACT INVOLVEMENT.   The principle problems in urinary tract involvement are renal failure and fluid retention. The former is treated by methods designed to restrict fluid retention until function can be restored. They include fluid restriction and oral administration of salts. If recovery does not occur within a few days or if blood creatine rises, dialysis should be carried out. Urine retention can be treated by catheterization.

INVOLVEMENT OF THE GI TRACT.   Involvement of the GI tract can include vomiting, diarrhea, and distension of the abdomen. Although the first is often initially beneficial, vomiting eventually causes a loss of fluid balance. It can be treated by glucose administered IV in saline until vomiting stops, followed by dry foods in small quantity, followed by fluids. If drugs such as chlorpromazine or promethazine are not contraindicated by the nature of the poison or by other medical considerations, the treating physician may prescribe them to be given orally or in suppositories.

Similarly, diarrhea may affect fluid balance, which must also be corrected by IV glucose while food intake is restricted to liquids or low-residue foods. Drugs used include codeine or atropine; pectin–kaolin mixtures may also be effective.

Distension of the abdomen is usually due to gas; it can be released by proper use of a rectal or colonic tube or intestinal intubation.

HEPATIC INVOLVEMENT.   Liver damage can be acute, as is often the case with chloroform, carbon tetrachloride, etc., or chronic, as may occur with ethanol. Characteristically, liver enzymes are found at elevated levels in the serum, eg, glutamic-oxalacetic transaminase, glutamic-pyruvic transaminase, lactic dehydrogenase, and alkaline phosphatase. In addition, the blood bilirubin level is increased and bilirubin is also found in the urine. Urine urobilinogen is also increased. Usually, all drugs are discontinued and the patient is maintained under conditions of complete bed rest. Other symptoms such as vomiting are controlled; the diet, when eating can be resumed, is one with low protein, low fat, and high carbohydrate content.

BLOOD SYSTEM INVOLVEMENT.   Methemoglobin formation is brought about by the oxidation of ferrous (Fe^{2+}) hemoglobin to ferric (Fe^{3+}) hemoglobin, usually as a result of such toxicants as nitrites, chlorates, etc. The reaction can be reversed by methylene blue. On an emergency basis, O_2 is also administered. Hemolytic reactions may occur, particularly in persons with glucose-6-phosphate dehydrogenase deficiency. Urine flow must be maintained; if renal failure is imminent (high serum hemoglobin), an exchange transfusion may be necessary.

11.4 SPECIFIC THERAPY

When the toxicant can be identified with certainty, a specific antidote or combination of antidotes may be available. Such therapies, when available, are often rapid and reliable. Unfortunately, for many toxicants specific antidotes are not known; in many poisoning cases, it is not clear precisely which toxicant is involved or whether a mixture of toxicants is involved. Finally, even with known toxicants for which a specific antidote is available, the damage may have reached a point at which the antidote is no longer effective.

11.4.1 Categories of Specific Therapy

Specific therapy may be based on activation and detoxication reactions, mode of action, or elimination of the toxicant. Examples of the types of specific therapy are presented in Table 11.3. The examples in Section 11.4.2 are chosen to illustrate the principles involved. In some cases, several antidotes, with different modes of action, are available for the same toxicant; this is also illustrated by specific examples.

11.4.2 Specific Examples

The structures of the toxicants and antidotes used as examples in this section are shown in Figure 11.1.

TABLE 11.3
Examples of Therapy Related to Mode of Action of Specific Toxicants

Mechanism	Poison	Therapeutic Agent
A. Metabolism of toxicant		
Competition for activation reaction	Methanol	Ethanol
Stimulation of detoxication mechanism	Cyanide	Thiosulfate
B. Direct effect of toxicant		
Complexing agents	Lead	CaEDTA
C. Effects on receptor site		
Competition for receptor	CO	O_2
Receptor blocking	Carbaryl	Atropine
D. Repair mechanism		
Reversal of toxic effect	Parathion	2-PAM
	Nitrite	Methylene blue
Bypass of toxic effect	Methotrexate	Thymidine adenine and glycine
E. Facilitation of excretion		
Administration of physiologically similar molecules	Bromide	Chloride

2-PAM, N-methypiridinium 2 aldoxime.

11.4.2.1 Methanol

Methanol is a common cause of poisoning and results in a number of deaths annually. The acute effects appear to be due to the formation of formaldehyde by the action of alcohol dehydrogenase and subsequently formic acid by the action of aldehyde oxidase. Formaldehyde has been shown to affect the retina and is probably the cause of the blindness associated with methanol poisoning, whereas formic acid causes the acute acidosis also associated with this toxicant.

Various nonspecific treatments include induction of vomiting with syrup of ipecac and the use of gastric lavage; acidosis is countered by administration of sodium bicarbonate, and urine flow is maintained by oral or IV fluids. If the patient fails to respond to specific or nonspecific therapy, dialysis is performed.

The specific therapy for methanol poisoning is the administration of ethanol, initially orally and subsequently IV. The ethanol acts by competition for alcohol-metabolizing enzymes, thus permitting the excretion of methanol before it is activated to formaldehyde and formic acid. The toxicity of the acetaldehyde and acetic acid formed from ethanol is low as compared with that of formaldehyde and formic acid.

11.4.2.2 Cyanide

Hydrogen cyanide and its salts have a variety of uses, and cyanide ion may be released metabolically from a number of secondary plant chemicals. It acts primarily by inhibiting cytochrome oxidase, thus blocking cellular respiration (see Section 6.2.3.1a). Other enzymes are also inhibited by cyanide, but the effects are relatively unimportant as compared with those caused by the rapid,

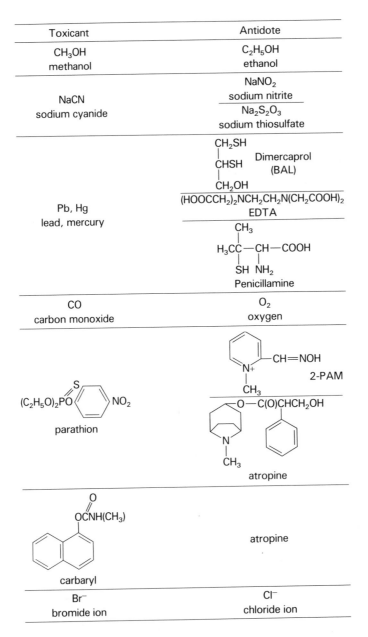

Toxicant	Antidote

FIGURE 11.1.
Toxicants and antidotes used in examples of specific therapy.

extensive, and high-affinity binding to cytochrome oxidase. Although the toxic dose is very small and the resultant poisoning is rapid and often fatal, chronic poisoning due to prolonged exposure to very small amounts is known.

Emergency measures for either inhaled or ingested cyanide include amyl nitrite, artificial respiration, and 100% O_2. In the case of ingestion, gastric lavage may also be used.

There are two forms of specific therapy. Sodium nitrite is administered to convert hemoglobin to methemoglobin. The latter then combines with cyanide to form cyanomethemoglobin. Although the affinity of cyanide for methemoglobin is less than its affinity for cytochrome oxidase, the large amount of hemoglobin available makes this a useful therapy. Methemoglobinemia itself is hazardous, however, and the nitrite dose must be so calculated to cause no more than 25–40% conversion of hemoglobin. In the second form of specific therapy, thiosulfate is administered to provide a sulfur donor for the reaction, catalyzed by the enzyme cyanide-thiosulfate sulfur transferase, which converts cyanide to thiocyanate (CN^- to SCN^-). Thus, the two specific therapies represent one case in which there is removal from the site of action by competition with another binding site, and one in which a detoxication mechanism is stimulated by providing a reactant that is normally rate-limiting in vivo. When these two specific antidotes are assessed in an experimental setting (eg, by their effect on the LD50 for cyanide) they are clearly synergistic, being much more than additive in their effect.

11.4.2.3 Heavy Metals (Lead and Mercury)

Although chronic lead poisoning is thought of as the most common and dangerous form, particularly among children, acute lead poisoning is also a hazard. In acute lead poisoning, the unabsorbed lead compound must be removed either by gastric lavage with dilute magnesium or sodium sulfate solution or by emesis. Subsequently, urine flow must be maintained, and chelation therapy must be started. Dimercaprol and CaEDTA both function by chelating the lead and rendering it excretable. These two drugs are given by injection; subsequently, penicillamine can be given orally. The treatment is monitored by following blood and urine lead concentrations.

Inorganic mercury, particularly in the form of mercuric salts, can be acutely toxic or can give rise to chronic toxicity. In acute poisoning, gastric lavage or emesis is used to remove unabsorbed material. Subsequently, dimercaprol is used to complex the mercury and render it excretable. Dialysis can be used to speed elimination if necessary. Dimercaprol is also used to treat chronic mercury poisoning.

Organic compounds of heavy metals, such as tetraethyl lead and methyl mercury, can also cause serious poisoning. They differ from the inorganic ions in uptake, toxicokinetics, mode of action, and therapy and should be treated separately.

11.4.2.4 Carbon Monoxide

Carbon monoxide (CO) is a common cause of poisoning, both deliberate, as in suicide attempts, and accidental. CO is produced by the incomplete combustion of fossil fuels, in automobiles, in industrial machinery, in home furnaces, etc., and exerts its toxic effects by binding reversibly, but with high affinity, to hemoglobin. It not only forms carboxyhemoglobin, thus occupying sites normally occupied by O_2, but also increases the affinity of unbound sites for O_2, thus impairing the release of O_2 to the tissues. Because the affinity of CO is 250 times that of O_2, it is imperative to remove the victim from the source of CO.

The patient is kept at rest to reduce O_2 demand. The specific therapy involves competition for the receptor, hemoglobin, by the physiological ligand, O_2. Respiration is maintained artificially, and either O_2 or a mixture of 95% O_2 and 5% CO_2 is administered. Because the affinity of CO is high, the use of high O_2 concentration is critical.

Although not often available, the use of a compression chamber at about two atmospheres is extremely helpful. Not only is more O_2 available to compete for hemoglobin, but the increased solubility allows some transport by the plasma.

11.4.2.5 Organophosphorus Cholinesterase Inhibitors

Organophosphorus cholinesterase inhibitors are compounds that exert their toxic effects by phosphorylating cholinesterase, thus bringing about its inhibition and preventing the breakdown of acetylcholine, giving rise to a situation in which the acetylcholine receptors remain occupied (see Section 6.2.2.1). Because death is the result of respiratory failure, the maintenance of an adequate airway and artificial respiration are of critical importance. Two forms of specific therapy are available. Atropine is used immediately since it competes with acetylcholine for the receptor site, thus preventing the toxic effects of an excess of this neurotransmitter. Subsequently, N-methylpyridinium 2-aldoxime (2-PAM) is used in conjunction with atropine since it reacts with the phosphorylated cholinesterase and removes the phosphorylating group, thus restoring the enzyme to normal activity. One should bear in mind that the use of two antidotes with different modes of action can be synergistic. In this case, the combination of 2-PAM and atropine can be 50 times as effective as might be expected from a simple additive effect.

11.4.2.6 Carbamate Cholinesterase Inhibitors

Although the overall mode of action is the same as that of organophosphorus compounds as noted above, the carbamylated cholinesterase is less stable than the phosphorylated enzyme, and its regeneration cannot be accelerated by 2-PAM. Thus, although the nonspecific therapy is the same, only atropine is used as a specific antidote, 2-PAM being without effect.

11.4.2.7 Bromide

Bromide ion is toxic, but its excretion can be stimulated by administering excess chloride. Excess chloride is normally excreted by the kidney, and the active transport mechanism cannot distinguish between the two ions. This is not a particularly rapid method, but fortunately bromide ion is neither particularly toxic nor particularly fast-acting.

11.5 CHRONIC TOXICITY

Chronic toxicity caused by chemicals is frequently not reversible nor susceptible to specific antidotes. The most extreme form, cancer, requires surgical intervention or the use of relatively nonspecific cellular poisons or radiation therapy. Certain forms of chronic toxicity involving the accumulation of chemicals that are not readily eliminated may be alleviated by therapy designed to facilitate excretion of the toxicant.

Treatment of neoplastic diseases depends on total destruction of the tumor cell type: if by surgery, all of the tumor must be removed; if by chemotherapy, all of the tumor cells must be killed, unlike in bacterial and virus diseases, in which a significant reduction in the causative organism permits the immune system to reassert its normal function. Thus, surgery alone is successful only when the tumor is discrete and readily removed in toto. Most chemotherapeutic drugs are cytotoxic but have been shown to affect tumor cells somewhat more readily than other cells. Toxic side effects are common, and the toxic dose is often close to the therapeutic one. Only the great benefit involved (saving life) justifies the risk. These chemotherapeutic agents include alkylating agents such as cyclophosphamide and antimetabolites such as methotrexate, as well as alkaloids, antibiotics, enzymes, and metal coordination complexes (eg, vincristine, asparaginase, and cisplatin, respectively). All appear to act at one or more points in the nucleic acid replication/protein synthesis cycles.

The use of chelation therapy as described for acute lead poisoning can also be used to facilitate excretion of accumulated lead in chronic lead poisoning. A dramatic example of the treatment of chronic toxicity by the facilitation of excretion is that developed for kepone (chlordecone) poisoning. Although the compound is readily excreted through the bile, it is reabsorbed from the intestine (enterohepatic circulation). Feeding cholestyramine, an ion-exchange resin that can bind kepone, interrupts the cycle and permits the excretion of kepone at a rate some sevenfold higher than in the untreated patient.

11.6 SUGGESTED FURTHER READING

Arena, J.M. Poisoning: Toxicology; Symptoms; Treatments. 4th ed. Springfield, Ill.: Charles C Thomas, 1979.

Dreisbach, R.H. Handbook of Poisoning. 11th Ed. Los Altos, Calif.: Lange Medical, 1983.

Goldsten, A., Aronow L., Kalman, S.M. Principle of Drug Action: The Basis of Pharmacology. New York: Wiley, 1974. (See Chapter 5 – Drug Toxicity.)

Guzelian, P.S. Chlordecone poisoning: A case study in approaches for detoxification of humans exposed to environmental chemicals. Drug Metab. Rev. 1982; 13:663–679.

Haddad, L.M., and Winchester, J.F. Clinical Management of Poisoning and Drug Overdose. Philadelphia: W.B. Saunders, 1983.

Loomis, T.A. Essentials of Toxicology. 3rd Ed. Philadelphia: Lea & Febiger, 1978. (See Chapter 11.)

Rumack, B.H., Peterson, R.G. Clinical Toxicology. Chapter 27. In Doull, J., Klaassen, C.D., Amdur, M.O. (eds.). Casarett and Doull's Toxicology. New York: Macmillan, 1980.

chapter twelve

LITERATURE OF TOXICOLOGY

Ernest Hodgson

12.1 INTRODUCTION

It should be evident by now that the literature of toxicology has, during the last decade, undergone an enormous expansion in all its aspects and that the task of keeping abreast of the literature currently being generated is a formidable one. Not only does it involve toxicology itself but also important related sciences such as chemistry, biochemistry, pharmacology, and statistics. Often from such related sciences new methodology and concepts arise that are of inestimable benefit in advancing the science of toxicology.

Although the recent expansion has given rise to textbooks and monographs, as well as review and primary journals, devoted exclusively to toxicology or one of its branches, the pattern of previous years was somewhat different. Journals devoted primarily to related sciences such as pharmacology or biochemistry mostly carried a small proportion of articles on toxicological subjects. This pattern has continued along with the newer, more specialized publications. An even more recent development, of great promise for the future, is the availability of readily accessed computer data bases and the technology necessary for the establishment of personal computer-based information retrieval systems. The sections that follow give examples of all of the various sources through which information on toxicology, in all its aspects, is obtained. The reader is referred to *Information Resources in Toxicology* by Phillip Wexler, an excellent resource in itself, in which all aspects of this subject are developed in considerable detail.

12.2 TEXTBOOKS

Although many monographs are in print or in press, some of which are, of necessity, used as textbooks, few toxicology books are written specifically for the classroom. Casarett and Doull's *Toxicology* is probably the best example of such a monograph and it is used widely as a textbook. Textbooks in toxicology include the following:

Ariens, E.J., Simonis, A.M., Offermeier, J. Introduction to General Toxicology. New York: Academic Press, 1976. An abbreviated treatment of toxicology in general. Now somewhat out of date but still useful as a starting point.

Brusick, D. Principles of Genetic Toxicology. New York: Plenum Press, 1980. Covers the area of genetic toxicology in a comprehensive manner, including mutagenesis tests and testing protocols.

Guthrie, F.E., Perry, J.J. Introduction to Environmental Toxicology. New York: Elsevier, 1980. A general introduction to environmental toxicology with case histories as well as principles.

Hodgson, E., Guthrie, F.E. Introduction to Biochemical Toxicology. New York: Elsevier, 1980. A general introduction to the biochemical principles involved in absorption, transport, metabolism, mode of action, and excretion of toxicants.

Lippman, M., Schlesinger, R.B. Chemical Contamination and the Human Environment. New York: Oxford University Press, 1979.

Loomis, T.A. Essentials of Toxicology. Philadelphia: Lea & Febiger, 1978. 3d ed. A concise introduction to the field, probably the most popular of the short treatments.

Purdom, P.W. Environmental Health. New York: Academic Press, 1980. A textbook that covers the effects of the environment on humans, including infection, toxic chemicals, and physical effects.

Timbrell, J.A. Principles of Biochemical Toxicology, London: Taylor and Francis, 1982.

12.3 MONOGRAPHS, CONFERENCE PROCEEDINGS, REVIEW AND PRIMARY RESEARCH JOURNALS

The following sections are arranged by subject matter and contain examples that are in print at the time of writing. A limited number of monographs and conference proceedings are presented, with a more detailed list of review and primary journals. Series of monographs grouped together by the publisher are not considered review journals; each is considered a separate monograph. The reader should always bear in mind that many publications could, with some justification, be placed in several different sections but that, in the interest of space, a choice was made.

12.3.1 General Toxicology

12.3.1.1 Monographs

Doull, J., Klaassen, C.D., Amdur, M.O. Casarett and Doull's Toxicology. New York: Macmillan, 1980. The most comprehensive and widely used monograph in general toxicology.

Gralla, E.J. Scientific Considerations in Monitoring and Evaluating Toxicological Research, Washington, D.C.: Hemisphere, 1981. Stresses quality control and accuracy throughout the entire scope of toxicological testing.

Hayes, A.W. Principles and Methods of Toxicology. New York: Raven Press, 1982. Although nominally a methodology book, this also contains much general toxicology.

Homburger, F., Hayes, J.A., Pelikan, E.W. (eds.). A Guide to General Toxicology. Basel: Karger Press, 1983.

12.3.1.2 Conference Proceedings

Galli, C.L., Murphy, S.D., Paoletti, R. Principles and Methods in Modern Toxicology. Amsterdam: Elsevier/North Holland, 1980. Proceedings of an international course on the principles and methods of modern toxicology held at Belgirate, Italy, in 1979.

Mehlman, M.A., Shapiro, R.E., Cranmer, M.F., Norvell, R.J. Hazards from Toxic Chemicals, Park Forest, Ill.: Pathotox, 1978. Proceedings of the Second Annual Conference on the Status of Predictive Tools in Application to Safety Evaluation.

Plaa, G.L., Duncan, W.A.M. Proceedings of the First International Congress on Toxicology: Toxicology as a Predictive Science. Lancaster, England: MTP Press, 1979; also New York: Academic Press, 1978.

12.3.1.3 Review Journals

CRC Critical Reviews in Toxicology. Boca Raton, Fla: Chemical Rubber Co. 1971 –.

Environmental Health Perspectives. Research Triangle Park, N.C.: National Institute of Environmental Health. 1972 –.

Toxicology Annual. Dekker, New York, 1974 –.

Reviews of general toxicological interest are also found in such general journals as Annual Reviews of Pharmacology and Toxicology, Pharmacology and Therapeutics, etc.

12.3.1.4 Primary Research Journals

Archives of Toxicology

Drug and Chemical Toxicology

Fundamental and Applied Toxicology

Journal of Applied Toxicology

Journal of Environmental Pathology and Toxicology

Journal of Toxicology and Environmental Health

Risk Analysis

Toxicologic Pathology

Toxicology

Toxicology and Applied Pharmacology

Toxicology Letters

Articles of toxicological interest appear in many pharmacology, biochemistry, and pathology journals as well as journals of general science.

12.3.2 Agricultural Chemicals

12.3.2.1 Monographs

Hayes, W.J. Toxicology of Pesticides. Baltimore: Williams & Wilkins, 3d ed. 1975.

Hayes, W.J. Pesticides Studied in Man. Baltimore: Williams & Wilkins, 1982.

Matsumura, F. Toxicology of Insecticides. New York: Plenum Press, 1975.

Wilkinson, C.F. Insecticide Biochemistry and Physiology. New York: Plenum Press, 1976.

12.3.2.2 Conference Proceedings

Khan, M.A.Q., Lech, J.J., Menn, J.J. Pesticide and Xenobiotic Metabolism in Aquatic Organisms. Washington, D.C.: American Chemical Society, 1979.

Moreland, D.M., St. John, J.B., Hess, F.D. Biochemical Responses Induced by Herbicides. Washington, D.C.: American Chemical Society, 1982.

Rosen, J.D., Magee, P.S., Casida, J.E. Sulfur in Pesticide Action and Metabolism. Washington, D.C.: American Chemical Society, 1981.

Chambers, J.E., Yarbrough, J.D. Effects of Chronic Exposures to Pesticides on Animal Systems. New York: Raven Press, 1982.

12.3.2.3 Review Journals

Residue Reviews. New York: Springer-Verlag, 1962.

12.3.2.4 Primary Research Journals

Journal of Environmental Sciences and Health, Part B: Pesticides, Food Contaminants, and Agricultural Wastes

Pesticide Biochemistry and Physiology

12.3.3 Analytical Toxicology

12.3.3.1 Monographs

Baselt, R.C. Biological Monitoring Methods for Industrial Chemicals. Davis, Calif.: Biomedical Publications, 1980.

Sunshine, I. Methodology for Analytical Toxicology. Boca Raton, Fla.: CRC Press, 1975.

Thoma, J.J., Bondo, P.B., Sunshine, I. Guidelines for Analytical Toxicology Programs. 2 vols. Boca Raton, Fla.: CRC Press, 1977.

12.3.3.2 Conference Proceedings

Schuetzle, D. Monitoring Toxic Substances. Washington, D.C.: American Chemical Society, 1979.

12.3.3.3 Primary Research Journals

Journal of Analytical Toxicology

12.3.4 Behavioral Toxicology

12.3.4.1 Conference Proceedings

Weiss, B., Laties, V. B. Behavioral Toxicology. New York: Plenum Press, 1972. Collection of papers presented at the Fifth Rochester International Conferences on Environmental Toxicity, University of Rochester, 1972.

Xintaras, C., Johnson, B.L., de Groot, I. Behavioral Toxicology: Early Detection of Occupational Hazards, Washington, D.C.: Government Printing Office, 1974. Proceedings of a behavioral toxicology workshop sponsored by the US Department of Health, Education and Welfare, Public Health Service, Center for Disease Control and the National Institute for Occupational Safety and Health.

12.3.4.2 Primary Research Journals

Neurobehavioral Toxicology

12.3.5 Biochemical Toxicology

12.3.5.1 Monographs

de Bruin, A. Biochemical Toxicology of Environmental Agents. Amsterdam: Elsevier/North Holland, 1976. Although now somewhat outdated, this is an extensive compendium with a particularly comprehensive list of references.

Caldwell, J., Jakoby, W.B. Biological Basis of Detoxication. New York: Academic Press, 1983.

Jakoby, W.D. Enzymic Basis of Detoxication. New York: Academic Press, 1980. 2 vols.

Jakoby, W.B., Bend, J.R., Caldwell, J. Metabolic Basis of Detoxication. New York: Academic Press, 1982.

See also Hodgson and Guthrie, as well as Timbrell (Section 11.2).

12.3.5.2 Conference Proceedings

Boobis, A.R., Caldwell, J., DeMatteis, F., Elcombe, C.R. Microsomes and Drug Oxidations. London: Taylor and Francis, 1985. Proceedings of a conference held in Brighton, England, 1984.

Coon, M.J., Cooney, A.H., Estabrook, R.W., Gelboin, H.V., Gillette, J.R., O'Brien, P.J. Microsomes, Drug Oxidations and Chemical Carcinogenesis.

New York: Academic Press, 1980. Proceedings of an International Symposium held at Ann Arbor, Michigan, in 1979.

Gustaffson, J., Carlstedt-Duke, J., Mode, A., Rafter, J. Biochemistry, Biophysics and Regulation of Cytochrome P-450. Amsterdam: Elsevier/North Holland, 1980.

Snyder, R., Parke, D.V., Kocsis, J.J., Jallow, D.J., Gibson, C.G., Witmer, C.M. Biological Reactive Intermediates II. New York: Plenum Press, 1982, Parts A and B. Proceedings of the 2nd International Symposium on Biological Reactive Intermediates held at Guilford, Surrey, England, in 1980.

12.3.5.3 Review Journals

Foreign Compound Metabolism in Mammals. London: The Chemical Society, 1970–.

Reviews in Biochemical Toxicology. New York: Elsevier, 1979–.

Reviews in the general area of biochemical toxicology are frequently found in such review journals as the *Annual Review of Pharmacology and Toxicology, Drug Metabolism Reviews,* and *Pharmacology and Therapeutics.*

12.3.5.4 Primary Research Journals

Chemico-Biological Interactions

Xenobiotica

Research articles in biochemical toxicology are frequently found in such journals as *Biochemical Pharmacology, Drug Metabolism and Disposition,* and *Molecular Pharmacology.*

12.3.6 Carcinogenesis, Mutagenesis, and Teratogenesis

12.3.6.1 Monographs

de Serres, F.J., Ashby, J. Evaluation of Short-Term Tests for Carcinogenesis. New York: Elsevier, 1981. Extensive consideration of all aspects of mutagenesis testing and short-term tests for carcinogenesis.

Grover, P.L. Chemical Carcinogenesis and DNA. Boca Raton, Fla.: CRC Press, 1979. Thorough coverage of the title topic with excellent literature citations.

Juchau, M.R. The Biochemical Basis of Chemical Teratogenesis. New York: Elsevier, 1981. Extensive review of the mechanisms by which chemicals affect development.

12.3.6.2 Conference Proceedings

Demopoulus, H.B., Mehlman, M.A. Cancer and the Environment: an Academic Review of the Environmental Determinants of Cancer Relevant to Prevention. Park Forest South, Ill.: Pathotox, 1980. A symposium held in conjunction with the American Cancer Society.

De Serres, F.J., Fouts, J.R., Bend, J.R., Philpot, R.M. In Vitro Metabolic

Activation in Mutagenesis Testing. New York: Elsevier, 1976. A symposium held in Research Triangle Park, N.C., by the National Institute of Environmental Health Sciences.

Emmelot, P., Kriek, E. Environmental Carcinogenesis: Occurrence, Risk Evaluation and Mechanisms. Amsterdam: Elsevier/North Holland, 1979. Proceedings of an international conference on environmental carcinogenesis held in Amsterdam in 1979.

12.3.6.3   Primary Research Journals

Carcinogenesis

Environmental Mutagenesis

Mutation Research

Teratogenesis, Carcinogenesis and Mutagenesis

Teratology

12.3.7   Clinical and Human Toxicology

12.3.7.1   Monographs

Arena, J.M. Poisoning: Toxicology-Symptoms — Treatment. Springfield, Ill.: Charles C Thomas, 1979. 4th ed. In-depth treatment of both common and unusual poisons.

Dreisbach, R.H. Handbook of Poisoning: Diagnosis and Treatment. Los Altos, Calif.: C.A. Lange, 1983. 11th ed. Well-referenced summary of important poisons.

Gosselin, R.E., Hodge, H.C., Smith, R.P., Gleason, M.N. Clinical Toxicology of Commercial Products. Baltimore: Williams & Wilkins, 1976. 4th ed. An extensive compendium of all aspects of poisoning by chemicals. This is updated monthly and is regarded by many as the definitive reference in clinical toxicology.

12.3.7.2   Primary Research Journals

Clinical Toxicology

Clinical Toxicology Consultant

International Journal of Clinical Pharmacology, Therapy and Toxicology

Human Toxicology

12.3.8   Drugs and Cosmetics

12.3.8.1   Monographs

Gorrod, J.W. Drug Toxicity. London: Taylor and Francis, 1979.

Grundmann, E. Drug-Induced Pathology. New York: Springer-Verlag, 1980.

Opdyke, D.L.J. Monographs on Fragrance Raw Materials. Oxford: Pergamon Press, 1979.

12.3.8.2 Conference Proceedings

Schwarz, R.H., Yaffe, S.J. Drugs and Chemical Risks to the Fetus and New-born. New York: Liss, 1980. Symposium held in New York in 1979.

Soda, T. Drug-Induced Suffering: Medical, Pharmaceutical and Legal Aspects. Amsterdam: Excerpta Medica, 1980. Proceedings of a symposium held in Kyoto, Japan, in 1979.

12.3.8.3 Review Journals

Drug Metabolism Reviews. New York; Dekker, 1972–.

Side Effects of Drugs Annual. Amsterdam: Excerpta Medica, 1977–.

12.3.8.4 Primary Research Journals

Drug and Chemical Toxicology

Drug Metabolism and Disposition

Food and Cosmetics Toxicology (also contains short reviews)

Food, Drug and Cosmetic Law Journal

12.3.9 Environmental Toxicology

12.3.9.1 Monographs

McKinney, J.D. Environmental Health Chemistry: The Chemistry of Environmental Agents as Potential Human Hazards. Ann Arbor, Mich.: Ann Arbor Science, 1981.

Rand, G.M., Petrocelli, S.R. Fundamentals of Aquatic Toxicology. Washington, D.C.: Hemisphere, 1985.

Vershueren, K. Handbook of Environmental Data on Organic Chemicals. 2d ed. New York: Van Nostrand Reinhold, 1983.

12.3.9.2 Conference Proceedings

Eaton, J.G., Parrish, P.R., Hendricks, A.C. Aquatic Toxicology. American Society for Testing Materials, Philadelphia, Pennsylvania, 1980. Proceedings of the Third International Symposium on Aquatic Toxicology held in New Orleans in 1978.

Fouts, J.R., Gut, I. Industrial and Environmental Xenobiotics: In Vitro Versus In Vivo Biotransformation and Toxicity. Medica, Amsterdam, 1978, Proceedings of an international congress held in Prague in 1977.

Hammond, E.C., Selikoff, I.J. Public Control of Environmental Hazards. New York: New York Academy of Science, 1979.

12.3.9.3 Review Journals

Environmental Health Perspectives. Research Triangle park, N.C.: National Institute of Environmental Health Sciences, 1972–.

Reviews in Environmental Toxicology. Amsterdam: Elsevier Biomedical Press, 1984 –.

Toxicological and Environmental Chemistry Reviews. New York: Gordon & Breach, 1972.

12.3.9.4 Primary Research Journals

Aquatic Toxicology

Archives of Environmental Contamination and Toxicology

Archives of Environmental Health

Bulletin of Environmental Contamination and Toxicology

Ecotoxicology and Environmental Safety

Environmental Research

Environmental Toxicology and Chemistry

International Archives of Occupational and Environmental Health

Journal of Environmental Pathology and Toxicology

Journal of Environmental Sciences and Health. (Part C has been discontinued as Environmental Health Sciences and is now Environmental Carcinogenesis Reviews.)

Journal of Toxicology and Environmental Health

12.3.10 Food Additive Toxicology

12.3.10.1 Monographs

Graham, H.D. The Safety of Foods. 2d ed. Westport, Conn.: AVI, 1980.

Furia, T.E. Handbook of Food Additives. Boca Raton, Fla.: CRC Press, Vol. 1, 1972; vol. 2, 1980.

Vettarazzi, G. Handbook of International Food Regulatory Toxicology. Jamaica, N.Y.: Spectrum, 1980.

12.3.10.2 Conference Proceedings

Galli, C.L., Paoletti, R., Vettorazzi, G. Chemical Toxicology of Foods. Amsterdam: Elsevier/North Holland, 1978. Proceedings of an international symposium held in Milan.

12.3.11 Forensic Toxicology

12.3.11.1 Monographs

Curry, A.S. Advances in Forensic and Clinical Toxicology. Boca Raton, Fla.: CRC Press, 1972.

Curry, A.S. Poison Detection in Human Organs. 3rd ed. Springfield, Ill.: Charles C Thomas, 1976.

12.3.11.2 Conference Proceedings

> Oliver, J.S. Forensic Toxicology. Croom Helm, London, 1980. Proceedings of the European Meeting of the International Association of Forensic Toxicologists.

12.3.12 Legislative and Societal Aspects of Toxicology

12.3.12.1 Monographs

> Environmental Law Handbook. 7th ed. Washington, D.C.: Government Institute, 1983. Reference book and important introduction to many aspects of environmental law.

> Environmental Statutes. Washington, D.C.: Government Institute, 1980. The complete text of all important statues in the area of environmental law.

> Vettorazzi, G. International Regulatory Aspects for Pesticide Chemicals. Boca Raton, Fla.: CRC Press, 1979.

12.3.12.2 Conference Proceedings

> Miller, M.L. Toxic Control in the 80's. Washington, D.C.: 1980. Government Institutes, Proceedings of the 4th Toxic Control Conference held in Washington, D.C., in 1979.

12.3.12.3 Review Journals

> Environmental Law. Portland, Oregon: Northwestern School of Law, Lewis and Clark College, 1970–.

12.3.12.4 Primary Research Journals

> Columbia Journal of Environmental Law
> Ecology Law Quarterly
> Environmental Management
> Food, Drug and Cosmetic Law Journal
> Hazardous Materials Management Journal
> Regulatory Toxicology and Pharmacology

12.3.13 Metal Toxicology

12.3.13.1 Monographs

> Berman, E. Toxic Metals and Their Analysis. London: Heydon, 1980.

> Friberg, L., Nordberg, G.F., Vouk, V.B. Handbook on the Toxicology of Metals. Amsterdam: Elsevier/North Holland, 1979.

> Nriagu, J.O. A series of titles, including the following:

>> The Biogeochemistry of Mercury in the Environment. Amsterdam: Elsevier/North Holland, 1979;

The last four in the series were published by Wiley, New York, 1980.

Cadmium in the Environment;

Copper in the Environment;

Nickel in the Environment;

Zinc in the Environment.

12.3.14 Nutritional Toxicology

12.3.14.1 Monographs

Calabrese, E.J. Nutrition and Environmental Health: The Influence of Nutritional Status on Pollutant Toxicity and Carcinogenicity. New York: Wiley, 1980. 2 vols.

Wurtman, R.J. Toxic Effects of Food Constituents on the Brain. New York: Raven Press, 1979.

12.3.14.2 Primary Research Journals

Many papers related to nutritional toxicology appear in nutrition journals such as the *Journal of Nutrition.*

12.3.15 Occupational Health and Industrial Hygiene

12.3.15.1 Monographs

Anderson, K.E., Scott, R.M. Fundamentals of Industrial Toxicology. Ann Arbor, Mich.: Ann Arbor Science, 1981. Summary of most essential areas of industrial toxicology.

Calabrese, E.J. Methodological Approaches to Deriving Environmental and Occupational Health Standards. New York: Wiley, 1978.

Patty's Industrial Hygiene and Toxicology. 3rd ed. Rev. Volume I — General Principles, 1978; Volume II — Toxicology, 1980; and Volume III — Theory and Rationale of Industrial Hygiene Practice, 1979. New York: Wiley. Many editors and authors, the most complete reference work for industrial hygiene and health.

12.3.15.2 Review Journals

Recent Advances in Occupational Health. Edinburgh: Churchill Livingstone, 1981.

12.3.15.3 Primary Research Journals

American Industrial Hygiene Association Journal

American Journal of Industrial Medicine

Hazardous Materials Management Journal

International Archives of Occupational and Environmental Health

Journal of Occupational Medicine

12.3.16 Organ Toxicity

12.3.16.1 Monographs

Hook, J.B. Toxicology of the Kidney. New York: Raven Press, 1981.

Mitchell, C.L. Nervous System Toxicology. New York: Raven Press, 1981.

Plaa, G.L., Hewitt, W.R. Liver Toxicity. New York: Raven Press, 1981.

von Stee, E.W. Cardiovascular Toxicology. New York: Raven Press, 1981.

Witschi, H., Nettersheim, P. Mechanisms in Respiratory Toxicology. Boca Raton, Fla.: CRC Press, 1981.

12.3.16.2 Conference Proceedings

Chambers, P.L., Gunzel, P. Mechanisms of Toxic Action on Some Target Organs. Berlin: Springer-Verlag, 1979. A supplement to Archives of Toxicology consisting of the proceedings of a meeting of the European Society of Toxicology held in Berlin in 1978.

Environmental Health Perspectives. Research Triangle Park, N.C.: National Institute of Environmental Health Sciences. Although nominally a general journal in the title area, this journal has included a long series of special volumes, each of which consists of the proceedings of a conference on the toxicology of a particular organ or organ system.

Manzo, L. Advances in Neurotoxicology, Oxford: Pergamon Press, 1980. Proceedings of an International Congress of Neurotoxicology held in Varese, Italy, in 1979.

12.3.16.3 Primary Research Journals

Neurotoxicology

12.3.17 Physical Agents

12.3.17.1 Monographs

Harm, W. Biological Effects of Ultraviolet Radiation. Cambridge: Cambridge University Press, 1980.

Prasad, H.N. Human Radiation Biology. Hagerstown, Md.: Harper & Row, 1974.

Tobias, J.V., Jansen, G., Ward, W.D. Noise as a Public Health Hazard. Rockville, Md.: American Speech-Language-Hearing Association, 1980.

12.3.17.2 Conference Proceedings

Illinger, K.H. Biological Effects of Ionizing Radiation. Washington, D.C.: American Chemical Society, 1981.

12.3.17.3 Primary Research Journals

Health Physics

International Journal of Radiation Biology and Related Studies in Physics, Chemistry and Medicine

Radiation Research

12.3.18 Toxins

12.3.18.1 Monographs

Bucherl, W., Buckley, E.E., Devlofue, V. Venomous Animals and Their Venoms. 3 vols. New York: Academic Press, 1968–1971.

Habermeyl, G.G. Venomous Animals and Their Toxins. Berlin: Springer-Verlag, Berlin, 1981.

Hayes, W.A. Mycotoxin Teratogenicity and Mutagenicity. Boca Raton, Fla.: CRC Press, 1981.

Kingsbury, J.M. Poisonous Plants of the United States and Canada. Englewood Cliffs, N.J.: Prentice-Hall, 1964.

Uraguchi, K., Yamazaki, M. Toxicology, Biochemistry and Pathology of Mycotoxins. New York: Halstead, 1978.

12.3.18.2 Conference Proceedings

Eaker, D., Wadstrom, T. Natural Toxins. Oxford: Pergamon Press, 1980. Proceedings of the 6th International Symposium on Animal, Plant and Microbial Toxins held at Uppsala, Sweden, in 1979.

12.3.18.3 Primary Research Journals

Toxicon

12.3.19 Veterinary Toxicology

12.3.19.1 Monographs

Buck, W.B., Osweiler, G.D., VanGelder, G.A. Clinical and Diagnostic Veterinary Toxicology. 2nd ed. Dubuque, Iowa: Kendall/Hunt, 1976.

Clarke, E.G.C., Clarke, M.L. Veterinary Toxicology. London: Bailliere Tindall, 1975.

Osweiler, G.D., Carson, T.L., Buck, W.B., VanGelder, G.A. Clinical and Diagnostic Veterinary Toxicology. 3d ed. Dubuque, Iowa: Kendall/Hunt, 1985.

12.3.19.2 Conference Proceedings

Keeler, R.F., van Kampen, K.R., James, L.F. Effects of Poisonous Plants on Livestock. New York: Academic Press, 1978. Proceedings of a joint US—Australian symposium on poisonous plants held at Logan, Utah in 1978.

12.3.19.3 Primary Research Journals

Veterinary and Human Toxicology

12.4 JOURNALS IN RELATED AREAS

The reader should always keep in mind that much toxicology is to be found in journals not specifically toxicological in nature. The number of such journals is too large to permit easy listing, but they can be classified into two general types.

The first group contains specialty journals serving other related disciplines, particularly, but not only, pharmacology and biochemistry. The following journals are examples of this category.

Advances in Pharmacology and Chemotherapy

Fate of Drugs in the Organism

Journal of the National Cancer Institute

Cancer Research

Journal of Nutrition

Pharmacology and Therapeutics

Drug Metabolism Reviews

Journal of Biological Chemistry

Archives of Biochemistry and Biophysics

Biochimica et Biophysica Acta

The second group contains journals in general science that occasionally carry articles of toxicological interest. Some of these, such as *Science* or *Nature,* are highly selective and of wide circulation and, as a result, the toxicology in them, although infrequent, is likely to be of importance. The following journals are examples.

Experientia

Naturwissenschften

Journal of the American Medical Association

Lancet

12.5 INTERNATIONAL DOCUMENTS, GOVERNMENT DOCUMENTS, AND MISCELLANEOUS SOURCES OF INFORMATION

12.5.1 International Documents

The principal origin of international documents relative to toxicology is various agencies of the United Nations. The most important of these are:

Environmental Health Criteria. A series of documents released at intervals since 1976 that include studies of metals: eg, mercury, 1976; lead, 1977; tin and organotin compounds, 1980; pesticides, eg, DDT and its derivatives, 1979; atmospheric pollutants, eg, oxides of nitrogen, 1977; and other toxicants.

International Agency for Research on Cancer (IARC). Monographs on the evaluation of the carcinogenic risk of chemicals to humans. A long series of reports evaluating such compounds as polycyclic aromatic hydrocarbons, organochlorine pesticides, aromatic azo compounds, asbestos, polychlorinated biphenyls, (PCBs) and polybrominated biphenyls. Series also includes supplements summarizing earlier volumes.

IARC Scientific Publications. Another extensive series covering various aspects of carcinogenesis including screening tests, epidemiology, chemical carcinogenesis in the laboratory, directories of ongoing carcinogenesis research, etc.

12.5.2 National Documents

National documents are a mixture of both well-known and relatively obscure sources of information. One of the more important is the series entitled "Medical and Biological Effects of Environmental Pollutants" published by the National Academy of Sciences. This long series includes comprehensive reports on such pollutants as arsenic, copper, lead, nitrogen oxides, polycyclic organic matter, etc.

Among the annual and other reports, those of the National Toxicology Program are the most comprehensive, summarizing the status of chemicals being tested for carcinogenesis as well as the results of completed tests. Others of importance include the status reports of CIIT, the Chemical Industries Institute for Toxicology, and various other reports of the Environmental Protection Agency, including those on TSCA, the Toxic Substances Control Act. The annual listing of threshold limit values (TLVs) by the American Conference of Governmental Industrial Hygienists is also of importance, as are the criteria documents issued by the National Institute for Occupational Safety and Health (NIOSH) and the Occupational Safety and Health Administration (OSHA).

Other sources of information for toxicologists are the many organizations that promote either the field in general or some specialized aspect of it. They include the following:

Society of Toxicology. The most important organization in toxicology; it offers student membership and has both regional and speciality sections. National and regional meetings.

American College of Toxicology. Recently formed, has national meetings.

International Society for the Study of Xenobiotics.

Society of Environmental Toxicology and Chemistry.

The American Chemical Society has several sections that are directly applicable to toxicology, including: Agricultural and Food Chemistry; Agrochemicals; Environmental Chemistry.

The following organizations are more specialized.

American Academy of Clinical Toxicology

American Society of Forensic Science

American College of Veterinary Toxicology

American Industrial Hygienists Association

International Society on Toxicology

12.6 ABSTRACTS, INDEXES, AND COMPUTER SERVICES

In view of the enormous amount of literature available in toxicology, the rate at which literature appears, and the wide diversity of outlets through which it is released, toxicologist must rely on some combination of abstracting or indexing services and computer data bases to supplement the information obtained from journals to which they or their library subscribes.

12.6.1 Abstracting Services

The most important general abstracting publications are *Biological Abstracts, Chemical Abstracts,* and *Excerpta Medica.*

Biological Abstracts. Philadelphia: Bioservices Information Service of Biological Abstracts, 1926 –. Covers most if not all the biological literature. Sections of particular interest to toxicologists are Pesticides, Pharmacology, Public Health, and Toxicology. Cross-indexed by author, biosystematics, concepts, and subject key words.

Chemical Abstracts. Columbus, Ohio: Chemical Abstracts Service of the American Chemical Society, 1907 –. Very broad coverage of chemistry and related sciences. Sections of particular interest to toxicologists are Pharmacodynamics, Biochemical Interactions, Toxicology, Agrochemicals. Includes author, patent, and key word indexes.

Excerpta Medica. Amsterdam: Excerpta Medica. Some sections of particular interests are Cancer, Developmental Biology and Teratology, Environmental Health and Pollution Control, Occupational Health and Industrial Medicine, Pharmacology, and Toxicology.

In addition to these general abstracting services, specific services are devoted to specific areas of toxicology. They include:

Abstracts on Health Effects of Environmental Pollutants. Philadelphia: Biosciences Information Service of Biological Abstracts, 1972 –.

Environmental Abstracts. New York Environment Information Center, 1974 –.

Industrial Hygiene Digest. Pittsburgh: Industrial Health Foundation, 1937 –.

Pesticide Abstracts. Washington, D.C.: Technical Services Division of the Office of Pesticide Programs, Environmental Protection Agency, 1974 –.

Toxicology Abstracts. London: Information Retrieval Ltd., 1978 –.

TOX/TIPS, US Toxicology Information Program, National Library of Medicine, 1976 –.

12.6.2 Indexes

Current Contents. Philadelphia: Institute for Scientific Information. The most rapid service. Weekly publication consisting of the table of contents of journals published very soon after they appear. Each edition, of which *Life Sciences* is most appropriate to toxicology, has an author and a key word index, as well as the author's address.

Index Medicus. Bethesda, Md.: National Library of Medicine. Probably most useful in clinical areas.

Monthly Catalogue of United States Government Publications. Washington, D.C.: Government Printing Office.

Science Citation Index. Philadelphia: Institute for Scientific Information. Articles throughout the scientific literature are indexed with cross-references to all of their citations to other publications. Probably most useful for literature searches conducted before the initiation of new projects.

Chemical Mutagenesis. Oak Ridge, Tennessee: Oak Ridge National Laboratory.

The Environmental Index. New York: Environmental Information Center.

Teratology Lookout. Stockholm: Karolinska Institute.

12.6.3 Computer Data Bases

One of the most interesting and potentially the most important recent development in literature searching is the introduction of on-line, interactive, computer-based data systems that can provide the user with rapid access either to bibliographic information or directly to factual information on the topic in question. Generally, the costs are low, and many university libraries either can or do subscribe; at present, however, industrial and regulatory toxicologists seem to make greatest use of these systems. If these systems continue to expand and develop at the same rate as in the last few years, one can foresee the day when most toxicologists will have access to them from terminals at their desks.

The following are among the most important bibliographic data bases, producing either references or, in some cases, references and abstracts.

BIOSIS Previews. Produced by Biosciences Information Service and supplied by Bibliographic Retrieval Services, Lockheed Information Services and Systems Development Corporation, this service is based on Biological Abstracts.

CA Search. Produced by Chemical Abstracts Service and supplied by Lockheed Information and Systems Development Corporation, this system is based on Chemical Abstracts.

MEDLINE. Produced and supplied by the National Library of Medicine, this service offers broad coverage of medicine and life sciences.

NIOSHTIC (National Institute for Occupational Safety and Health Technical Information Center). Produced and supplied by NIOSH, this data base covers occupational safety and health in the broadest sense, including journals, symposia, NIOSH documents, etc.

SCISEARCH. Produced by the Institute for Scientific Information and supplied by Lockheed Information and Services and Bibliographical Retrieval Services, this service is based on the Science Citation index and can also search references cited as well as the articles themselves.

TOXLINE. Produced and supplied by the National Library of Medicine, this service is probably the most important bibliographic data base devoted to toxicology. It consists of a merged set of several previous files on several different aspects.

Nonbibliographic data can supply a variety of information on toxic compounds or other aspects of toxicology, including chemical structures, synonyms and properties, hard data from toxicity tests, information on tests, animals, etc. Several of the more important are listed below.

CHEMDEX (Chemical Abstracts Service and Systems Development Corporation).

CHEMLINE (National Library of Medicine) and CHEMNAME (Chemical Abstracts Service and Lockheed Information Services). All are different forms of a chemical dictionary.

Laboratory Animal Data Bank. Produced and supplied by Battelle Columbus Laboratories, this system provides data on animal husbandry, breeds and strains, pathology, testing protocols, etc.

NIH-EPA Chemical Information System. Produced and supplied by Interactive Sciences Corporation, this system consists of many linked files covering many aspects of chemistry and toxicology, including mass spectral data, x-ray crystallographic data, toxic effects, etc.

RTECS (Registry of the Toxic Effects of Chemical Substances). Produced by NIOSH and supplied by the Interactive Sciences Corporation and the National Library of Medicine. This system contains information on more than 35,000 compounds and can be searched by name, chemical class, CA number, etc. This is also a part of the NIH-EPA Chemical Information System already described.

Toxicology Data Base. Produced and supplied by the National Library of Medicine, this service is an outgrowth of the NIH Toxicology Study Section. All information on the toxicity of chemicals is peer-reviewed before being entered into the data base. This is the most important nonbibliographic data base devoted to toxicology.

TSCA. Produced by the Environmental Protection Agency and supplied by Lockheed Information Services, this system includes the list of chemicals in the initial inventory of the Toxic Substances Control Act.

12.7 PERSONAL INFORMATION STORAGE AND RETRIEVAL SYSTEMS

Most scientific careers evolve, with regard to literature in a particular field, from a small pile of reprints on a convenient corner of a desk, to a large and disorganized pile of reprints that threatens to engulf the desk itself, through a variety of index card systems that seldom prove adequate for long, leaving the scientist with an abiding distaste for protracted literature searches.

The principal problem is that the number of references in the system always grows faster than had been anticipated, giving rise to a situation in which the research worker and teacher continually work with an obsolete system and are faced with the problem of adopting a new system and transferring all the old material that is still relevant. With any of the index card-based systems, this involves not only the construction of new categories and/or the deletion of old categories, but also the preparation of new cards—a tedious and often postponed task. The method mentioned next, personal computer-based information storage and retrieval systems, can avoid this, since the program itself can be written in such a way that new categories can be introduced and references transferred into them by the computer itself. Although the choice of system depends primarily on the expected size of the data base, it is probably wise to assume that ultimately it will be large. Three systems are described below.

1. Small numbers of references, possibly several hundred, can be conveniently organized on numbered index cards containing the complete reference with or without an abstract, numbered and stored in the sequence in which they are added to the data base. The numbers are then used in cross-indexing files that can vary in number and complexity according to individual need or desire. Subject and author indexes are essential; however, storing in alphabetical order ignores the authors other than the first, a serious limitation. Other indexes that might be useful include: experimental animal, chemical class, enzyme or other preparation, and organ system. Special and possibly temporary cross-indexes can be set up for special writing projects such as reviews, grant proposals, textbooks, etc.

2. Larger numbers, possibly as many as 1,000 or 2,000, can be accommodated on a punched card system. Precut holes in the cards are coded and punched out to form notches corresponding to the characteristics of the reference. When a steel rod is run through a particular hole and the pile is picked up, the cards so notched fall out. These cards can then be resorted according to another characteristic. For example, a search for references related to the microsomal metabolism of piperonyl butoxide in mammalian liver might be carried out first for synergists in the chemical-use class section; the cards thus obtained might then be screened for mammals in the experimental animal section, followed by liver in the organ section, and microsomes in the section on enzyme preparations.

3. As the number of references in the data base becomes large, the above system becomes unwieldy, and a computer-based system should be considered. Most research workers now have access to large, shared-time computer systems or a choice of the many microcomputers and minicomputers available at moderate prices. The advantages are many: The computer can search several cross-indexes simultaneously, no bulky card files are necessary, and the computer can be programmed to change categories as needed and to reclassify the references in the data base to suit new categories.

Under the circumstances, it is recommended that the reader consider a computer-based system initially. Although this is not yet common, the great flexibility and increasing availability of both hardware and software make it attractive; some packaged programs are available and, for those not familiar with computer programs and programming, most institutions have trained personnel who can help. Although the esoteric nature of computers gave rise to a generation of programmers who could talk to machines but could rarely communicate effectively with people, they are yielding to a new generation who interface effectively between computer and potential user.

As an example, the following is a brief description of a system developed in the author's laboratory. Initially, the data was stored on-line on the shared-time computer of the Triangle Universities Computing Center, and the program was based on the language FAMULUS. It could be accessed by all laboratory personnel on a remote terminal in the laboratory. All personnel could add to the data base and, as described below, could use the entire data base or their own personal data base as required.

References were entered by the following categories:

a. AUTH: All authors

b. TITL: Title in full

c. JOUR: Journal citation or book title

d. CHEM: Classification used is a use classification (drugs, insecticides, synergists, etc.) Eventually, a structure notation will be added.

e. ANIM: The experimental animal is identified by common name (rat, rabbit, etc.) or taxonomic group (insects, fish, etc.)

f. ORGN: Organ or organ system

g. PREP: Enzyme or other preparation (microsomes, hepatocytes, perfused organ, etc.)

h. SUBJ: A numerical subject classification arranged in a hierarchical manner similar to that of the chapters of this text is used. For example, 3 would retrieve all references on the metabolism of toxicants; 4 would retrieve only those on nutritional effects. Further subdivisions can be created as desired, and references can be added to them by adding the numbers to the reference in the data base.

i. APPL: For special applications. For example, references for a textbook under preparation could have a special classification in this category. Individuals can append their own initials and can then restrict a search to references added to the data base by themselves.

Recently, we transferred this system essentially as described above to the SCI-MATE program developed by the Institute for Scientific Information. We use an Apple IIe microcomputer with hard-disk storage. One of the advantages of such a system is the dedicated computer; another advantage is that the system provides access to ISI's large data base, permitting references to be transferred directly to the user's personal data file.

Any combination of terms can be searched for, and operation of the system is relatively simple. After access to the program is acquired, the user is asked which of various actions will be made: search, add to data base, etc. If search is indicated, the list of categories listed above is given, with a request to list which of these will be involved. On being given this, the computer asks for a search formula, that is, which items within the categories are to be searched for; the computer then lists all references that include all of these items. Variations in the program enable these references to be listed in several ways, alphabetically, chronologically, etc. Last, but of considerable importance, is the storage of all hard copy (reprints, xerox copies, etc., with coding sheet attached) in close proximity to the terminal, entering only material that is available as hard copy and has been read and coded by a member of the laboratory group and permitting the borrowing of hard copy only under controlled conditions.

12.8 CONCLUSIONS

The available information in toxicology, as outlined above, is extensive and appears in a variety of forms. Furthermore, in order to keep pace with developments, the toxicologist must also be concerned with literature in related fields and in sources that are more general in nature. This is particularly true in the case of methodology, an area that is frequently the key to further advances. Despite these problems, the practicing toxicologist can, by a judicious choice of primary research journals, review journals, abstracting and indexing services, and computer-based retrieval systems, keep abreast of current thinking and advances while still carrying out research and/or teaching functions.

12.9 SUGGESTED FURTHER READING

Cosmides, G.J. Proceedings of the Symposium on Information Transfer in Toxicology. Sponsored by the Department of Health and Human Services Committee to Coordinate Environmental and Related Programs and the Interagency Toxic Substances Data Committee, 1981. Available from the National Technical Information Service, accession no. PB-283 164.

Wexler, P. Information Resources in Toxicology. New York, Elsevier, 1982.

GLOSSARY

ACID DEPOSITION. Wet and dry air pollutants that lower the pH of deposition and subsequently the pH of the environment. ACID RAIN with a pH of 4 or lower refers to the wet components. Normal rain has a pH of about 5.6. Sulfuric and nitric acids, from sulfur and nitrogen oxides, respectively, are the major contributors. In lakes in which the buffering capacity is low, the pH becomes acidic enough to cause fish kills, and the lakes cannot support fish populations. A contributing factor is the fact that acidic conditions concurrently release toxic metals, such as aluminum, into the water.

ACID RAIN. *See* ACID DEPOSITION.

ACTIVATION (BIOACTIVATION). In toxicology, this term is used to describe metabolic reactions of a xenobiotic in which the product is more toxic than the substrate. Such reactions are most commonly monooxygenations, the products of which are electrophiles that, if not detoxified by phase II (conjugation) reactions, may react with nucleophilic groups on cellular macromolecules such as proteins and DNA.

ACTIVE OXYGEN. Used to describe various short-lived, highly reactive intermediates in the reduction of oxygen. Active oxygen species such as superoxide anion ($O_2 \dot{-}$) and hydroxyl radical ($OH^\bullet$) are known or believed to be involved in several toxic actions. Superoxide anion is detoxified by superoxide dismutase.

ACUTE TOXICITY. Refers to adverse effects on, or mortality of, organisms following soon after a brief exposure to a chemical agent. Either a single exposure or multiple exposures within a short time period may be involved, and an acute effect is generally regarded as an effect that occurs within the first few days after exposure, usually less than two weeks.

ACUTE TOXICITY TESTS. The most common tests for acute toxicity are the LC50 and LD50 tests which are designed to measure mortality in response to an acute toxic insult. Other tests for acute toxicity include dermal irritation tests, dermal sensitization tests, eye irritation tests, photoallergy tests, and phototoxicity tests. *See also* EYE IRRITATION TESTS; LC50; and LD50.

ADAPTATION TO TOXICANTS. Refers to the ability of an organism to show insensitivity or decreased sensitivity to a chemical that normally causes deleterious effects. The terms resistance and tolerance are closely related and have been used in several different ways. However, a concensus is emerging to use RESISTANCE to mean that situation in which a change in the genetic constitution of a population in response to the stressor chemical enables a greater number of individuals to resist the toxic action than were able to resist it in the previous, unexposed population. Thus, an essential feature of resistance is selection and then inheritance by subsequent generations. In microorganisms this frequently involves mutations and induction of enzymes by the toxicant: in higher organisms it usually involves selection for genes already present in the population at low frequency. TOLERANCE is then reserved for situations in which individual organisms acquire the ability to resist the effect of a toxicant, usually as a result of prior exposure.

Ah LOCUS. A gene(s) controlling the trait of responsiveness for induction of enzymes by aromatic hydrocarbons. In addition to aromatic hydrocarbons such as the polycyclics, the chlorinated dibenzo-p-dioxins, dibenzofurans, and biphenyls, as well as the brominated biphenyls, are also involved. This trait, originally defined by studies of induction of hepatic aryl hydrocarbon hydroxylase activity following 3-methylcholanthrene treatment, is inherited by simple autosomal dominance in crosses and backcrosses between C57BL/6 (Ah-responsive) and DBA/2 (Ah-nonresponsive) mice.

Ah RECEPTOR (TCDD BINDING PROTEIN). A protein coded for by a gene of the Ah locus. The initial location of the Ah receptor is believed to be in the cytosol, although recent evidence suggests it may reside within the nucleus. Binding of aromatic hydrocarbons to the Ah receptor of mice is a prerequisite for the induction of many xenobiotic metabolizing enzymes, as well as for two responses to 2,3,7,8-tetrachlorodibenzo-p-dioxin: epidermal hyperplasia and thymic atrophy. Ah responsive mice have a high-affinity receptor while the Ah nonresponsive mice appear to have a low-affinity receptor.

AIR POLLUTION. In general, the principal air pollutants are carbon monoxide, oxides of nitrogen, oxides of sulfur, hydrocarbons, and particulates. The principal sources are transportation, industrial processes, electric power generation, and the heating of buildings. Hydrocarbons such as benzo(a)pyrene are produced by incomplete combustion and are associated primarily with the automobile. They are usually not present at levels high enough to cause direct toxic effects but are important in the formation of photochemical air pollution, formed as a result of interactions between oxides of nitrogen and hydrocarbons in the presence of ultraviolet light, giving rise to lung irritants such as peroxyacetyl nitrate, acrolein, and formaldehyde. Particulates are a heterogeneous group of particles, often seen as smoke, that are important as carriers of absorbed hydrocarbons and as irritants to the respiratory system.

ALKYLATING AGENTS. These are chemicals that can add alkyl groups to DNA, a reaction which can result either in mispairing of bases or in chromosome breaks. The mechanism of the reaction involves the formation of a reactive carbonium ion (eg, CH_3^+) that combines with electron rich bases in DNA. Thus alkylating agents such as dimethylnitrosomine are frequently carcinogens and/or mutagens.

AMES TEST. An in vitro test for mutagenicity utilizing mutant strains of the bacterium *Salmonella typhimurium,* which is used as a preliminary screen of chemicals for assessing potential carcinogenicity. Several strains are available that cannot grow in the absence of histidine because of metabolic defects in histidine biosynthesis. Mutagens and presumed carcinogens can cause mutations that enable the strains to regain their ability to grow in a histidine deficient medium. The test can be performed in the presence of the S-9 fraction from rat liver to allow metabolic activation of promutagens. There is a high correlation between bacterial mutagenicity and carcinogenicity of chemicals.

ANTAGONISM. In toxicology, antagonism is usually defined as that situation in which the toxicity of two or more compounds administered together is less than that expected from consideration of their toxicities when administered alone. Although this includes lowered toxicity resulting from induction of detoxifying enzymes, this is frequently considered separately because of the time that must elapse between treatment with the inducer and subsequent treatment with the toxicant. Antagonism not involving induction is often at a marginal level of detection and is consequently difficult to explain. Such antagonism may involve competition for receptor sites or nonenzymatic combination of one toxicant with another to reduce the toxic effect. Physiological antagonism, in which two agonists act on the same physiological system but produce opposite effects, may also occur.

BEHAVIORAL TOXICITY. Behavior may be defined as an organism's motor or glandular response to changes in its internal or external environment. Such changes may be simple or highly complex, innate or learned, but in any event represent one of the final integrated expressions of nervous function. Behavioral toxicity is adverse or potentially adverse effects on such expression brought about by exogenous chemicals.

BINDING, COVALENT. *See* COVALENT BINDING.

BIOACTIVATION. *See* ACTIVATION.

BIOASSAY. This term is used in two distinct ways. The first and most appropriate is the use of a living organism to measure the amount of a toxicant present in a sample or the toxicity of a sample. This is done by comparing the toxic effect of the sample with that of a graded series of a known standard. The second, and less appropriate, meaning is in the use of animals to investigate the toxic effects of chemicals as in chronic toxicity tests.

CARCINOGEN, EPIGENETIC. Cancer causing agents that exert their carcinogenic effect by mechanisms other than genetic, such as by immunosuppression, hormonal imbalance, or cytotoxicity; they may act as cocarcinogens or promoters. Epigenetic carcinogenesis is not as well understood a phenomenon as genotoxic carcinogenesis.

CARCINOGEN, PROXIMATE. *See* CARCINOGEN, ULTIMATE.

CARCINOGEN, ULTIMATE. Many, if not most, chemical carcinogens are not intrinsically carcinogenic but require metabolic activation to express their carcinogenic potential. The terms PRECARCINOGEN, PROXIMATE CARCINOGEN, and ULTIMATE CARCINOGEN are used to describe respectively the initial reactive compound, its more active products, and the product that is actually responsible for carcinogenesis by its interaction with DNA.

CARCINOGENESIS. This is the process encompassing the conversion of normal cells to neoplastic cells and the further development of these neoplastic cells into a tumor. This process results from the action of specific chemicals, certain viruses, or radiation from ultraviolet light, x-rays, or α- and β-particles. Chemical carcinogens have been classified into those that are genotoxic and those that are epigenetic (i.e., not genotoxic).

CHRONIC TOXICITY. This term is used to describe adverse effects manifested after a long time period of uptake of small quantities of the toxicant in question. The dose is small enough so that no acute effects are manifested, and the time period is frequently a significant part of the expected normal lifetime of the organism. The most serious manifestation of chronic toxicity is carcinogenesis, but other types of chronic toxicity are also known, e.g., reproductive effects and behavioral effects.

CHRONIC TOXICITY TESTS. Chronic tests are those conducted over the greater part of the lifespan of the test species or, in some cases, more than one generation. The most important are carcinogenicity tests and the most common test species are rats and mice.

COCARCINOGENESIS. Cocarcinogenesis is the enhancement of the conversion of normal cells to neoplastic cells. This process is manifested by enhancement of carcinogenesis when the agent is administered either before or together with a carcinogen. Cocarcinogenesis should be distinguished from promotion as, in the latter case, the promoter must be administered after the initiating carcinogen.

COMPARTMENT. In pharmaco(toxico)kinetics a compartment is a hypothetical volume of an animal system wherein a chemical acts homogeneously in transport and transformation. A single mathematical compartment may be one, two, or more physiological tissues or entities. Compartmental models are mathematical depictions of physiological reality. Transport into, out of, or between compartments is described by rate constants which are used in models of the intact animal.

CONJUGATION REACTIONS. *See* PHASE II REACTIONS.

COVALENT BINDING. This involves the covalent bond or "shared electron pair" bond. Each covalent bond consists of a pair of electrons shared between two atoms and occupying two stable orbitals, one of each atom. Although this is distinguished from the ionic bond or ionic valence, in fact chemical bonds may show both covalent and ionic character. In toxicology the term covalent binding is used in a less precise way to refer to the binding of toxicants or their reactive metabolites to endogenous molecules (usually macromolecules) to produce stabile adducts resistant to rigorous extraction procedures. A covalent bond between ligand and macromolecule is generally assumed. Many forms of chronic toxicity involve covalent binding of the toxicant to DNA or protein molecules within the cell.

CROSS RESISTANCE, CROSS TOLERANCE. These terms describe the situation in which either resistance or tolerance to a particular toxicant (as defined under adaptation to toxicants) is induced by exposure to a different toxicant. This is commonly seen in resistance of insects to insecticides in which selection with one insecticide brings about a broad spectrum of resistance to insecticides of the same or different chemical classes. Such cross resistance is usually caused by the inheritance of a high level of nonspecific xenobiotic-metabolizing enzymes.

DELANEY AMENDMENT. *See* FOOD, DRUG AND COSMETICS ACT.

DETOXICATION. A metabolic reaction or sequence of reactions that reduces the potential for adverse effect of a xenobiotic. Such sequences normally involve an increase in water solubility that facilitates excretion and/or the reaction of a reactive product with an endogenous substrate (conjugation), thereby not only increasing water solubility but also reducing the possibility of interaction with cellular macromolecules. Not to be confused with DETOXIFICATION.

DETOXIFICATION. Treatment by which toxicants are removed from intoxicated patients or a course of treatment during which dependence on alcohol or other drugs of abuse is reduced or eliminated. Not to be confused with DETOXICATION.

DISTRIBUTION. The term distribution refers both to the movement of a toxicant from the portal of entry to the tissue and also to the description of the different concentrations reached in different locations. The first involves the study of transport mechanisms primarily in the blood, and both are subject to mathematical analysis in toxicokinetic studies.

DOSAGE. The amount of a toxicant drug or other chemical administered or taken expressed as some function of the organism, e.g., mg/kg body weight/day.

DOSE. Total amount of a toxicant, drug, or other chemical administered or taken by the organism.

DOSE RESPONSE. In toxicology, the quantitative relationship between the amount of a toxicant administered or taken and the incidence or extent of the adverse effect.

DOSE–RESPONSE ASSESSMENT. A step in the risk-assessment process to characterize the relationship between the dose of a chemical administered to a population of test animals and the incidence of a given adverse effect. It involves mathematical modeling techniques to extrapolate from the high-dose effects observed in test animals to estimate the effects expected from exposure to the typically low doses that may be encountered by humans.

DRAIZE TEST. *See* EYE IRRITATION TEST.

DRUGS OF ABUSE. Although all drugs may have deleterious effects on humans, drugs of abuse either have no medicinal function or are taken at higher than therapeutic doses. Some drugs of abuse may affect only higher nervous functions (mood, reaction time, and coordination) but many produce physical dependence and have serious physical effects, with fatal overdose being a common occurrence. The drugs of abuse include central nervous system depressants such as ethanol, methaqualone (quaalude), and secobarbital; central nervous system stimulants such as cocaine, methamphetamine (speed), caffeine, and nicotine; opioids such as heroin and morphine, hallucinogens such as lysergic acid diethylamide (LSD), phencyclidine (PCP), and tetrahydrocannabinol, the most important active principle of marijuana.

DRUGS, THERAPEUTIC. All therapeutic drugs can be toxic at some dose. The danger to the patient is dependent upon the nature of the toxic response, the dose necessary to produce the toxic response, and the relationship between the therapeutic and the toxic dose. Drug toxicity is affected by all of those factors that affect the toxicity of xenobiotics, including (genetic) variation, diet, age, and the presence of other exogenous chemicals. The risk of toxic side effects from a particular drug must be weighed against the expected benefits; the use of a quite dangerous drug with only a narrow tolerance between the therapeutic and toxic doses might well be justified if it is the sole treatment for an otherwise fatal disease. For example, cytotoxic agents used in the treatment of cancer are known carcinogens.

ELECTRON TRANSPORT SYSTEM (ETS). This term is often restricted to the mitochondrial system although it applies equally well to others, including that of microsomes and chloroplasts. The mitochondrial ETS (RESPIRATORY CHAIN, CYTOCHROME CHAIN) consists of a series of cytochromes and other electron carriers arranged in the inner mitochondrial membrane. These components transfer the electrons from NADH or $FADH_2$ generated in metabolic oxidations to oxygen, the final electron acceptor, through a series of alternate oxidations and reductions. The energy which these electrons lose during these transfers is used to pump $H+$ from the matrix into the intermembrane space, creating an electrochemical proton gradient that drives oxidative phosphorylation. The energy is conserved as ATP.

ELECTRON TRANSPORT SYSTEM INHIBITORS. The three major respiratory enzyme complexes of the mitochondrial electron transport system can all be blocked by inhibitors. For example, rotenone inhibits the NADH dehydrogenase complex, antimycin A inhibits the b-c complex, and cyanide and carbon monoxide inhibit the cytochrome oxidase complex. While oxidative phosphorylation inhibitors prevent phosphorylation while allowing electron transfers to proceed, electron transport system inhibitors prevent both electron transport and ATP production.

ELECTROPHILIC. Electrophiles are chemicals that are attracted to and react with electron-rich centers in other molecules in reactions known as electrophilic reactions. Many activation reactions produce electrophilic intermediates such as epoxides, which exert their toxic action by forming covalent bonds with cellular macromolecules such as DNA or proteins.

ENDOPLASMIC RETICULUM. The endoplasmic reticulum (ER) is an extensive branching and anastomosing double membrane distributed in the cytoplasm of eucaryotic cells. The ER is of two types: rough ER contains attached ribosomes on the cytosolic surface and smooth ER is devoid of ribosomes. The ribosomes are involved in protein biosynthesis, and RER is abundant in cells specialized for protein synthesis. Many xenobiotic-metabolizing enzymes are integral components of both SER and RER, such as the cytochrome P-450–dependent monooxygenase system and the FAD-containing monooxygenase, although the specific content is usually higher in SER. When tissue or cells are disrupted by homogenization, the ER is fragmented into many smaller (c. 100 nm diameter) closed vesicles called microsomes, which can be isolated by differential centrifugation.

ENTEROHEPATIC CIRCULATION. This term describes the excretion of a compound into the bile and its subsequent reabsorption from the small intestine and transport back to the liver, where it is available again for biliary excretion. The most important mechanism is conjugation in the liver, followed by excretion into the bile. In the small intestine the conjugation product is hydrolyzed, either nonenzymatically or by the microflora and the compound is reabsorbed to become a substrate for conjugation and reexcretion into the bile.

ENVIRONMENTAL TOXICOLOGY. This is concerned with the movement of toxicants and their metabolites in the environment and in food chains and the effect of such toxicants on population of organisms.

EPIGENETIC CARCINOGEN. *See* CARCINOGEN, EPIGENETIC.

EXPOSURE ASSESSMENT. A component of risk assessment. The number of individuals likely to be exposed to a chemical in the environment or in the workplace is assessed, and the intensity, frequency, and duration of human exposure are estimated.

EYE IRRITATION TESTS (DRAIZE TEST). Eye irritation tests measure irritancy of compounds applied topically to the eye. These tests are variations of the Draize test, and the experimental animal used is the albino rabbit. The test consists of adding the material to be tested directly into the conjunctival sac of one eye of each of several albino rabbits, the other eye serving as the control. This test is probably the most controversial of all toxicity tests, being criticized primarily on the grounds that it is inhumane. Moreover, since both concentrations and volumes used are high, and show high variability, it has been suggested that these tests cannot be extrapolated to humans. However, since visual impairment is a critical toxic endpoint, tests for ocular toxicity are essential. Attempts to solve the dilemma have taken two forms: to find substitute in vitro tests and to modify the Draize test so that it becomes not only more humane but also more predictive for humans.

FEDERAL INSECTICIDE, FUNGICIDE AND RODENTICIDE ACT (FIFRA). This law is the basic U.S. law under which pesticides and other agricultural chemicals distributed in interstate commerce are registered and regulated. First enacted in 1947, FIFRA placed the regulation of agrichemicals under control of the U.S. Department of Agriculture. In 1970, this responsibility was transferred to the newly created Environmental Protection Agency (EPA). Subsequently, FIFRA has been extensively revised by the Federal Environmental Pesticide Control Act (FEPCA) of 1972 and by the FIFRA amendments of 1975, 1978, and 1980. Under FIFRA all new pesticide products used in the United States must be registered with the EPA. This requires the registrant to submit information on the composition, intended use, and efficacy of the product, along with a comprehensive data base establishing that the material can be used without causing unreasonable adverse effects on humans or the environment.

FETAL ALCOHOL SYNDROME (FAS). FAS refers to a pattern of defects in children born to alcoholic mothers. Three criteria for FAS are: prenatal or postnatal growth retardation; characteristic facial anomalies such as microcephaly, small eye opening, and thinned upper lip; central nervous system dysfunction such as mental retardation and developmental delays.

FOOD ADDITIVES. Chemicals may be added to food as preservatives (either antibacterial or antifungal compounds or antioxidants), to change the physical characteristics, for processing, or to change the taste or odor. Although most food additives are safe and without chronic toxicity, many were introduced when toxicity testing was relatively unsophisticated, and some have been shown subsequently to be toxic. The most important inorganic additives are nitrate and nitrite. Well-known examples of food additives include the antioxidant butylatedhydroxyanisole (BHA), fungistatic agents such as methyl p-benzoic acid, the emulsifier propylene glycol, sweeteners such as saccharin and aspartame, and dyes such as tartrazine and Sunset Yellow.

FOOD CONTAMINANTS (FOOD POLLUTANTS). Food contaminants, as opposed to food additives, are those compounds included inadvertantly in foods, either raw, cooked, or processed. They include bacterial toxins such as the exotoxin of *Clostridium botulinum,* mycotoxins such as aflatoxins from *Aspergillus flavus,* plant alkaloids, animal toxins, pesticide residues, residues of animal food additives such as diethylstilbestrol and antibiotics, and a variety of industrial chemicals such as polychlorinated biphenyls and polybrominated biphenyls.

FOOD, DRUG AND COSMETICS ACT. The federal Food, Drug and Cosmetic Act is administered by the FOOD AND DRUG ADMINISTRATION (FDA). It establishes limits for food additives, sets criteria for drug safety for both humans and animal use, and requires proof both of safety and efficacy. This act contains the DELANEY AMENDMENT which states that food additives that cause cancer in humans or animals at any level shall not be considered safe and are, therefore, prohibited. This law also empowers the FDA to establish and modify the GRAS ("Generally Recognized as Safe") list and to establish Good Laboratory Practice (GLP) rules.

FORENSIC TOXICOLOGY. Forensic toxicology is concerned with the medico-legal aspects of the adverse effects of chemicals on humans and animals. Although primarily devoted to the identification of the cause and circumstances of death and the legal issues arising therefrom, forensic toxicologists also deal with sublethal poisoning cases.

FREE RADICALS. Molecules that have unpaired electrons. Free radicals may be produced metabolically from xenobiotics and, since they are extremely reactive, may be involved in interactions with cellular macromolecules, giving rise to adverse effects. Examples include the trichloromethyl radical ($\cdot CCL_3$) produced from carbon tetrachloride or the carbene radical ($>C\colon$) produced by oxidation of the acetal carbon of methylenedioxyphenyl synergists.

GENOTOXICITY. Genotoxicity is an adverse effect on the genetic material (DNA) of living cells that, upon the replication of the cells, is expressed as a mutagenic or a carcinogenic event. Genotoxicity results from a reaction with DNA which can be measured either biochemically or in short-term tests with end points that reflect DNA damage.

GENOTOXIC CARCINOGEN. *See* CARCINOGEN, GENOTOXIC.

GOOD LABORATORY PRACTICES. In the United States, this is a code of laboratory procedures laid down under the law and to be followed by laboratories undertaking toxicity tests, the results of which will be used for regulatory or legal purposes.

GRAS LIST. *See* FOOD, DRUG AND COSMETICS ACT.

HAZARD IDENTIFICATION. Considered the final step in risk assessment, hazard identification involves the qualitative determination of whether exposure to a chemical causes an increased incidence of an adverse effect, such as cancer or birth defects, in a population of test animals and an evaluation of the relevance of this information to the potential for causing similar effects in humans.

HEPATOTOXICITY. Hepatotoxicants are those chemicals causing adverse effects on the liver. The liver may be particularly susceptible to chemical injury because of its anatomic relationship to the most important portal of entry, the GI tract, and its high concentration of xenobiotic-metabolizing enzymes. Many of these enzymes, but particularly the cytochrome P-450–dependent monooxygenase system, metabolize xenobiotics to produce reactive intermediates which can react with endogenous macromolecules such as proteins and DNA to produce adverse effects.

IMMUNOTOXICITY. This term can be used in either of two ways, the first referring to toxic effects mediated by the immune system such as dermal sensitivity reactions to compounds like 2,4-dinitrochlorobenzene. The second and currently most acceptable definition refers to toxic effects which impair the functioning of the immune system, for example, the ability of a toxicant to impair resistance to infection.

INDUCTION. The process of causing a quantitative increase in an enzyme due to de novo protein synthesis following exposure to an inducing agent. This can occur either by a decrease in the degradation rate, an increase in the synthesis rate, or both. Increasing the synthesis rate is the most common mechanism for induction by xenobiotics. Coordinate (pleiotypic) induction is the induction of multiple enzymes by a single inducing agent. For example, phenobarbital can induce both cytochrome P-450 isozymes and glutathione S-transferase.

INDUSTRIAL TOXICOLOGY. A specific area of environmental toxicology dealing with the work environment; it includes risk assessment, establishment of permissible levels of exposure, and worker protection.

INHIBITION. In its most general sense, inhibition means a restraining or a holding back. In biochemistry and biochemical toxicology, inhibition is a reduction in the rate of an enzymatic reaction, and an inhibitor is any compound causing such a reduction. Inhibition of enzymes important in normal metabolism is a significant mechanism of toxic action of xenobiotics, while inhibition of xenobiotic-metabolizing enzymes can have important consequences in the ultimate toxicity of their substrates. Inhibition is sometimes used in toxicology in a more general, and rather ill-defined, way to refer to the reduction of an overall process of toxicity, as in the inhibition of carcinogenesis by a particular chemical.

INITIATION. The initial stage of carcinogenesis involving the conversion of a normal cell to a neoplastic cell. Initiation is considered to be a rapid, essentially irreversible change involving the interaction of the ultimate carcinogen with DNA; this change primes the cell for subsequent neoplastic development via the promotion process.

INTOXICATION. In the general sense this term refers primarily to inebriation with ethyl alcohol, secondarily to causing excitement or delirium by other means, including other chemicals. In the clinical sense it refers to poisoning or becoming poisoned. In toxicology, it is sometimes used as a synonym for activation, i.e., the production of a more toxic metabolite from a less toxic parent compound. This latter use of intoxication is ambiguous and should be abandoned in favor of the aforementioned general meanings, and activation or bioactivation used instead.

IN VITRO TESTS. Literally, these are tests conducted outside of the body of the organism. In toxicity testing they would include studies using isolated enzymes, subcellular organelles, or cultured cells. While technically the term would not include tests involving intact eukaryotes (e.g., the Ames test), it is frequently used by toxicologists to include all short-term tests for mutagenicity that are normally used as indicators of potential carcinogenicity.

ISOZYMES (ISOENZYMES). Isozymes are multiple forms of a given enzyme that occur within a single species or even a single cell and which catalyze the same general reaction but are coded for by different genes. Different isozymes may occur at different life stages and/or in different organs and tissues or they may coexist within the same cell.

The first well-characterized isozymes were those of lactic dehydrogenase. Several xenobiotic-metabolizing enzymes exist in multiple isozymes, including cytochrome P-450 and glucuronosyltransferase.

LC50 (MEDIAN LETHAL CONCENTRATION).   The concentration of a test chemical that, when a population of test organisms is exposed to it, is estimated to be fatal to 50 percent of the organisms under the stated conditions of the test. Normally used in lieu of the LD50 test in aquatic toxicology and inhalation toxicology.

LD50 (MEDIAN LETHAL DOSE).   The quantity of a chemical compound which, when applied directly to test organisms, is estimated to be fatal to 50 percent of those organisms under the stated conditions of the test. The LD50 value is the standard for comparison of acute toxicity between toxicants and between species. Since the results of LD50 determinations may vary widely it is important that both biological and physical conditions be narrowly defined (e.g., strain, sex, and age of test organism, time and route of exposure, environmental conditions). The value may be determined graphically from a plot of log. dose against mortality expressed in probability units (probits) or, more recently, by using one of several computer programs available.

LETHAL SYNTHESIS.   This term is used to describe the process by which a toxicant, similar in structure to an endogenous substrate, is incorporated into the same metabolic pathway as the endogenous substrate, ultimately being transformed into a toxic or lethal product. For example, fluroacetate simulates acetate in intermediary metabolism being transformed, via the tricarboxylic acid cycle to fluorocitrate, which then inhibits aconitase, resulting in disruption of the TCA cycle and energy metabolism.

LIPOPHILIC.   The physical property of chemical compounds that causes them to be soluble in nonpolar solvents (e.g., chloroform and benzene) and, generally, relatively insoluble in polar solvents such as water. This property is important toxicologically since lipophilic compounds tend to enter the body easily and to be excretable only when they have been rendered less lipophilic by metabolic action.

MAXIMUM TOLERATED DOSE (MTD).   The MTD has been defined for testing purposes by the U.S. Environmental Protection Agency as the highest dose that causes no more than a 10 percent weight decrement, as compared to the appropriate control groups, and does not produce mortality, clinical signs of toxicity, or pathologic lesions (other than those that may be related to a neoplastic response) that would be predicted to shorten the animals' natural life span. It is an important concept in chronic toxicity testing; however, the relevance of results produced by such doses has become a matter of controversy.

MEMBRANES.   Membranes of tissues, cells, and cell organelles are all basically similar in structure. They appear to be bimolecular lipid leaflets with proteins embedded in the matrix and also arranged on the outer polar surfaces. This basic plan is present despite many variations, and it is important in toxicological studies of uptake of toxicants by passive diffusion and active transport.

MICROSOMES. Microsomes are small closed vesicles (c. 100 nm in diameter) that represent membrane fragments formed from the endoplasmic reticulum when cells are disrupted by homogenization. Microsomes are separated from other cell organelles by differential centrifugation. The cell homogenate contains rough microsomes which are studded with ribosomes and are derived from rough endoplasmic reticulum, and smooth microsomes which are devoid of ribosomes and are derived from smooth endoplasmic reticulum. Microsomes are important preparations for studying the many processes carried out by the endoplasmic reticulum, such as protein biosynthesis and xenobiotic metabolism.

MONOOXYGENASE (MIXED-FUNCTION OXIDASE). An enzyme for which the cosubstrates are an organic compound and molecular oxygen. In reactions catalyzed by these enzymes one atom of a molecule of oxygen is incorporated into the substrate while the other is reduced to water. Monooxygenases of importance in toxicology include cytochrome P-450 and the FAD-containing monooxygenase, both of which initiate the metabolism of lipophilic xenobiotics by the introduction of a reactive polar group into the molecule. Such reactions may represent detoxication or may generate reactive intermediates of importance in toxic action.

MUTAGENICITY. Mutations are heritable changes produced in the genetic information stored in the DNA of living cells. Chemicals capable of causing such changes are known as MUTAGENS and the process as MUTAGENESIS.

MYCOTOXINS. Toxins produced by fungi. Many, such as aflatoxins, are particularly important in toxicology.

NEPHROTOXICITY. A pathologic state which can be induced by chemicals (NEPHROTOXICANTS) and in which the normal homeostatic functioning of the kidney is impaired. It is often associated with necrosis of the proximal tubule and may involve either the excretion of large volumes of very dilute urine or excretion of minimal amounts of urine.

NEUROTOXICITY. This is a general term referring to all toxic effects on the nervous system including those measured as behavioral abnormalities. Since the nervous system is complex, both structurally and functionally, and has considerable functional reserve, the study of neurotoxicity is a many-faceted branch of toxicology. It involves electrophysiology, receptor function, pathology, behavior, and other aspects.

NO OBSERVED EFFECT LEVEL (NOEL). This is the highest dose level of a chemical that, in a given toxicity test, causes no observable effect in the test animals. The NOEL for a given chemical varies with the route and duration of exposure and the nature of the adverse effect (i.e., the indicator of toxicity).

The NOEL for the most sensitive test species and the most sensitive indicator of toxicity is usually employed for regulatory purposes. Effects considered are usually adverse effects, and this value may be called the NO OBSERVED ADVERSE EFFECTS LEVEL (NOAEL).

OCCUPATIONAL SAFETY AND HEALTH ADMINISTRATION (OSHA). In the United States, OSHA is the government department concerned with health and safety in the workplace. OSHA sets the standards for worker exposure to specific chemicals, for air concentration values, and for monitoring procedures. OSHA is also concerned with research (through the National Institute for Occupational Safety and Health [NIOSH]), information, education, and training in occupational safety and health.

ONCOGENES. Oncogenes are genes that, when activated in cells, can transform the cells from normal to neoplastic. Sometimes oncogenes are carried into normal cells by infecting viruses, particularly RNA viruses, or retroviruses. In some cases, however, the oncogene is already present in the normal human cell, and it needs only a mutation or other activating event to change it from a harmless, and possible essential gene, called a proto-oncogene, into a cancer-producing gene. More than 30 oncogenes have been identified in humans.

OXIDATIVE PHOSPHORYLATION. The conservation of chemical energy extracted from fuel oxidations by the phosphorylation of adenosine diphosphate (ADP) by inorganic phosphate to form adenosine triphosphate (ATP) is accomplished in several ways. The majority of ATP is formed by respiratory chain-linked oxidative phosphorylation associated with the electron transport system in the mitochondrial inner membrane. The oxidations are tightly coupled to phosphorylations through a chemiosmotic mechanism in which H+ are pumped across the inner mitochondrial membrane. Uncouplers of oxidative phosphorylation serve as H+ ionophores to dissipate the H+ gradient and thus uncouple the phosphorylations from the oxidations.

PARTITION COEFFICIENT. This is a measure of the relative lipid solubility of a chemical and is determined by measuring the partitioning of the compound between a lipid phase and an aqueous phase (e.g., octanol and water). The partition coefficient is important in studies of the uptake of toxicants since compounds with high coefficients (lipophilic compounds) are usually taken up more readily by organisms and tissues.

PHASE I REACTIONS. These reactions introduce a reactive polar group into lipophilic xenobiotics. In most cases this group becomes the site for conjugation during phase II reactions. Such reactions include microsomal monooxygenations, cytosolic and mitochondrial oxidations, cooxidations in the prostaglandin synthetase reaction, reductions, hydrolyses, and epoxide hydrolases. The products of phase I reaction may be potent electrophiles which can be conjugated and detoxified in phase II reaction or which may react with nucleophilic groups on cellular constituents, thereby causing toxicity.

PHASE 2 REACTIONS. Reactions that involve the conjugation with endogenous substrates of phase I products and other xenobiotics which contain functional groups such as hydroxyl, amino, carboxyl, epoxide, or halogen. The endogenous metabolites include sugars, amino acids, glutathione, and sulfate. The conjugation products, with rare exceptions, are more polar, less toxic, and more readily excreted than their parent compounds. There are two general types of conjugations: type I (e.g., glycoside and sulfate formation), in which an activated conjugating agent combines with the substrate to yield the conjugated product; and type II (e.g., amino acid conjugation), in which the substrate is activated and then combines with an amino acid to yield a conjugated product.

POISON (TOXICANT).   A poison (toxicant) is any substance that causes a harmful effect when administered to a living organism. Due to a popular connotation that poisons are, by definition, fatal in their effects and that their administration is usually involved with attempted homicide or suicide, most toxicologists prefer the less prejudicial term *toxicant.* Poison is a quantitative concept. Almost any substance is harmful at some dose and, at the same time, is harmless at a very low dose. There is a range of possible effects, from subtle long-term chronic toxicity to immediate lethality.

POLLUTION.   This is contamination of soil, water, food, or the atmosphere by the discharge or admixture of noxious materials. A POLLUTANT is any chemical or substance contaminating the environment and contributing to pollution.

PORTALS OF ENTRY.   The sites at which xenobiotics enter the body are referred to as portals of entry. They include the skin, the gastrointestinal tract, and the respiratory system.

POTENTIATION.   *See* SYNERGISM AND POTENTIATION.

PRECARCINOGEN.   *See* CARCINOGEN, ULTIMATE.

PROMOTION.   The facilitation of the growth and development of neoplastic cells into a tumor. This process is manifested by enhancement of carcinogenesis when the agent is given after a carcinogen.

PULMONARY TOXICITY.   This term refers to the effects of compounds that exert their toxic effects on the respiratory system, primarily the lungs.

QSAR (QUANTITATIVE STRUCTURE ACTIVITY RELATIONSHIPS). The relationship between the physical and/or chemical properties of chemicals and their ability to cause a particular effect, enter into particular reactions, etc. The goal of QSAR studies in toxicology is to develop procedures whereby the toxicity of a compound can be predicted from its chemical structure by analogy with the properties of other toxicants of known structure and toxic properties.

REACTIVE INTERMEDIATES (REACTIVE METABOLITES). Chemical compounds, produced during the metabolism of xenobiotics, that are more chemically reactive than the parent compound. Although they are susceptible to detoxication by conjugation reactions, these metabolites, as a consequence of their increased reactivity, have a greater potential for adverse effects than the parent compound. A well-known example is the metabolism of benzo(a)pyrene to its carcinogenic dihydrodiol epoxide derivative as a result of metabolism by cytochrome P-450 and epoxide hydrolase. Reactive intermediates involved in toxic effects include epoxides, quinones, free radicals, reactive oxygen species, and a small number of unstable conjugation products.

RESISTANCE.   *See* ADAPTATION TO TOXICANTS.

RESOURCE CONSERVATION AND RECOVERY ACT (RCRA).
Administered by the EPA, the Resource Conservation and Recovery
Act is the most important act governing the disposal of hazardous
wastes in the United States; it promulgates standards for identification
of hazardous wastes, their transportation and their disposal. Included in
the latter are siting and construction criteria for landfills and other
disposal facilities as well as the regulation of owners and operators of
such facilities.

RISK (TOXICOLOGIC).   The probability that some adverse effect will
result from a given exposure to a chemical is known as the risk. It is the
estimated frequency of occurrence of an event in a population and may
be expressed in absolute terms (e.g., one in one million) or in terms of
relative risk, i.e., the ratio of the risk in question to that in an
equivalent unexposed population.

RISK ANALYSIS (RISK ASSESSMENT).   The process by which the
potential adverse health effects of human exposure to chemicals are
characterized; it includes the development of both qualitative and
quantitative expressions of risk. The process of risk assessment may be
divided into four major components: hazard identification, dose–
response assessment (high-dose to low-dose extrapolation), exposure
assessment, and risk characterization.

SAFETY FACTOR (UNCERTAINTY FACTOR).   A number by which
the no observed effect level (NOEL) is divided to obtain the acceptable
daily intake (ADI) of a chemical for regulatory purposes. The safety
factor is intended to account for the uncertainties inherent in estimating
the potential effects of a chemical on humans from results obtained
with test species. The safety factor allows for possible differences in
sensitivity between the test species and humans, as well as for variations
in the sensitivity within the human population. The size of safety factor
(e.g., 100–1,000) varies with confidence in the data base and the nature
of the adverse effect. Small safety factors indicate a high degree of
confidence in the data, an extensive data base, and/or the availability of
human data. Large safety factors are indicative of an inadequate,
uncertain data base and/or the severity of the unexpected toxic effect.
The use of safety factors is restricted to noncarcinogenic toxicants.

SELECTIVITY (SELECTIVE TOXICITY).   A characteristic of the
relationship between toxic chemicals and living organisms whereby a
particular chemical may be highly toxic to one species but relatively
innocuous to another. The search for and study of selective toxicants is
an important aspect of comparative toxicology since chemicals toxic to
target species but innocuous to nontarget species are extremely valuable
in agriculture and medicine. The mechanisms involved vary from
differential penetration rates through different metabolic pathways, to
differences in receptor molecules at the site of toxic action.

SLEEPING TIME.   A test used to assess the ability of one xenobiotic to
affect the metabolism of another. It is usually carried out with mice as
the test species and using the drug hexobarbital. Hexobarbital-induced

sleep is highly dependent upon the blood concentration of hexobarbital which, in turn, is dependent upon the rate of metabolism of hexobarbital by monooxygenases. Inhibitors of cytochrome P-450 prolong hexobarbital-induced sleep while it is shortened by inducers of this enzyme.

SOLVENTS. In toxicology this term usually refers to industrial solvents. These belong to many different chemical classes and a number of these are known to cause problems of toxicity to humans. They include: aliphatic hydrocarbons (e.g., hexane), halogenated aliphatic hydrogens (e.g., methylene chloride), aliphatic alcohols (e.g., methanol), glycols and glycol ethers (e.g., propylene and propylene glycol), and aromatic hydrocarbons (e.g., toluene).

SUBCHRONIC TOXICITY. Toxicity due to chronic exposure to quantities of a toxicant which do not cause any evident acute toxicity for a time period that is extended but is not so long as to constitute a significant part of the lifespan of the species in question. In subchronic toxicity tests using mammals a 30–90 day period is considered appropriate.

SYNERGISM AND POTENTIATION. The terms synergism and potentiation have been variously used and defined but in any case involve a toxicity that is greater when two compounds are given simultaneously or sequentially than would be expected from a consideration of the toxicities of the compounds given alone.

In an attempt to make uniform the use of these terms, it is suggested that, insofar as toxic effects are concerned, they be used as defined as follows; i.e., both involve toxicity greater than would be expected from the toxicities of the compounds administered separately, but in the case of synergism one compound has little or no intrinsic toxicity administered alone, whereas in the case of potentiation both compounds have appreciable toxicity when administered alone.

TERATOGENESIS. This term refers to the production of defects in the reproduction process resulting either in reduced productivity due to fetal or embryonic mortality or in the birth of offspring with physical, mental or behavioral, or developmental defects. Compounds causing such defects are known as TERATOGENS.

THERAPY. Poisoning therapy may be nonspecific or specific.

Nonspecific therapy is treatment for poisoning that is not related to the mode of action of the particular toxicant. It is designed to prevent further uptake of the toxicant and to maintain vital signs. Specific therapy, on the other hand, is that related to the mode of action of the toxicant and not simply to the maintenance of vital signs by treatment of symptoms. Specific therapy may be based on activation and detoxication reactions, on mode of action, or on elimination of the toxicant. In some cases more than one antidote, with different modes of action, is available for the same toxicant.

THRESHOLD DOSE. The dose of a toxicant below which no adverse effect occurs. The existence of such a threshold is based on the fundamental tenet of toxicology that, for any chemical, there exists a range of doses over which the severity of the observed effect is directly related to the dose, the threshold level representing the lower limit of this dose range. Although practical thresholds are considered to exist for most noncarcinogenic adverse effects, it has been argued that there is no threshold dose for carcinogens.

THRESHOLD LIMIT VALUE (TLV).   Upper permissive limits of airborne concentrations of substances. They represent conditions under which it is believed that nearly all workers may be repeatedly exposed day after day without adverse effect. Threshold limits are based on the best available information from industrial experience, from experimental human and animal studies, and, when possible, from a combination of the three.

THRESHOLD LIMIT VALUE – CEILING (TLV – C).   This is the concentration that should not be exceeded even momentarily. For some substances (e.g., irritant gases) only one TLV category, the TLV-ceiling, may be relevant. For other substances, two or three TLV categories may need to be considered.

THRESHOLD LIMIT VALUE – SHORT-TERM EXPOSURE LIMIT (TLV – STEL).   This is the maximal concentration to which workers can be exposed for a period up to 15 minutes continuously without suffering from (1) irritation, (2) chronic or irreversible tissue change, or (3) narcosis of sufficient degree to increase accident proneness, impair self-rescue, or materially reduce work efficiency, provided that no more than four excursions per day are permitted, that at least 60 minutes elapse between exposure periods, and provided that the daily TLV – TWA is not exceeded.

THRESHOLD LIMIT VALUE – TIME WEIGHTED AVERAGE (TLV – TWA).   This is the TWA concentration for a normal 8-hour workday or 40-hour workweek to which nearly all workers may be repeatedly exposed, day after day, without adverse effect. Time-weighted averages allow certain permissible excursions above the limit provided they are compensated by equivalent excursions below the limit during the workday. In some instances, the average concentration is calculated for a workweek rather than for a workday.

TOLERANCE.   *See* ADAPTATION TO TOXICANTS.

TOXIC SUBSTANCES CONTROL ACT (TSCA).   This act was enacted in 1976 and provides the EPA with the authority to require testing and to regulate chemicals, both old and new, entering the environment. It was intended to supplement sections of the Clean Air Act, the Water Act, and the Occupational Safety and Health Act which already provide for regulation of chemicals. Manufacturers are required to submit information to allow the EPA to identify and evaluate the potential hazards of a chemical prior to its introduction into commerce. The act also provides for the regulation of production, use, distribution, and disposal of chemicals.

TOXICANT.   *See* POISON.

TOXICODYNAMICS (TOXICOKINETICS).   This is the study of the quantitative relationship between absorption, distribution, and excretion of toxicants and their metabolites. It involves the derivation of rate constants for each of these processes and their integration into mathematical models that can predict the distribution of the chemical throughout the body compartments on any time point after administration.

TOXICOLOGY.   Toxicology is defined as that branch of science that deals with poisons (toxicants) and their effects; a poison is defined as any substance which causes a harmful effect when administered, either by accident or design, to a living organism. There are difficulties in bringing a more precise definition to the meaning of poison and in the definition and measurement of toxic effect. The range of deleterious effects is wide and varies with species, sex, developmental stage, etc., while the effects of toxicants are always dose dependent.

TOXIN.   A toxin is a toxicant produced by a living organism.

TRANSPORT.   In toxicology this term refers to the mechanisms that bring about movement of toxicants and their metabolites from one site in the organism to another. Transport usually involves binding to either blood albumins or blood lipoproteins.

ULTIMATE CARCINOGEN.   *See* CARCINOGEN, ULTIMATE.

VENOM.   A venom is a toxin produced by an animal specifically for the poisoning of other species via a mechanism designed to deliver the toxin to its prey. Examples include the venom of bees and wasps, delivered by a sting, and the venom of snakes, delivered by fangs.

WATER POLLUTION.   Water pollution is of concern in both industrialized and nonindustrialized nations. Chemical contamination is most common in industrialized nations, while microbial contamination is more important in nonindustrialized areas. Surface water contamination has been the primary cause for concern but, since the discovery of insecticides in ground water, contamination of water from this source is also a problem. Water pollution may arise from run-off of agricultural chemicals, from sewage, or from specific industrial sources. Agricultural chemicals found in water include insecticides, herbicides, fungicides, and nematocides; fertilizers, while less of a toxic hazard, contribute to such environmental problems as eutrophication. Other chemicals of concern include low-molecular-weight halogenated hydrocarbons such as chloroform, dichloroethane, and carbon tetrachloride; polychlorinated biphenyls (PCBs); chlorophenols; 2,3,7,8-tetrachlorodibenzo-p-dioxin (TCDD); phthalate ester plasticizers; detergents; and a number of toxic inorganics.

XENOBIOTIC.   A general term used to describe any chemical interacting with an organism that does not occur in the normal metabolic pathways of that organism. The use of this term in lieu of "foreign compound," etc., is gaining wide acceptance.

INDEX

A

Absorption of toxicants, 23–40. *See also* Penetration
    dermal, 32
    distribution, 40
    endocytosis, 29
    filtration, 29
    gastrointestinal, 36
    ionization, 26–27
    membranes, 24–26
    partition coefficient, 27–28
    passive transport, 28
    rates, 30
    references, 50
    respiratory, 38
    special transport, 29
    toxicodynamics, 46
Abstracts, 350
Acceptable daily intake (ADI), 281
Acetaminophen
    hepatotoxicity, 137–138, 172–173
    structure, 138
Acetanilide, metabolism, 104
2-Acetylaminofluorene
    activation, 136–137
    N-hydroxylation, 63, 137
    species variation, 94–95
    structure, 63, 137
Acetylation, 82
    fast acetylators, 103, 219
    isoniazid, 103, 219
    slow acetylators, 103, 219
Acetylcholinesterase (AChE), 139–141. *See also* Cholinesterase inhibition
Acid deposition, 189, 192, 195
Acid rain. *See* Acid deposition
Aconitase, 145

Activation. *See* Metabolic activation
Acute toxicity, 139–145
    definition, 139
Acylation reactions, 81–82
Adenine, structure, 157
Adenosine-5′-phosphosulfate (APS), 76
S-Adenosyl methionine (SAM), 76–77
ADI (acceptable daily intake), 281
Adrenal hormones, effect on metabolism, 90
Aflatoxin B1, 116, 136
    activation, 135–136
    epoxidation, 61, 135
    structure, 17, 61, 135
Aflatoxins, 16–17
Aging, 141
Agricultural chemicals, 4, 21–22
    literature, 338
Ah locus, 103, 104, 116
Air pollution, 7–8, 185–192, 315–316
    environmental effects, 190–192
    gases, 187–188
    health effects, 189–190
    measurements, 288–291
    particulates, 187–188
    sources, 188–189
    types of pollutants, 186–188
Alcohol. *See also* Ethanol
    isopropanol, 228–229
    methanol, 135, 228, 329
    toxicity, 227–229, 329
Alcohol dehydrogenases, 65–66
Aldehyde dehydrogenase, 67
Aldehyde reduction, 70
Aldicarb (Temik), LD50 and structure, 211
Aldrin
    epoxidation, 61

375

Aldrin: *(cont.)*
LD50, 209
structure, 61, 209
Aldrin epoxidase, 100
Algal bloom, 194
Alimentary canal, drawing, 37
Alimentary elimination, 130–131
Aliphatic epoxidation, 60
Aliphatic hydroxylation, 60
Alkaloids, 16–17
Alkylating agents, 155–156, 158
Allylisopropylacetamide, 111
structure, 107
Altitude, 119
Ames test, 269–270
Amidase, 70–71
Amine oxidases, 67–68
Amino acid conjugation, 82–83
O-Aminoazotoluene
reduction, 69
structure, 69
Aminopeptidases, 80
Aminopterin, 165
Aminopyrine, metabolism, 104
Amphetamine (Benzedrine), structure, 214
Amphetamines, 216
Amphipathic molecules, 127
Amygdalin, 142
Analytical toxicology, 3
literature, 338–339
Aniline hydroxylation, species variation,
94–95
Animal toxins, 18–20
Antabuse (Disulfiram)
effects, 108
structure, 107
Antagonism, 112
Antibiotics, nephrotoxicity, 175–176
Anticonvulsants, 218
Antidepressants, 216
Antioxidants, 198–199
APS (adenosine-5'-phosphosulfate), 76
Arachidonic acid, biosynthesis of
prostaglandin and structure, 68
Arochlor 1254, 114
Aromatic hydroxylation, species variation,
94–95
Artificial sweeteners, 201–202
Asbestos, 149, 207–208
Asbestosis, 177, 207–208
Aspartame, 201–202
structure, 201
ATP sulfurylase, 75
Atrazine, structure, 15
Atropine, 141, 332
structure, 330
Azaguanine, 102
Azide, 143
Azo reduction, 70

B

Bacterial toxins, 17–18
Barbital, structure, 214
Barbiturates (Barbitals), 214

Barbituric acid, structure, 214
Batrachotoxin, 142
structure, 20
Bee venom, 20
Behavioral tests, 263–264
Behavioral toxicology, 3, 179–182
literature, 339
Benzene, 230
toxicity, 207
Benzidine, acetylation and structure, 81
Benzodiazepines, 215
Benzoic acid, conjugation with CoASH and
structure, 81
Benzo(a)pyrene, 116
activation, 59–60
7,8-diol-9,10-epoxide, 59
oxidation, 59–60
structure, 16, 59
ultimate carcinogen, 60
Benzo(e)pyrene, structure, 16
BHA, structure, 199
BHT, structure, 199
Bile formation and secretion, 126–127
Bioaccumulation, 48–50, 194
Bioactivation, 133–138. *See also* Metabolic
activation
Bioassay, 305–307
Biochemical toxicology, 3
literature, 339
Biologic limit value (BLVs), 204
Biomathematics and statistics, 4
Biphenyl 2-hydroxylase, 100
Biphenyl 4-hydroxylase, 100
Bis(chloromethyl)ether, structure, 152
Bloom's syndrome, 158
Botulinum toxins, 142
Bromide toxicity, 332
Bromobenzene
activation, 173
hepatotoxicity, 172
structure, 173
5-Bromouracil, 155
n-Butanol, 18
structure, 18

C

Cadaverine, oxidation and structure, 67
Cadmium
nephrotoxicity, 175
soil and water contamination, 193–194
toxicity, 193, 205–206
Caffeine, structure, 11
Calcium propionate, structure, 200
Carbamate insecticides, 210–211
AChE inhibition, 140–141, 332
Carbaryl (Sevin)
LD50, 211
structure, 15, 211, 330
Carbene formation, 64–65
Carbon monoxide, 144, 190, 331
Carbon tetrachloride, 93, 226
activation, 171
hepatotoxicity, 171–172

Carbonylcyanide trifluoromethoxyphenylhy-
drazone, structure, 144
Carbophenothion, structure, 69
Carbophenothion sulfoxide, reduction and
structure, 69
Carboxylesterases, 70–71, 111–112, 209
Carcinogenesis, 3, 145–154
bioactivation, 150–152
cocarcinogenesis, 149–150
covalent binding, 151–152, 265–266
DNA repair, 152
epigenetic carcinogens, 150
genotoxin carcinogens, 150
history, 145–146
initiation and promotion, 147–149
literature, 340–341
liver, 170
mutagenesis, 158–159
nitrites, 200–201
occupational, 204–205
oncogenes, 153
radiation, 152–153
risk assessment, 281–282
testing, 252–253, 277
testing protocol, 278
vinyl chloride, 227
Cell mutation test, 271
Cell necrosis, 169–170
Cell transformation, 277
Chinese hamster ovary, test, 271
Chloramphenicol, inhibition of cytochrome
P-450 and structure, 107
Chlordane, LD50 and structure, 209
Chlorfenvinphos, dealkylation and structure,
62
Chlorinated hydrocarbons, 195, 225–227
p-Chlorobenzaldehyde, reduction and
structure, 69
p-Chlorobenzylamine, oxidation and
structure, 67
1-Chloro-2,4-dinitrobenzene, conjugation
with GSH and structure, 80
Chloroform
metabolism, 226
toxicity, 225–226
p-Chlorothiophenol, methylation and
structure, 77
Cholestasis, 170
Cholinesterase inhibition, 139–141, 210,
330–332
Chromatography, 296–301
column, 296–297
GLC, 297–301
HPLC, 301
paper, 296
TLC, 296
Chromium, toxicity, 206
Chromosomal abnormalities, 158, 163,
274–276
Chrysene, structure, 16
Cigarette smoke, 115, 149, 150, 177, 208
Cirrhosis, 170
Citric acid cycle, inhibition by fluoroacetate,
145

Clara cells, 178
Clastogenesis, 158
Clean Air Act, 310
Clean Water Act, 310
Clinical drugs. *See* Therapeutic drugs
Clinical toxicology, 4
literature, 341
Cocaine, 220–221
structure, 11
Cocarcinogenicity, 107–108, 149–150
Colchicine, 158, 164
Color Additive Amendment, 196
Combustion products, 5
Compound 1080, 144
Computer data bases, 351–352
Conjugation reactions, 73–83, 97–99
species variation, 96–98
Consumer Products Safety Act, 310
Controlled Substances Act, 310
Cooxidation, 68
Cosmetics, 15–16
literature, 341
Coumarin 7-hydroxylase, 100
Covalent binding, 134, 136, 139, 151–152,
171, 219, 227
testing, 265–266
Cretinism, 161
Critical periods, 160–161
Curare, 141
Cyanide, poisoning and treatment, 142–143,
329
Cycasin
carcinogenicity, 137–138
structure, 138
Cyclamate, 149, 201–202
structure, 201
Cyclophosphamide, 116
Cysteine conjugate β-lyase, 81
Cysteinyl glycinase, 78
Cytidine, structure, 155
Cytochrome b5, 54
Cytochrome P-448 (P_1-450), 114
Cytochrome P-450, 52–64
distribution, 54, 56
housefly, 105
induction (*see* Cytochrome P-450 induction)
inhibitors, 107, 173
insecticide resistance, 104–105
isozymes, 136, 138
kidney, 174
lung, 178–179
mechanism, 54–55
placenta, 115, 117
purification and reconstitution, 56–57
reactions, 57–64
role in bioactivation, 133–138
species variation, 100–101
spectra, 52–53
spectra, housefly, 105
Cytochrome P-450 spectra, 52–53
Cytochrome P-450 induction, 113–118, 138,
172–173, 214
biphasic effects, 117
genetics, 115–116

Cytochrome P-450 induction: *(cont.)*
  by insecticides, 117
  mechanism, 115–116
  by PCN, 114
  by phenobarbital, 113–114
  by TCDD, 113–114, 116
  by 3-MC, 113, 114
Cytochrome P-450 reductase, 53
Cytosine, structure, 157

D

Daphnia
  bioassay, 305–306
  testing, 279
DDE, formation and structure, 73
DDT, 21
  DDE formation, 73
  eggshell thinning, 93
  fat and milk storage, 130
  induction of cytochrome P-450, 117
  LD50, 209
  structure, 73, 209
DDT-dehydrochlorinase, 72–73
Deacetylation, 83
N-Dealkylation, 61
O-Dealkylation, 60
S-Dealkylation, 61
Delayed neuropathy, 93
  testing, 261–263
O-Demethylation, 60
Dermal irritation tests, 244–245
DES (diethylstilbestrol), 168
Desulfuration, 63–64
Detoxication, 120
Development, enzyme changes, 87–89
Diagnosis. *See* Treatment of toxicity
Diamine oxidases, 67
Diazepam (Valium), structure, 214
Diazinon, LD50 and structure, 210
Dibenzo(a,h)acridine, structure, 16
Dibenzo(a,h)anthracene, structure, 16
2,4-Dichlorophenoxyacetic acid (2,4-D),
  structure, 212
Dicrotaline, structure, 19
Dicumarol, structure, 144
Dieldrin, structure, 61
Diethylene glycol, structure, 229
Diethylmaleate, conjugation with GSH and
  structure, 80
Diethylnitrosamine, structure, 146
Diethylpyrocarbonate (DEPC), 200–201
  structure, 200
Dilantin, 218
Dimethoate, 95, 101
4-Dimethylaminoazobenzene, structure, 146
Dimethylaniline, oxidation by FMO and
  structure, 66
7,12-Dimethylbenz(a)anthracene, 148
Dimethyl carbamyl chloride, structure, 152
1,2-Dimethylhydrazine (DMH), structure, 156
N,N-Dimethyl-p-nitrophenyl carbamate
  dealkylation, 62
  structure, 62

Dimethylnitrosamine (DMN)
  alkylating agent, 155–156
  structure, 156
3,3-Dimethyl-1-phenyl triazene, structure, 156
Dimethylsulfate, structure, 152
Dimethyltryptamine (DMT), 224
  structure, 221
Dinitrophenol, structure, 144
Dioxane, structure, 229
Dioxins. *See* TCDD
Diphenylmethylphosphine, oxidation by
  FMO and structure, 66
Distribution of toxicants, 40–49
Disulfide reduction, 70
Disulfiram (Antabuse)
  effects, 108
  reduction, 69
  structure, 69, 107
Disulfoton, LD50 and structure, 210
DNA adducts, 156–157, 265
DNA repair, 152, 156–157, 273–274
Dominant lethal test, 276
Down's syndrome, 158
Draize test, 243–244
Drosophila (tests), 271–272
Drugs. *See also* Therapeutic drugs
  literature, 341
Drugs of abuse, 4, 9–11, 220–224

E

Ebers papyrus, 6
Electron transport inhibitors, 142
Electrophile, 134,148, 151, 155
Elimination of toxicants, 123–131
  alimentary, 130
  bile, 96, 126–128
  egg, 130
  enterohepatic circulation, 128
  fetus, 130
  hepatic, 126–128
  kidneys, 124–125
  liver, 126–128
  lungs, 128–129
  milk, 129–130
  obscure, 131
  pulmonary, 128
  references, 131
  renal, 124–125
Endocytosis, 29–30
Endoplasmic reticulum, 52
Enterohepatic circulation, 37, 128–129
Environmental movement of toxicants, 21–22
Environmental pollution, 315–316
  measurement, 292
Environmental toxicology, 4
  literature, 342–343
Epidemiology, 4
Epigenetic carcinogens, 150–152
EPN
  carboxylesterase inhibition, 111, 112
  structure, 107
Epoxidation, 59–60

Epoxide hydrolase, 60, 72
species variation, 100
1,2-Epoxy-3-(p-nitrophenoxy)propane,
conjugation with GSH and structure, 80
Ergotamine, structure, 17
Esterases, 71–72
Estrone, structure and sulfate conjugation, 76
Ethanol
effect of disulfiram, 108
elimination, 129
structure, 11
teratogenicity, 166–167
Ethionine, structure, 146
2-Ethoxybiphenyl deethylase, 100
4-Ethoxybiphenyl deethylase, 100
Ethylene glycol
structure, 229
toxicity, 229–230
Ethyleneimine, structure, 152
Ethylmorphine
N-demethylation, 62, 100
structure, 62
Excretion. *See* Elimination
Eye irritation test, 243–244

F

FAD-containing monooxygenase, 61, 64–66
Falconi's anemia, 158
Fatty liver, 168
FD&C lakes, 196
Federal Food, Drug and Cosmetic Act,
310–311
Federal Insecticide, Fungicide and
Rodenticide Act. *See* FIFRA
Fenvalerate
LD50, 211
structure, 15, 211
Fetal alcohol syndrome, 167
Fick's law, 30
FIFRA, 278, 311–312
Fluoracetamide, 95
N-2-fluorenylacetamide, 116
Fluoride toxicity, 191
Fluoroacetate, 95, 144–145, 213
5-Fluorouracil, 165
Folic acid antagonists, 165
Fonofos, activation and structure, 135
Food Additive Amendment, 196
Food additives, 4, 8–9, 195–202
Food additive toxicology, literature, 343
Food colorings, 196–198
Food pollutants, 7–8, 202
Forensic toxicology, 4
literature, 343–344
S-9 fraction, 269–270
Frameshift mutations, 156–157
Freund's adjuvant, 245
Fumigants, 213
Fungicides, 213

G

GABA, 219
Galen, 6

Genetic polymorphism, 103
Genotoxic, 150–152
German measles, 167
Glomerular filtration, 124
Glucoside formation, 75
Glucosinolates, structure, 19
Glucuronide formation, 73–74
genetic differences, 104
species variation, 97–98
Glutamyltranspeptidase, 79
Glutathione, protective role, 134, 137, 139,
172–174
Glutathione conjugation, 78–79
species variation, 101–102
Glutathione transferases, 78–79
developmental pattern, 88
Glycols, 229–230
Glycoside conjugation, 73–75
Government documents, 348–349
GRAS, 196
Greenhouse effect, 192
Griseofulvin, structure, 147
Guanine, structure, 157
Gunn rats, 104

H

Halogenated hydrocarbons, 225–227
Halothane, metabolism and structure, 135
Hepatic excretion, 126–128
Hepatitis, 170
Hepatotoxicity, 168–174
acetaminophen, 137–138
aflatoxin, 136
Herbicides, 212
Heroin, structure, 11
Hexobarbital sleeping time, 94, 103, 104, 106,
116
genetic variation, 103, 104
metabolism, 104
Hippuric acid, formation and structure, 81
Hormones
effect on metabolism, 90–91
teratogenesis, 165–166
Human toxicology, literature, 341
Hydrocarbons, 225
Hydrolysis reactions, 70–72
Hydroxyacetanilide, methylation and
structure, 77
3-Hydroxyxanthine, structure, 146

I

Imipramine, structure, 214
Immediately Dangerous to Life or Health
(IDLH), 204
Immune system, 267
Immunotoxicity, testing, 266–268
Indexes, 350–351
Indomethacin, 96
Induction, 113–118. *See also* Cytochrome
P-450 induction
AHH activity, 103
phenobarbital, 112–113
Industrial chemicals, 4

Industrial toxicology, 4, 8–9, 202–208,
    314–315
  literature, 345
Information storage (personal), 352–354
Inhibition
  competitive, 110
  effect on metabolism, 106–113
  irreversible, 110
  kinetics, 110
  noncompetitive, 110
  uncompetitive, 110
Initiation, 147–149
Insecticides. *See also* Pesticides
  protein binding, 42
Insecticide resistance, 103, 104–105
Insulin, effect on metabolism, 90
International documents, 348–349
Intoxication, 120
In vitro metabolism, 108–109
In vivo metabolism, 93
In vivo toxicity, 93, 103
4-Ipomeanol, activation and structure, 178
Isoniazid (INH), 103, 219
  liver toxicity, 219
  metabolism, 212, 219
  structure, 219
Isopropyl alcohol, 228–229
Isozymes, 120
  constitutive, 114
Itai-Itai, 175, 193

K

Ketone reduction, 70
Kidney
  nephron structure, 124
  renal excretion, 124–126
Kidney injury. *See* Nephrotoxicity
Klinefelter's syndrome, 158
Ks, 53

L

Laetrile, 142
LC50
  definition, 239
  tests, 239–243
LD50, 2
  definition, 239
  tests, 239–243
Lead
  air pollution, 190
  nephrotoxicity, 175
  toxicity, 206–207
Legal aspects, 5. *See also* Regulation
Legislative toxicology. *See also* Regulation
  literature, 344
Lethal synthesis, 144–145
Light, effects on metabolism, 119
Lindane, LD50 and structure, 209
Lipid peroxidation, 134, 171–172
Literature of toxicology, 335–355
  abstracts, 350
  agricultural chemicals, 338
  analytical, 338–339
  behavioral, 339
  biochemical, 339–340

carcinogenesis, 340–341
clinical and human, 341
computer data bases, 351
cosmetics, 342
documents, government, 349
documents, international, 349
drugs, 341
environmental, 342–343
food additives, 343
forensic, 343–344
general, 336–338
human, 341
indexes, 350
industrial, 345
legislative, 344
metal toxicology, 344
mutagenesis, 340–341
nutritional, 345
occupational, 345
organ toxicity, 346
personal information storage, 352
physical agents, 346
regulatory, 344
societal, 344
teratogenesis, 340–341
textbooks, 335
toxins, 347
veterinary, 347
Lithium, 220
Liver
  bile formation, 126
  diagram, 126
  hepatic excretion, 126–128
Liver injury. *See* Hepatotoxicity
LSD (Lysergic Acid Diethylamide), 221–223
  structure, 11, 221
Lung
  alveolar region, 39
  pulmonary excretion, 128–129
Lung toxicity. *See* Pulmonary toxicity

M

Malathion, 111
  LD50, 210
  potentiation by EPN, 112
  selective toxicity, 95, 102, 209
  structure, 15, 210
Marijuana, 224
  THC structure, 11
Maximum tolerated dose (MTD), 252
Measurement of toxicants, 287–307
  AA spectroscopy, 302
  air pollutants, 288–290
  bioassay, 305–306
  chemical and physical methods, 287–305
  chromatography, 296
  column chromatography, 296
  data handling, 305
  environmental, 292
  extraction, 294–295
  forensic studies, 293
  GLC, 297
  HPLC, 301
  identification, 295–304
  MS, 303

NMR, 304
paper chromatography, 296
references, 307
sampling, 288–294
separation, 295
soil pollutants, 291
SR, 303
tissues, 292
TLC, 296
UV/VIS, 304
water pollutants, 291
Membranes, function and structure, 24–26
Menaphthyl sulfate, conjugation with GSH
    and structure, 80
Meperidine (Demerol), structure, 11, 217
Mercapturic acid formation, 78–79, 102
Mercury
    Minamata Bay, 193
    nephrotoxicity, 175
    toxicity, 193, 207, 331
Mescaline, 223
    structure, 221
Metabolic activation, 133–138. *See also*
        Bioactivation
    carcinogens, 150–152
    definition, 133
    kidney, 174–176
    liver, 170–172
    lungs, 178
Metabolism
    age effects, 87–88
    chemical effects on, 105–118
    comparative effects, 91–92
    disease effects, 91
    diural rhythms, 91
    effect of disulfiram, 108
    environmental effects, 118–119
    genetic effects, 91–92
    hormone effects, 90–91
    induction effects, 113–119
    inhibition effects, 106–113
    nutritional effects, 85–87
    physiological effects, 87–88
    pregnancy, 91
    sex differences, 89–90
    variations among taxonomic groups,
        92–101
Metabolism of toxicants, 51–84
    activation, 133–138
    acylation, 81–82
    alcohol dehydrogenase, 65–66
    aldehyde dehydrogenase, 67, 108
    amine oxidase, 67
    biomethylation, 78
    conjugations, 73–82
    cysteine conjugation, 81
    cytochrome P-450 monooxygenase system,
        52–56
    cytochrome P-450 reactions, 57–64
    DDT-dehydrochlorinase, 72
    dealkylations, 60
    deamination, 61
    desulfuration, 63
    epoxidation, 59–60
    epoxide hydrolyase, 60, 72

FAD-containing monooxygenase, 64
glucoside conjugation, 74
glucuronide conjugation, 73
glutathione conjugation, 78–80
hydrolysis, 70
hydroxylations, 59–60
MDP oxidation, 64–65
mercapturic acids, 78–80
methyl transferase, 76
N-oxidation, 61
P-oxidation, 63
S-oxidation, 62
phase I reactions, 51–72
phase II reactions, 73–83
phosphate conjugation, 83
prostaglandin synthase, 68
reduction reactions, 69–70
references, 83
sulfate conjugation, 75
Metabolism–modification, 85–120
    chemical effects, 105–118
    disease, 91
    diurnal rhythms, 91
    environmental, 118–119
    genetic effects, 91–104
    hormonal effects, 90
    induction, 113–117
    inhibition, 106
    nutritional effects, 85–87
    physiological effects, 87–91
    potentiation, 111
    pregnancy, 91
    references, 120
    sex effects, 89
    synergism, 111
Metal toxicology, literature, 344–345
Metcalf model ecosystem, 279
Methadone, structure, 217
Methamphetamine, structure, 11
Methanol
    metabolism, 135
    toxicity and treatment, 228, 329
Methaqualone, structure, 11
Methemoglobin, 143, 194, 331
2-Methoxybiphenyl demethylase, 100
4-Methoxybiphenyl demethylase, 100
Methoxychlor, LD50 and structure, 209
Methylation reactions
    biomethylation, 78
    N-methylation, 76–77
    O-methylation, 77
    S-methylation, 77–78
    methylmercury, 78
Methyl chloride, 226
3-Methylcholanthrene
    carcinogenicity, 145
    structure, 16, 146
Methylene chloride, 226
Methylenedioxyphenyl compounds, 53
    induction of cytochrome P-450, 117–118
    metabolite inhibitory complex, 109–111
    oxidation to carbene, 64–65
N-Methyl-N-formylhydrazine, structure, 147
2-Methylfuran, activation and structure,
    135

Methyl mercury. *See also* Mercury toxicity
  teratogenicity, 167
Methylmethanesulfonate (MMS), structure,
  152, 156
Methyl-N'-nitro-N-nitrosoguanidine
  (MNNG), structure, 156
Methyl-N-nitrosourea (MNU), structure, 156
Methyl paraben, structure, 200
Methylthiolation, 78
Methyltransferases, 76–78
Metyrapone, 110
  structure, 107
Microbial toxins, 17–18
Micronucleus test, 275–276
Microsomes, 52
Miller, Elizabeth and James, 150–151
Minamata bay, 193
Minamata disease, 167
Mirex, LD50 and structure, 209
Mitomycin C, structure, 147
Monoamine oxidases, 67
Monocrotaline, 116, 178
Monooxygenations, 52–65
Morphine, structure, 11, 217
MTD (maximum tolerated dose), 252
Mustard gas, structure, 152
Mutagenesis, 3, 154–159, 163
  literature, 340–341
  testing, 268–277
  testing protocol, 278
Mutation, 154–159
Mycotoxins, 16–17

N

Naphthalene
  epoxide formation, 59
  oxidation, 59–60
  structure, 59
1-Naphthol
  glucuronide formation, 74
  structure, 74
2-Naphthylamine, 116
  carcinogenicity, 98, 146
  glucuronide formation, 74
  structure, 74, 76, 146
  sulfate conjugation, 76
Narcotic, 217–218
National documents, 349
National Environmental Policy Act, 311
Natural substances, 5
Natural toxins, 16–19
Nephrotoxicity, 174–176
Nervous system toxicants, 139–142
Neurotoxicity, testing, 261–263
Neurotoxins, 141–142
Nicotine, 65, 93
  formation, 77
  oxidation by FMO, 66
  structure, 11, 66, 77
NIOSH, 311
Nitrates
  food preservatives, 200–201
  in soil and water, 194
  toxicity, 194

Nitrites, carcinogenicity and food
  preservatives, 200–201
o-Nitroanisole, metabolism, 104
p-Nitroanisole, 62
p-Nitroanisole O-demethylase, 100
Nitrobenzene, reduction and structure, 69
Nitrogen mustard, structure, 152
Nitrogen oxides, 187–192
p-Nitrophenol
  glucoside formation, 74
  structure, 74
4-Nitroquinoline-1-oxide
  activation, 135
  structure, 135, 146
Nitro reduction, 69
Nitrosobenzene, 69
Nitroso compounds, carcinogenesis, 200–201
Nitrous acid, 155
NOEL (no observable effect level), 245, 281
Nornicotine
  nicotine formation, 77
  structure, 77
Nucleophile, 149, 151, 155
Nutritional toxicology, 3
  literature, 345

O

Occupational Safety and Health Act, 311
Occupational toxicology. *See also* Industrial
  toxicology
  literature, 345
Oncogenes, 153–154
Opiates, 217–218
Orfila, 6
Organ toxicity, 3, 168–179
  literature, 346
Organochlorine insecticides, 208–209
Organophosphates, 208–210
  AChE inhibition, 140–141
Ornithine conjugation, 96, 98
OSHA, 311
N-Oxidation, 61
P-Oxidation, 63, 66
S-Oxidation, 62, 66
Oxidative deamination, 61
Oxidative dearylation, 63–64
Oxidative phosphorylation, inhibition,
  142–144
Ozone, 190, 191

P

2-PAM, 141, 329, 333
  structure, 330
PAPS (3'-phospho-adenosine-
  5'-phosphosulfate), 75–76
Paracelsus, 6
Paraquat, 102, 213
  activation, 178–179
  lung toxicity, 178–179
  structure, 178
Paraquat dichloride, structure, 15
Parathion
  AChE inhibition, 140–141, 332
  LD50, 210
  paraoxon formation, 64

structure, 64, 210, 330
toxicity, 89
treatment of poisoning, 141, 329–330, 332
Parathion desulfurase, 100
Partition coefficient, 27–28
Passive transport, 28–29
PCBs (polychlorinated biphenyls), 195
    fat and milk storage, 130
    induction of cytochrome P-450, 114
PCP. *See also* Phencyclidine
    structure, 11, 221
Penetration. *See also* Absorption
    gastrointestinal (GI), 36–37
    kinetics, 30–34
    pesticides, 31
    respiratory, 38–40
    routes, 32–40
    skin, 32–36
Pentachlorophenol, structure, 144
Percutaneous absorption, 34–35
Personal information storage, 352–354
Pesticides
    carbamates, 210
    chlorinated hydrocarbons, 208
    classification, 12–15
    herbicides, 212
    organophosphates, 208–210
    penetration, 31
    poisoning and treatment, 139–141,
        330–332
    protein binding, 42
    pyrethrins, 211–212
    soil and water pollution, 7, 194
Petroleum, pollution, 193–195
Peyote, 223
Phagocytes, 28
Phagocytosis, 29
Pharmacokinetics, 46–48
Phase one reactions, 51–72, 120, 133–139,
    170–173, 178–179
    alcohol dehydrogenase, 65–66
    aldehyde dehydrogenase, 67
    amine oxidase, 67–68
    DDT-dehydrochlorinase, 72–73
    dealkylation, 60–61
    deamination, 61–62
    desulfuration, 63–64
    epoxidation, 59–60
    epoxide hydrolase, 72
    esterases, 70–72
    hydrolysis, 70–72
    hydroxylations, 59–60
    methylenedioxyphenyl oxidation, 64–65
    N-oxidation, 61, 66
    P-oxidation, 63, 66
    S-oxidation, 62, 66
    prostaglandin synthetase, 68
    reductions, 69–70
Phase two reactions, 72–83, 87, 120,
    133–139, 170–173
    acylation, 81–83
    amino acid conjugation, 82–83
    cysteine conjugate β-lyase, 81
    deacetylation, 83
    glucoside conjugation, 75

glucuronide conjugation, 73–74
glutathione conjugation, 78–80
glutathione transferases, 78–80
mercapturic acids, 78–80
methyltransferases, 76–78
phosphate conjugation, 83
sulfate conjugation, 75–76
Phencyclidine (PCP), structure, 11, 221–222
Phenobarbital, structure, 214
Phenol
    in vivo metabolism, 99
    species variation, 99
    structure, 99
Phenylcyclidine (PCP), 221–222
Phenylketonuria (PKU), 202
Phenytoin, 218
Phocomelia, 166, 258
Phorate
    oxidation by FMO, 66
    structure, 66
Phosphate conjugation, 83
Phosphates, in soil and water, 194
3′-Phospho-adenosine-5′-phosphosulfate
    (PAPS), 75–76
PHP,1-(1-phenylcyclohexyl)pyrrolidine,
    structure, 221
Physical agents, literature, 346–347
Pinocytosis, 29
Piperonyl butoxide, 111. *See also*
    Methylenedioxyphenyl compounds
    induction of cytochrome P-450, 117–118
    inhibition effect, 107–109
    structure, 107
pKa, 26–27
Plant toxins, 18
Point mutations, 154
Pollution, air, water, land, food, 7–8, 19–22,
    185–202, 315–316
Polycyclic aromatic hydrocarbons (PAH),
    15–16
Polyethylene glycols, structure, 229
Polyploidy, 158, 164
Portal of entry, 23
Potentiation, 111, 262
Pott, Sir Percivall, 145
Preservatives (food), 8–9, 199–200
Prevention of toxicity, 308–317
    air, water, land, 315–316
    education, 316–317
    environment, 315–316
    home, 313–314
    legislation, 308–313
    references, 317
    regulation, 308–313
    workplace, 314–315
Promotion, 147–149
β-Propiolactone
    structure, 152
Propoxur (Baygon), LD50 and structure,
    211
Propoxyphene (Darvon), structure, 217
Propylene glycol
    structure, 229
    toxicity, 230
Propyl gallate, structure, 199

Prostaglandin synthase reaction, 68
Proto-oncogenes, 153
Psilocybin, 223
　structure, 221
Puffer fish, 142
Pulmonary excretion, 128–129
Pulmonary toxicity, 177–179
Pyocyanine, structure, 18
Pyrethrins
　insecticides, 12–15, 211–212
　LD50, 211
　structure, 211
Pyrollizidine alkaloids, 178
　structure, 147

Q

Quercetin, structure, 147

R

Radiation, effects on metabolism, 118–119
Radiation carcinogenesis, 152
Radiation toxicology, literature, 346–347
Ramazzini, 6
RCRA (Resource Conservation and Recovery
　Act), 311
Reactive metabolite formation. *See*
　Bioactivation and Metabolic activation
Reduction reactions, 69
Regulation of toxic chemicals, 234–235
Regulation of toxic substances, 309–312
　Clean Air Act, 310
　Clean Water Act, 310
　Consumer Products Safety Act, 310
　Controlled Substances Act, 310
　Federal Food, Drug and Cosmetic Act,
　　310–311
　Federal Insecticide, Fungicide and
　　Rodenticide Act, 311
　National Environmental Policy Act, 311
　Occupational Safety and Health Act, 311
　Resource Conservation and Recovery Act,
　　311
　Toxic Substance Control Act, 311–312
Regulatory toxicology, literature, 344
Rehn, Ludwig, 145
Renal excretion, 124–126
Reproductive toxicity testing, 253–256
Resource Conservation and Recovery Act, 311
Rhodanese, 143. *See also* Cyanide poisoning
Ricinine, structure, 19
Risk assessment, 5, 233, 281–283
Rodenticides, 14, 213

S

Saccharin, 149, 201–202
　structure, 201
Safrole, structure, 19, 147
SAM (S-adenosyl methionine), 76–77
Sassafrass. *See* Safrole
Saxitoxin, structure, 20
Scatchard plot, 44–45
SCE. *See* Sister chromatid exchange
Scheele, Karl Wilhelm, 142
Secobarbital, structure, 11

Silicosis, 177
Sister chromatid exchange (SCE), 274–275
SKF-525A, 53, 111
　inhibition effect, 107–109
　structure, 107
Skin, structure, 33
Skin irritation. *See* Dermal irritation
Sleeping time. *See* Hexobarbital sleeping time
Smog, 7, 186, 190
Snake venoms, 19
Societal toxicology, literature, 344
Sodium benzoate, structure, 200
Soil pollutants, measurement, 291
Soil pollution, 7, 192–195, 315–316
Solanine, structure, 19
Solvents, 14, 224–230
Sorbic acid, structure, 200
Sources of toxic compounds. *See* Toxic
　compounds, sources of
Special transport, 29
Spectroscopy, 301–305
　AA, 302–303
　IR, 303–304
　MS, 303
　NMR, 304
　UV/VIS, 304
Stilbestrol, 96
Stress effects, 119
Structure-activity study, 3
Strychnine, 26
Styrene 7, 8-oxide, hydrolysis and structure, 72
Succinylsulfathioazole, 96
Suicide substrates, 109, 111
Sulfate conjugation, 75–76
Sulfone formation, 62, 66
Sulfotransferases, 75, 136–137
Sulfoxide formation, 62, 66, 135
Sulfoxide reduction, 70
Sulfur oxides, 187–192
Synergism, 111, 262

T

TCDD (2,3,7,8-tetrachlorodibenzo-p-dioxin),
　195
　bioaccumulation, 48–50
　induction of cytochrome P-450, 113–114,
　　116
　structure, 212
　toxicity, 212
Temperature effects, 118
Teratogenesis, 3, 159–168, 258–260
　behavioral, 180–181
　critical periods, 160–161
　history, 159
　human, 165–168
　literature, 340–341
　mechanisms, 160–165
　phenytoin, 218
　testing, 253, 256–260
Testing. *See* Toxicity testing
Tetracycline, 102
Tetraethylpyrophosphate (TEPP), 209
Tetrahydrocannabinol (THC).
　structure, 11

Tetrodotoxin, 93, 142
Tetrodoxin, structure, 20
Thalidomide, 160, 166
Therapeutic drugs, 10–11, 213–220
Therapy. *See* Treatment of toxicity
Thioacetamide, activation and structure, 135
Thiobenzamide
    oxidation by FMO, 66
    structure, 66
Thiophenol
    glucuronide formation, 74
    structure, 74
Thiourea, structure, 146
Threshold-limit values (TLVs), 203–204,
    314–315
    TLV-ceiling (TVL-C), 203–208
    TLV-short-term exposure limit
      (TLV-STEL), 203
    TLV-time-weighted average (TLV-TWA),
      203
Thymine, structure, 157
Thyroid hormone, effect on metabolism, 90
Titanium dioxide, 196, 198
Tobacco smoke. *See* Cigarette smoke
Toluene
    structure, 229
    toxicity, 230
Torrey canyon, 193
Toxic compounds, sources of, 7–20, 185–231
    air pollutants, 7, 185–189
    animal toxins, 18, 141–142
    bacterial toxins, 17, 142
    cosmetics, 15
    drugs of abuse, 9, 220–224
    food additives, 7–8, 195–202
    inorganic chemicals, 19, 194
    microbial toxins, 17, 142
    mycotoxins, 16
    pesticides, 12, 208–213
    plant toxins, 18, 141–142
    polycyclic aromatic hydrocarbons, 15–16
    solvents, 14, 224–230
    therapeutic drugs, 10, 213–220
    water pollutants, 7, 192–195
    workplace, 8, 202–208
Toxicity, genetic differences, 103
Toxicity testing, 3, 233–285
    acute toxicity, 239
    Ames test, 269–270
    behavioral, 181, 263–264
    carcinogenesis, 252–253
    cell mutation, 271
    cell transformation, 277
    chromosome aberrations, 274–276
    chronic tests, 251–260
    covalent binding, 265–266
    dermal irritation, 244–245
    dominant lethal, 276
    Drosophilia, 271–272
    environmental tests, 278–281
    eye irritation, 243–244
    future of testing, 283
    immunotoxicity, 266–268
    in vitro tests, 268–278
    in vivo tests, 239–268
    LC50, 239–243
    LD50, 239–243
    micronucleus, 275–276
    neurotoxicity, 261–262
    90-day feeding, 246
    potentiation, 262
    reproductive tests, 253–256
    risk analysis, 281–283
    routes of exposure, 235–238
    sister chromatid exchange (SCE), 274–275
    special tests, 268
    subchronic tests, 245–251
    summary of tests, 236
    teratogenesis, 256–260
    30-day dermal, 251
    30–90 day inhalation, 237–238, 251
    toxicokinetics, 262–263
    unscheduled DNA synthesis, 273–274
Toxicodynamics, 46–50
Toxicokinetic models, 48
Toxicokinetics, 46–49, 262
Toxicological pathology, 3
Toxicology
    definition and scope, 1–5
    history, 6–7
    relation to other sciences, 5–6
    sources of toxic compounds, 7–20
Toxic Substances Control Act, 311
T-2 toxin, structure, 17
Toxins, 16–19, 141–142
    animal, 18
    literature, 347
    microbial, 17–18
    mycotoxins, 16–17
    plant, 18
Tranquilizers, 214–215
Transplacental carcinogenesis, 168
Transport of toxicants, 40–49
Treatment of toxicity, 318–333
    carbon monoxide, 330–331
    cyanide, 142–143, 329–330
    diagnosis, 319–322
    emergency management, 323–324
    first aid, 323–324
    life support, 324
    maintenance therapy, 325–328
    metals, 330–331
    methanol, 228, 329–330
    pesticides, 139–141, 330, 332
    systemic examination, 322–323
Trichloroethylene, 226
2,4,5-Trichlorophenoxyacetic acid (2,4,5-T),
    structure, 212
Tricothecenes, 17
Trimethylacetophenone imine, N-
    hydroxylation and structure, 63
Tubocurarine, 141–142
Tubular reabsorption, 124
Tubular secretion, 125
Turner's syndrome, 158
Type I ligands, 53
Type II ligands, 53
Type III ligands, 53

U

UDPG (uridine diphosphate glucose), 73–74
UDPGA (uridine diphosphate glucuronic acid), 73–74
Ultimate carcinogen, 60, 147–148, 151
Uncoupling agents, 144
Unscheduled DNA synthesis, 273–274
Uranium, nephrotoxicity, 175
Uranium dust, 149
Urethan, structure, 146
Uridine, structure, 155
Uridine diphosphate glucose (UDPG), 73–74
Uridine diphosphate glucuronic acid (UDPGA), 73–74

V

Veterinary toxicology, 4
    literature, 347
Vincristine, 158, 164

Vinyl chloride, carcinogenicity and metabolism, 227
VLDL (very-low-density-lipoprotein), 168

W

Warfarin, structure, 15
Water pollution, 7–8, 192–195, 315–316
    measurement, 291–292
Workplace, toxic chemicals in, 8–9, 202, 314–315

X

Xylene, 230
    structure, 229
o-Xylene, structure, 229

Z

Zoxazolamine paralysis time, 106, 116
    structure, 152